# NATURAL KILLER CELLS

Edited by **Mourad Aribi**

**Natural Killer Cells**
http://dx.doi.org/10.5772/66568
Edited by Mourad Aribi

**Contributors**

May Sabry, Mark Lowdell, Haiyan Liu, Bo Hu, Rajiv Saxena, Yui Harada, Hiroshi Ban, Yoshikazu Yonemitsu, Minori Ishii, Koji Teraishi, Lynda Addou-Klouche, Gordana Konjevic, Ana Vuletic, Katarina Mirjacic Martinovic, Radan Dzodic, Hend M. El Tayebi, Yasumitsu Nishimura, Naoko Kumagai-Takei, Hidenori Matsuzaki, Suni Lee, Kei Yoshitome, Takemi Otsuki, Mourad Aribi

**Published by InTech**
Janeza Trdine 9, 51000 Rijeka, Croatia



**Publishing Process Manager** Maja Bozicevic
**Technical Editor** SPi Global
**Cover** InTech Design team

First published December, 2017
Printed in Croatia
Legal deposit, Croatia: National and University Library in Zagreb

Additional hard copies can be obtained from orders@intechopen.com

Natural Killer Cells, Edited by Mourad Aribi
p. cm.
Print ISBN 978-953-51-3671-2
Online ISBN 978-953-51-3672-9

For EU product safety concerns:
IN TECH d.o.o., Prolaz Marije Krucifikse Kozulić 3, 51000 Rijeka, Croatia,
info@intechopen.com or visit our website at intechopen.com.

# Meet the editor

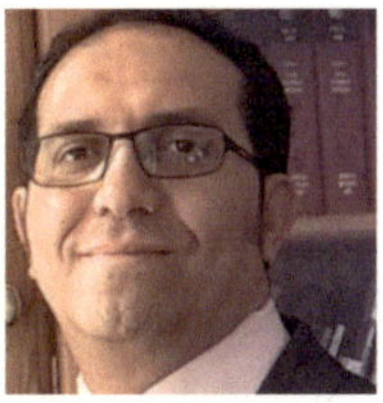

Dr. Mourad Aribi, PhD, Dr. Hab., is a professor of Immunology at the University of Tlemcen (Algeria). He is also the founder and director of the Laboratory of Applied Molecular Biology and Immunology. His current research focuses on the modulation of cell-mediated and inflammatory immune responses in autoimmune diseases, cancer diseases, and infectious diseases. Thanks to his interdisciplinary skills, he was able to develop numerous high-level collaboration projects, notably with CNRS and INSERM partners (Institut de Génétique Humaine, UMR 9002 CNRS-University of Montpellier (formerly UPR 1142 CNRS), Montpellier, France,; INSERM U1090, Luminy, Aix-Marseille University, Marseille, France; and INSERM U866, Burgundy, France). He is a reviewer in several international journals and is also a member of the Editorial Board of *Frontiers in Immunology* (the official journal of the International Union of Immunological Societies, IUIS).

# Contents

# Preface

As a result of collective work, this book addresses in a clear and comprehensive way for readers and through as many sensuous details as possible the most and various fundamental aspects of natural killer (NK) cells, as well as their clinical applications in cancer immunotherapy. It consists of nine chapters.

The introductory chapter provides a general overview on NK cells. It is mainly devoted for a pedagogic and academic context.

Chapter 2 is mainly focused on the description of mechanisms of inhibition and activation of NK cells, the mechanisms of immune evasion by tumors, and NK cell–based cancer immunotherapy.

Chapter 3 specifically explores the immunobiological and functional aspects of NK cells, especially in tumor immune surveillance.

Chapter 4 describes the substantial roles of NK cells in tumor immune surveillance and their applications for cancer immunotherapy.

The main purpose of Chapter 5 is to describe alterations in the expression of NK cell receptors, particularly in cancer patients, which could be potential therapeutic targets.

Chapter 6 focuses more specifically on the therapeutic applications of NK cells. It first addresses the fundamental aspects of such cells, in particular the various receptors, before treating their therapeutic use.

In addition to the description of NK cell immunobiology and functions, as well as the induction of memory-like NK cells and their education, Chapter 7 aims to review the present state of donor NK cell therapy during allogeneic hematopoietic stem cell transplantation and its future direction.

Chapter 8 focuses on the impacts of carbon nanotubes on NK cell immune effector functions.

Chapter 9 provides a simple method for statistically evaluating the activity of NK cells in human peripheral blood mononuclear cells.

My great desire is that this book will serve as an invaluable resource and pedagogical support for clinicians, researchers, basic scientists, and immunology and immunopathology lecturers, as well as for students in biology and medicine, especially the ones with an advanced understanding of immunology.

I would like to take this opportunity to kindly thank all collaborators who contributed in this book. I would also like to address a special word of thanks to Maja Bozicevic, Publishing Process Manager, and all the team of InTechOpen Publishing House, for their trust, their patience, and their help in making this book.

**Prof. Mourad Aribi**
Laboratory of Applied Molecular Biology and Immunology BIOMOLIM, W0414100
University of Tlemcen, Algeria

Chapter 1

# Introductory Chapter: A Brief Overview on Natural Killer Cells

Mourad Aribi

Additional information is available at the end of the chapter

http://dx.doi.org/10.5772/intechopen.72328

## 1. Introduction

Natural killer (NK) cells represent about 5–15% of circulating lymphocytes [1] and belong to the innate immune system, in particular due to their invariant antigen receptors. Morphologically, as opposed to "small lymphocytes," most of them are typically large azurophilic granules containing lymphocytes (LGL) [2], characterized by high cytoplasmic:nuclear ratio. They have initially been referred to as k or null lymphocytes (non-B and non-T cells), with the highest cytotoxic capacity [3, 4], because they lack conventional T-cell membrane markers and the surface membrane immunoglobulin (smIg) [5, 6]. NK cells mediate resistance against intracellular pathogens, mainly viral-infected, bacteria-infected and protozoa-infected cells, and have the potential to restrain cancer and metastasis. They are also able to contribute to the activation and the regulation of the immune responses, as well as the orientation of adaptive immune responses [7, 8]. More recently, NK cells were recognized as a subtype of type 1 innate lymphoid cells (ILC1), which express the transcription factor T-box expressed in T cells (T-bet), and defined by the production of the T helper cell type 1 (Th1)-associated cytokine interferon gamma (IFN-γ) and the inability to produce Th2 cell-associated and Th17 cell-associated cytokines [9]. As a result of collective work, this book has therefore the ultimate purpose to address the most fundamental aspects of NK cells, as well as their clinical applications for cancer immunotherapy.

## 2. Lineage of NK cells

NK cells constitute a third lymphoid line derived from a common T-cell and B-cell bone marrow precursor. Unlike T cells, NK cells do not have a specialized differentiating organ, are matured inside of bone marrow, and can develop even in athymic mice. The acquisition of their functions does not use recombination-activating gene (RAG) enzymes for rearrangement of their receptor genes or complete V(D)J recombination as is the case for T cells or B cells [10] and is considered as the only lymphocytes without a clonally specific receptor [11]. Additionally, in contrast to the conventional $\alpha\beta$ T cells, the genesis of NK cells appears to be independent of the self-major histocompatibility complex (MHC), although they have different recognition specificities of allogeneic MHC molecules.

Mature NK cells are able to self-renew and possibly persist in the host for months or years. Nevertheless, unlike long-lived $CD8^+$ and $CD4^+$ T cells that retain a "memory-like" phenotype and function after homeostatic proliferation, expanded NK cells return to a quiescent phenotype and respond with comparable kinetics against viral challenge [10].

## 3. Localization of NK cells

NK cells are present in the bloodstream and in the lymphatic vessels [12], as well as in placenta, spleen, liver, lungs, tonsils, peripheral ganglia, and bone marrow where they act as sentinels. Nevertheless, it appears that they have no access to other tissues apart from inflammatory responses. Of note, it has been reported that the homeostasis-driven NK cells can reside in both lymphoid and nonlymphoid organs for a long time [13].

## 4. LGL surface markers

### 4.1. $CD3^-$ LGL markers

In human, the LGL population can be separated into $CD3^+$ and $CD3^-$ subtypes. The majority of LGL $TCR^-CD3^-$ expresses CD16 (or Fc$\gamma$RIIIA, low-affinity receptor for the Fc portion of immunoglobulin G, 90%), CD56 (neural cell adhesion molecule [N-CAM], > 95%), and some markers of T cells, such as CD7 (100%), CD11b (80–80%), CD2 (70–80%), CD4 (<5%), and CD8 (15–20%).

### 4.2. $CD19^-CD3^-$ NK cell subsets

NK cells are $CD3^-CD19^-$ LGLs [14]. They thus lack two main markers of T cells ($CD3^+$) and B cells ($CD19^+$). In human peripheral blood, five NK cell subpopulations can be separated depending on the relative presence and expression levels of CD16 and CD56 markers [15]:

1. $CD56^{bright}$ $CD16^-$ (50–70% of $CD56^{bright}$)
2. $CD56^{bright}$ $CD16^{dim}$ (30–50% of $CD56^{bright}$)
3. $CD56^{dim}$ $CD16^-$ (small proportion)
4. $CD56^{dim}$ $CD16^{bright}$ (at least 90% of all peripheral blood NK cells)
5. $CD56^-$ $CD16^{bright}$ (small proportion)

| | NK cell subgroup | |
|---|---|---|
| | $CD16^{bright}CD56^{dim/+}$ NK cells | $CD16^{dim/-}CD56^{bright}$ NK cells |
| Proportion | ≥90% of PBNKCs | ≤10% of PBNKCs |
| Cytotoxic/lytic granules | +++ | + |
| ADCC function | +++ | + |
| LAK cell activity | +++ | +++ |
| Natural cytotoxicity | +++ | + |
| Cytokine production | + | +++ |
| Immunoregulation | + | +++ |
| NK cell migration | Migration to the sites of acute inflammation (arrive very early to the sites of inflammation) | Migration to the SLOs |

ADCC, antibody-dependent cell-mediated cytotoxicity; LAK, lymphokine-activated killer; NK, natural killer; PBNKCs, peripheral blood natural killer cells; SLO, secondary lymphoid organs.

**Table 1.** Key features of $CD16^{bright}CD56^{dim/+}$ and $CD16^{dim/-}CD56^{bright}$ NK cells.

The NK cells can also be separated into two subgroups according to the expression levels of the CD16 and CD56 markers in healthy individuals (**Table 1**).

## 5. Immune roles of NK cells

After maturation, NK cells migrate to the blood to provide innate defense against tumor cells and metastases, as well as infected cells by intracellular pathogens (such as viruses, bacteria, and protozoan parasites). Additionally, NK cells are also involved in the acute rejection of bone marrow transplants [16]. Finally, in addition to their ability to secrete various cytokines and regulate the immune response, activated NK cells are also involved in tissue remodeling through their ability to secrete matrix metalloproteinases (MMPs), in both physiological and pathological abnormalities, within the tumor microenvironment, through the cleavage of CD16 from the cell surface [17].

## 6. MHC I as molecular basis of target recognition by NK cells

The activation of NK cells does not require prior sensitization with an antigen. However, their activities are inversely correlated with the density of MHC class I molecules (MHC I), which are expressed on the surface of certain nucleated cell lines, with the exception of red blood cells and certain tissues such as salivary glands, brain, cornea, anterior chamber of the eye, liver, testis, fetotrophoblast, hair matrix, and proximal nail matrix [18].

## 7. "Missing self" hypothesis

NK cells lack antigen-specific receptors, but their activation can be blocked by an inhibitory signal generated by their recognition of MHC I alleles on host cells. However, the absence of MHC molecules I triggers an activating signal [19]. Nevertheless, the recognition of MHC I molecules would be one of the major causes of the tumor escape from NK cell immune surveillance and activation. Therefore, among the current therapeutic strategies is the use of monoclonal antibodies that target the NK cell inhibitory receptors.

## 8. NK cell-activating and inhibitory receptors

NK cells express two major types of receptors, inhibitory and activating receptors, that may belong to one of the following receptor categories:

(i) Immunoglobulin superfamily (IgSF) - activating or inhibitory - receptors.

(ii) C-type lectin family - activating or inhibitory - receptors.

(iii) Natural cytotoxicity - activating - receptors (NCRs).

NK cell receptors can be either MHC class I-dependent or MHC class I-independent receptors (**Table 2**).

### 8.1. MHC class I-dependent receptors

#### *8.1.1. Killer cell immunoglobulin-like receptors*

Killer cell immunoglobulin-like receptors (KIRs) are a family of type I transmembrane glycoproteins belonging to the immunoglobulin superfamily (IgSF) receptors and grouped together with other receptors of the same IgSF. KIR genes are found in a cluster on human chromosome 19q13.4 within the 1 Mb leukocyte receptor complex (LRC) [28].

KIR molecules are also expressed by some T-cell subtypes. The ligands for several KIRs are subsets of MHC I molecules.

##### *8.1.1.1. Dominant receptors on NK cells*

NK cell functions are regulated by a balance between activating and inhibitory signals [29]. Their receptors recognizing the same MHC I or other ligands are polymorphic and highly homologous and can induce two opposite signals, but one of them dominates signal transduction. Usually, the presence of MHC I molecules on a cell generates a dominant negative signal, but some ligands induced by abnormal or virus-encoded cell damage can stimulate activating receptors and generate a dominant positive signal. Additionally, the absence of MHC I molecules is not sufficient to induce a dominant activating signal, especially in normal cells. From the molecular point of view, it is the length of the cytoplasmic domain that determines the function of NK cells. Thus, long-tailed receptors (L) are associated with an inhibitory function upon ligand binding *via* an immune tyrosine-based inhibitory motif (ITIM), while short ones (S) lack the ITIM and instead associate with the TYRO protein tyrosine kinase-binding protein to transduce activating signals. In the rare situation where an NK cell co-expresses an inhibitory and an activating KIR (KAR) with the same specificity, the inhibitory receptors block activation signals at an early step [30].

| **NK cell receptors** | | | | | **Ligands** |
|---|---|---|---|---|---|
| Inhibitory NK cell receptors | MHC class I-dependent receptors | IgSF receptors | KIR2DL | (1) KIR2DL1/NKAT1 (CD158a) | HLA-Cw2, HLA-Cw4, HLA-Cw5, HLA-Cw6 |
| | | | | (2) KIR2DL2/NKAT6 (CD158b1) | HLA-Cw1, HLA-Cw3, HLA-Cw7, HLA-Cw8 |
| | | | | (3) KIR2DL3/NKAT2 (CD158b2) | HLA-Cw1, HLA-Cw3, HLA-Cw7, HLA-Cw8 |
| | | | | (4) KIR2DL5 (CD158f) | Unknown |
| | | | KIR3DL | (1) KIR3DL1/NKAT3 (CD158e1) | HLA-Bw4 |
| | | | | (2) KIR3DL2 (CD158k) | HLA-A3/ HLA-A11 |
| | | | | (3) KIR3DL3 (CD158z) | Unknown |
| | | | ILT | (1) IL-T2 (CD85j) | HLA-A, HLA-B, HLA-C, CMV UL-18 |
| | | | | (2) IL-T5 (CD85a) | Unknown |
| | | | | (3) IL-T8 (CD85c) | Ligand still needs to be identified |
| | | CTLRs | CD94-NKG2A/B | CD159a | HLA-E loaded with HLA-A, HLA-B, HLA-C, or HLA-G leader peptide |
| | MHC class I-independent receptors | CTLRs | KLRG1 | | E-cadherin |
| | | | NKR-P1A | CD161 | LLT1 |

| NK cell receptors | | | | | Ligands |
|---|---|---|---|---|---|
| Activating NK cell receptors/KARs | MHC class I-dependent receptors | IgSF receptors | KIR2DL | KIR2DL4/KIR103 (CD158d)* | HLA-G, HLA-Bw4 |
| | | | KIR2DS | (1) KIR2DS1 (CD158h) | HLA-Cw2, HLA-Cw4, HLA-Cw5, HLA-Cw6 |
| | | | | (2) KIR2DS2 (CD158j) | HLA-Cw1, HLA-Cw3, HLA-Cw7, HLA-Cw8 |
| | | | | (3) KIR2DS3/NKAT7 | With no detectable avidity for C1, C2, or any other HLA class I epitope |
| | | | | (4) KIR2DS4 (CD158i) | HLA-C (weak) |
| | | | | (5) KIR2DS5 (CD158g) | With no detectable avidity for C1, C2, or any other HLA class I epitope |
| | | | KIR3DS | KIR3DS1/NKB1 (CD158e2) | Ligand still needs to be identified (HLA-Bw4-I80, HLA-Bw4-T80, allotype HLA-B*2705?) |
| | | CTLRs | CD94-NKG2C | CD159c | HLA-E loaded with HLA-A, HLA-B, HLA-C, or HLA-G leader peptide |
| | | | CD94-NKG2E/H | CD159a | HLA-E loaded with HLA-A, HLA-B, HLA-C, or HLA-G leader peptide |
| | | | NKG2D | CD314 | MICA, MICB, ULBP1, ULBP2, ULBP3, ULBP4 |
| | MHC class I-independent receptors | IgSF receptors | NCR1 | NKp46 (CD335) | Viral HA and NDHN |
| | | | NCR2 | NKp44 (CD336) | Viral HA |
| | | | NCR3 | NKp30 (CD337) | BAT3, B7-H6 on human tumor cells |

Adapted from Ref. [20] and completed from Refs. [21–26]. Costimulatory NK cell receptors are not presented here.*An unusual activating KIR with L cytoplasmic and hybrid D0-D2 structure domains, displaying very weak inhibitory potential [27]. BAT3, B-associated transcript 3; B7-H6, B7 homolog 6; HLA, human leukocyte antigen; HLA-Bw4-I80, HLA-Bw4 molecules containing an isoleucine in position 80; ILTs, immunoglobulin-like transcripts; ILRs, immunoglobulin-like receptors; HA, hemagglutinin; IgSF, immunoglobulin superfamily; KAR, killer cell-activating receptors; KIR, killer cell immunoglobulin-like receptor; LLT1, lectin like transcript-1; CTLR, C-type lectin-like receptor; MICA/MICB, major histocompatibility complex class I-related chain A/B; KLRG1, co-inhibitory receptor killer cell lectin like receptor G1; NCR, natural cytotoxicity receptor; NK cell, natural killer cell; NDHN, Newcastle disease hemagglutinin-neuraminidase; NKAT, natural killer-associated transcript; ULBP, UL-16-binding proteins.

**Table 2.** Inhibitory and activating human NK cell receptors.

#### *8.1.1.2. Classification of KIR molecules*

KIR molecules are classified into two types according to the number of extracellular Ig-like domains (D), 2D and 3D, and by whether they have a long (L) or short (S) cytoplasmic domain (**Figure 1**) [31].

### *8.1.2. CD94-NKG2 C-type lectin receptor complex*

C-type lectin receptors are characterized by calcium-dependent carbohydrate recognition domain (CRD) and the presence of one or more C-type lectin-like (CTLD) domains. They play a crucial role in enabling NK cells to discriminate between self and nonself [32, 33]. The CD94-NKG2 C-type lectin receptors have been found to be expressed predominantly on the surface of a majority of NK cells and on subsets of $CD8^+$ T cells [34] and to be involved in NK cell-mediated recognition of MHC I molecules [35]. They are encoded by the NK gene complex (NKC) on human chromosome 12 (12p13.3–12p13.4). NKG2 receptors recognize the nonclassical MHC class I HLA-E molecule and can provide either an activating signal through their noncovalently association with the immunoreceptor tyrosine-based activation motif (ITAM)-containing DNAX adaptor protein of 12 kDa (DAP12) or an inhibitory signal when they contain an immunoreceptor tyrosine-based inhibitory motif (ITIM).

The cell surface molecule CD94 is a common invariant chain in five different disulfide-linked heterodimeric transmembrane glycoprotein complexes, including CD94-NKG2A, CD94-NKG2B, CD94-NKG2C, CD94-NKG2E, and CD94-NKG2H [36].

NKG2F is expressed in the cytosol and therefore does not form heterodimers with CD94. NKG2D (apparently not belonging to the NKG2 family) is expressed on the cell surface of NK cells, $\gamma\delta$ T cells, and subsets of $CD4^+$ and $CD8^+$ T cells as a homodimer. It lacks an ITIM sequence and is

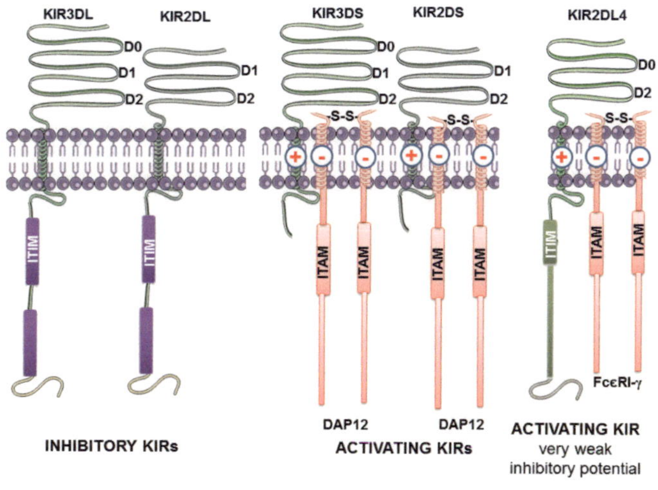


**Figure 1.** Structure of inhibitory and activating KIRs. DAP12, DNAX adaptor protein of 12 kDa; FcεRI-γ, high-affinity immunoglobulin epsilon receptor subunit gamma; ITAM, immunoreceptor tyrosine-based activation motif; ITIM, immunoreceptor tyrosine-based inhibitory motif; KIR, killer cell immunoglobulin-like receptor. This Figure was illustrated using image fragments from Servier Medical Art.

not associated with CD94. Its signaling is achieved by association with two dimers of DAP10, a transmembrane adaptor molecule containing a tyrosine-based signaling motif (YINM), carrying phosphatidylinositol-3 kinase-binding sites in their cytoplasmic tails and recruiting growth factor receptor-bound protein 2 (Grb2) [37].

Both NKG2A and NKG2B are alternative spliced products from a single gene. They can dimerize with CD94 to form inhibitory receptors through their cytoplasmic domains, which contain two ITIMs. Conversely, CD94-NKG2C, CD94-NKG2E, and CD94-NKG2H dimers and homodimer-forming NKG2D and the orphan receptor NKG2F activate NK cells [37–39].

### 8.2. MHC class I-independent receptors

There are at least three activating and two inhibitory MHC class I-independent receptors.

#### *8.2.1. Natural cytotoxicity receptors*

Natural cytotoxicity receptors (NCRs) are composed by a heterogeneous group of molecules belonging to IgSF and include NKp46 (NCR1), NKp44 (NCR2), and NKp30 (NCR3) activating receptors targeting most tumor cell lines. They are characterized by a type I transmembrane domain containing a positively charged amino acid residue and a short cytoplasmic tail. All these transmembrane type I receptors are expressed almost exclusively by NK cells. Binding of one or more of these receptors with a specific ligand leads to the increased NK cell activation and cytotoxicity [40]. It has been reported that these receptors can initiate tumor targeting by recognition of heparan sulfate on cancer cells [41].

#### *8.2.2. C-type lectin receptors*

C-type lectin receptors include mostly killer cell lectin-like receptor subfamily G member 1 (KLRG1) and KLRB1 (also known as NK1.1, NKR-P1A, or CD161), which inhibit the cytotoxicity of NK cells and therefore prevent tissue damage. NKR-P1A is encoded by the KLRB1 gene and recognizes lectin like transcript-1 (LLT1) as a functional ligand. Its signaling in NK cells has previously been known to involve the activation of acid sphingomyelinase, which represent the catabolic pathway for N-acyl-sphingosine generation as a second messenger for the induction of apoptosis, proliferation, and differentiation [42]. KLRG1 is expressed by antigen-experienced (memory) $CD4^+$ and $CD8^+$ T cells and by a large proportion of NK cells and naive phenotype $CD4^+$ and $CD8^+$ T cells in umbilical cord blood, as well as in a substantial subset of $\gamma\delta$ T cells [43]. KLRG1 can bind three of the classical cadherins (E, N, and R), which are ubiquitously expressed in vertebrates and mediate cell-cell adhesion by homotypic and heterotypic interactions [44]. It has also been postulated to be a marker of senescence [45].

## 9. NK cells in alarming situations

Situations related to cellular stress resulting from the presence of intracellular infectious agents and changes in self-elements (the presence of damaged-self [damage-associated molecular patterns (DAMPs)] or altered-self [tumor-associated molecular patterns (TAMPs)]) induce an increase in the expression of ligands that can "exclusively" stimulate activating receptors (major histocompatibility complex class I-related chain A [MICA], MICB, UL-16-binding proteins [ULBP]1, ULBP2, ULBP3, ULBP4, viral hemagglutinin, Newcastle disease hemagglutinin-neuraminidase, B7-H6, etc.) and consequently activate NK cell cytotoxicity.

## 10. NK cell-based immunotherapy in cancer

The main current therapeutic strategies, especially in allogeneic hematopoietic cell transplantation (HCT), are based on the use of NK cells through their education to render them alloreactive against tumor targets missing self-MHC ligand. In practice, autologous or haploidentical transplantation of NK cells requires obtaining of a very large number of pure and cytotoxic cells. Additionally, a favorable mismatch of the human leukocyte antigen class I (HLA I) molecules between donor and recipient tissues, or the absence of inhibitory KIR ligands in the recipient's HLA repertoire (KIR mismatch in the receptor-ligand model) allows NK cells in the graft to reduce its rejection by the host and the attack of residual leukemia cells, as well as the best prediction of the risk of relapse (**Figure 2**) [46, 47]. Finally, other promising approaches aim to induce an increase in their cytotoxic activities in the treatment of both hematopoietic and solid cancers by blocking inhibitory receptor signal transduction.

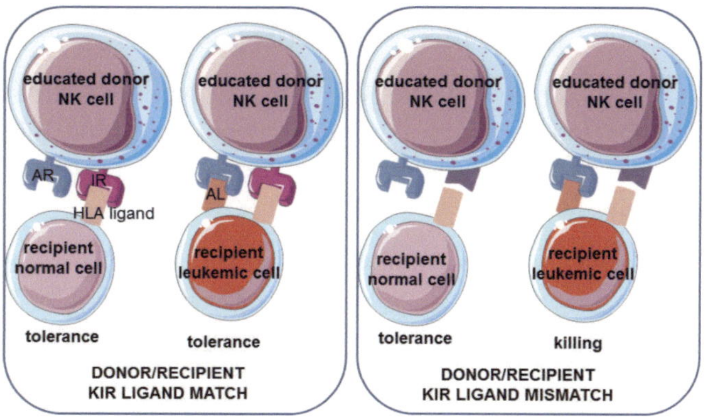


**Figure 2.** Role of KIR ligand mismatch in killing leukemic targets. AR, activating receptor; AL, activating ligand; IR, inhibitory receptor; KIR, killer cell immunoglobulin-like receptor. (Adapted from Ref. [26]. Images of cells are provided from Servier Medical Art.).

## 11. Conclusions

The specific structural and functional features of NK cells describe them as major players in innate antitumor immunosurveillance and in the fight against infection. Their availability at the proximity of cellular stress signals allows them to effectively control both the process of carcinogenesis and the development of infectious diseases. Nevertheless, their activities seem to be strongly immunomodulated by cell microenvironment factors. Therefore, one of the best therapeutic strategies should create an ideal microenvironment for NK cell infiltration within target tissues while decreasing functions of their inhibitory receptors and enhancing their cytotoxic activities. Such a strategy should contribute not only to substantially increase the efficacy of targeted immunotherapies but also to prevent relapse after transplantation.

## Author details

Mourad Aribi

Address all correspondence to: m_aribi@mail.univ-tlemcen.dz

Laboratory of Applied Molecular Biology and Immunology (BIOMOLIM, W0414100), University of Tlemcen, Tlemcen, Algeria

## References

[1] Cheent K, Khakoo SI. Natural killer cells: Integrating diversity with function. Immunology. 2009;**126**:449-457. DOI: 10.1111/j.1365-2567.2009.03045.x

[2] Tao X, Xu A. Basic Knowledge of Immunology. In: Amphioxus Immun. Elsevier; 2016. pp. 15-42. DOI: 10.1016/B978-0-12-849903-0.00002-6

[3] Lowell GH, Smith LF, Artenstein MS, Nash GS, MacDermott RP. Antibody-dependent cell-mediated antibacterial activity of human mononuclear cells. I. K lymphocytes and monocytes are effective against meningococi in cooperation with human imune sera. The Journal of Experimental Medicine. 1979;**150**:127-137

[4] Caraux J, Thierry C, Serrou B. Quantitative comparison of K cell potential in human T and null cells. European Journal of Immunology. 1978;**8**:806-812. DOI: 10.1002/eji.1830081111

[5] Haegert DG, Coombs RR. Do human B and null lymphocytes form a single immunoglobulin-bearing population? Lancet (London, England). 1979;**2**:1051-1053

[6] Clot J, Guilhou JJ, Meynadier J, Paradis B, Andary M. Immunologic aspects of psoriasis. III. Fc-gamma-receptor bearing mononuclear cells in peripheral blood. The British Journal of Dermatology. 1978;**99**:25-30

[7] Molgora M, Bonavita E, Ponzetta A, Riva F, Barbagallo M, Jaillon S, Popović B, Bernardini G, Magrini E, Gianni F, Zelenay S, Jonjić S, Santoni A, Garlanda C, Mantovani A. IL-1R8 is a checkpoint in NK cells regulating anti-tumour and anti-viral activity. Nature. 2017; **551**:110-114. DOI: 10.1038/nature24293

[8] Cruz-González DDJ, Gómez-Martin D, Baranda L, Abud-Mendoza C, Alcocer-Varela J, González-Amaro R, Monsiváis-Urenda AE. Analysis of the regulatory function of

NK cells from patients with systemic lupus erythematosus. Clinical and Experimental Immunology. 2017. DOI: 10.1111/cei.13073

[9] Spits H, Artis D, Colonna M, Diefenbach A, Di Santo JP, Eberl G, Koyasu S, Locksley RM, McKenzie ANJ, Mebius RE, Powrie F, Vivier E. Innate lymphoid cells—A proposal for uniform nomenclature. Nature Reviews. Immunology. 2013;**13**:145-149. DOI: 10.1038/nri3365

[10] Sun JC, Lanier LL. NK cell development, homeostasis and function: Parallels with $CD8^+$ T cells. Nature Reviews. Immunology. 2011;**11**:645-657. DOI: 10.1038/nri3044

[11] Cerwenka A, Lanier LL. Natural killer cells, viruses and cancer. Nature Reviews. Immunology. 2001;**1**:41-49. DOI: 10.1038/35095564

[12] Robertson MJ, Ritz J. Biology and clinical relevance of human natural killer cells. Blood. 1990;**76**:2421-2438

[13] Sun JC, Beilke JN, Bezman NA, Lanier LL. Homeostatic proliferation generates long-lived natural killer cells that respond against viral infection. The Journal of Experimental Medicine. 2011;**208**:357-368. DOI: 10.1084/jem.20100479

[14] Freud AG, Yokohama A, Becknell B, Lee MT, Mao HC, Ferketich AK, Caligiuri MA. Evidence for discrete stages of human natural killer cell differentiation in vivo. The Journal of Experimental Medicine. 2006;**203**:1033-1043. DOI: 10.1084/jem.20052507

[15] Poli A, Michel T, Thérésine M, Andrès E, Hentges F, Zimmer J. CD56bright natural killer (NK) cells: An important NK cell subset. Immunology. 2009;**126**:458-465. DOI: 10.1111/j.1365-2567.2008.03027.x

[16] Murphy WJ, Koh CY, Raziuddin A, Bennett M, Longo DL. Immunobiology of natural killer cells and bone marrow transplantation: Merging of basic and preclinical studies. Immunological Reviews. 2001;**181**:279-289

[17] Zhou Q, Gil-Krzewska A, Peruzzi G, Borrego F. Matrix metalloproteinases inhibition promotes the polyfunctionality of human natural killer cells in therapeutic antibody-based anti-tumour immunotherapy. Clinical and Experimental Immunology. 2013;**173**:131-139. DOI: 10.1111/cei.12095

[18] Campoli M, Ferrone S. HLA antigen and NK cell activating ligand expression in malignant cells: a story of loss or acquisition. Seminars in Immunopathology. 2011;**33**:321-334. DOI: 10.1007/s00281-011-0270-z

[19] Ljunggren HG, Kärre K. In search of the "missing self": MHC molecules and NK cell recognition. Immunology Today. 1990;**11**:237-244

[20] Gu J. Primary Liver Cancer: Challenges and Perspectives. Hangzhou/Heidelberg: Zhejiang University Press/Springer; 2012 http://site.ebrary.com/id/11045219 [Accessed 01-11-2017]

[21] Körner C, Altfeld M. Role of KIR3DS1 in human diseases. Frontiers in Immunology. 2012; **3**:326. DOI: 10.3389/fimmu.2012.00326

[22] Moesta AK, Graef T, Abi-Rached L, Older Aguilar AM, Guethlein LA, Parham P. Humans differ from other hominids in lacking an activating NK cell receptor that recognizes the C1 epitope of MHC class I. Journal of Immunology (Baltimore, Md.: 1950). 2010;**185**:4233-4237. DOI: 10.4049/jimmunol.1001951

[23] Lanier LL. DAP10- and DAP12-associated receptors in innate immunity. Immunological Reviews. 2009;**227**:150-160. DOI: 10.1111/j.1600-065X.2008.00720.x

[24] Della Chiesa M, Romeo E, Falco M, Balsamo M, Augugliaro R, Moretta L, Bottino C, Moretta A, Vitale M. Evidence that the KIR2DS5 gene codes for a surface receptor triggering natural killer cell function. European Journal of Immunology. 2008;**38**:2284-2289. DOI: 10.1002/eji.200838434

[25] Li Y, Hofmann M, Wang Q, Teng L, Chlewicki LK, Pircher H, Mariuzza RA. Structure of natural killer cell receptor KLRG1 bound to E-cadherin reveals basis for MHC-independent missing self recognition. Immunity. 2009;**31**:35-46. DOI: 10.1016/j.immuni.2009.04.019

[26] Foley B, Felices M, Cichocki F, Cooley S, Verneris MR, Miller JS. The biology of NK cells and their receptors affects clinical outcomes after hematopoietic cell transplantation (HCT). Immunological Reviews. 2014;**258**:45-63. DOI: 10.1111/imr.12157

[27] Rajagopalan S, Long EO. KIR2DL4 (CD158d): An activation receptor for HLA-G. Frontiers in Immunology. 2012;**3**:258. DOI: 10.3389/fimmu.2012.00258

[28] Liu WR, Kim J, Nwankwo C, Ashworth LK, Arm JP. Genomic organization of the human leukocyte immunoglobulin-like receptors within the leukocyte receptor complex on chromosome 19q13.4. Immunogenetics. 2000;**51**:659-669

[29] Brandstadter JD, Yang Y. Natural killer cell responses to viral infection. Journal of Innate Immunity. 2011;**3**:274-279. DOI: 10.1159/000324176

[30] Long EO, Kim HS, Liu D, Peterson ME, Rajagopalan S. Controlling natural killer cell responses: integration of signals for activation and inhibition. Annual Review of Immunology. 2013;**31**:227-258. DOI: 10.1146/annurev-immunol-020711-075005

[31] Traherne JA, Martin M, Ward R, Ohashi M, Pellett F, Gladman D, Middleton D, Carrington M, Trowsdale J. Mechanisms of copy number variation and hybrid gene formation in the KIR immune gene complex. Human Molecular Genetics. 2010;**19**:737-751. DOI: 10.1093/hmg/ddp538

[32] Redelinghuys P, Brown GD. Inhibitory C-type lectin receptors in myeloid cells. Immunology Letters. 2011;**136**:1-12. DOI: 10.1016/j.imlet.2010.10.005.

[33] Jacobs J, Braun J. The mucosal microbiome. In: Mucosal Immunol. Elsevier; 2015. pp. 63-77. DOI: 10.1016/B978-0-12-415847-4.00005-7.

[34] Borrego F, Masilamani M, Marusina AI, Tang X, Coligan JE. The CD94/NKG2 family of receptors: From molecules and cells to clinical relevance. Immunologic Research. 2006;**35**:263-278. DOI: 10.1385/IR:35:3:263

[35] López-Botet M, Carretero M, Pérez-Villar J, Bellón T, Llano M, Navarro F. The CD94/NKG2 C-type lectin receptor complex: involvement in NK cell-mediated recognition of HLA class I molecules. Immunologic Research. 1997;**16**:175-185

[36] Lanier LL. NK cell recognition. Annual Review of Immunology. 2005;**23**:225-274. DOI: 10.1146/annurev.immunol.23.021704.115526

[37] Posch P, Hurley C. Histocompatibility. In: Blood Bone Marrow Pathol. Elsevier; 2011. pp. 641-676. DOI: 10.1016/B978-0-7020-3147-2.00039-0.

[38] Natural Killer Cells. In: Immunol. Pharm. Elsevier; 2012. pp. 169-174. DOI: 10.1016/B978-0-323-06947-2.10021-5

[39] Orbelyan GA, Tang F, Sally B, Solus J, Meresse B, Ciszewski C, Grenier J-C, Barreiro LB, Lanier LL, Jabri B. Human NKG2E is expressed and forms an intracytoplasmic complex with CD94 and DAP12. Journal of Immunology (Baltimore, Md.: 1950). 2014;**193**:610-616. DOI: 10.4049/jimmunol.1400556

[40] Horton NC, Mathew PA. NKp44 and natural cytotoxicity receptors as damage-associated molecular pattern recognition receptors. Frontiers in Immunology. 2015;**6**:31. DOI: 10.3389/fimmu.2015.00031

[41] Hecht M-L, Rosental B, Horlacher T, Hershkovitz O, De Paz JL, Noti C, Schauer S, Porgador A, Seeberger PH. Natural cytotoxicity receptors NKp30, NKp44 and NKp46 bind to different heparan sulfate/heparin sequences. Journal of Proteome Research. 2009;**8**:712-720. DOI: 10.1021/pr800747c

[42] Pozo D, Valés-Gómez M, Mavaddat N, Williamson SC, Chisholm SE, Reyburn H. CD161 (human NKR-P1A) signaling in NK cells involves the activation of acid sphingomyelinase. Journal of Immunology (Baltimore, Md.: 1950). 2006;**176**:2397-2406

[43] Thimme R, Appay V, Koschella M, Panther E, Roth E, Hislop AD, Rickinson AB, Rowland-Jones SL, Blum HE, Pircher H. Increased expression of the NK cell receptor KLRG1 by virus-specific CD8 T cells during persistent antigen stimulation. Journal of Virology. 2005;**79**:12112-12116. DOI: 10.1128/JVI.79.18.12112-12116.2005

[44] Ito M, Maruyama T, Saito N, Koganei S, Yamamoto K, Matsumoto N. Killer cell lectin-like receptor G1 binds three members of the classical cadherin family to inhibit NK cell cytotoxicity. The Journal of Experimental Medicine. 2006;**203**:289-295. DOI: 10.1084/jem.20051986

[45] Gründemann C, Bauer M, Schweier O, von Oppen N, Lässing U, Saudan P, Becker K-F, Karp K, Hanke T, Bachmann MF, Pircher H. Cutting edge: Identification of E-cadherin as a ligand for the murine killer cell lectin-like receptor G1. Journal of Immunology (Baltimore, Md.: 1950). 2006;**176**:1311-1315

[46] Leung W, Iyengar R, Turner V, Lang P, Bader P, Conn P, Niethammer D, Handgretinger R. Determinants of antileukemia effects of allogeneic NK cells. Journal of Immunology (Baltimore, Md.: 1950). 2004;**172**:644-650

[47] Karre K. Immunology: A perfect mismatch. Science. 2002;**295**:2029-2031. DOI: 10.1126/science.1070538

Chapter 2

# NK Cells and Cancer

May Sabry and Mark W. Lowdell

Additional information is available at the end of the chapter

http://dx.doi.org/10.5772/intechopen.69658

**Abstract**

NK cells play an important role in host immunity against cancer by exerting cytotoxicity and secreting a wide variety of cytokines to inhibit tumour progression. Their effector functions are regulated by the integration of opposing signals from activating and inhibitory receptors, which determine NK cell activity against tumour targets. NK cell cytotoxicity requires successful progression through discrete activation events that begin with NK cell adhesion to a tumour target cell and culminate in the polarized release of cytotoxic granules into the immunological synapse. Tumour cells can evade NK cell attack through numerous mechanisms such as shedding of activating ligands, upregulation of inhibitory ligands, or stimulation of inhibitory regulatory T lymphocytes. A better understanding of specific NK cell responses to tumour targets can generate better NK cell-based immunotherapeutic strategies for cancer. This chapter discusses NK cell immunosurveillance of cancer, NK cell tumour recognition strategies, cancer immune evasion from NK cells, and different approaches to NK cell modulation for cancer therapy.

**Keywords:** natural killer, cancer, cytokines, target recognition

## 1. Introduction: cancer immunosurveillance by NK cells

Natural killer (NK) cells were discovered more than four decades ago and were the focus of some of the earliest trials of cancer immunotherapy. With our more sophisticated understanding of their functional requirements, NK cells are once again attracting attention for their potential in cancer therapy [1]. Initially thought to be an artefact in cytotoxicity assays, NK cells are now known to play an important role in host immunity against tumourigenesis. The theory of cancer immunosurveillance was proposed by Burnet and Thomas in 1957, postulating that immune cells continuously monitor the body such that any threat to the immune system is detected and eliminated [2]. In 1975, NK cells were discovered in mice as a subpopulation of lymphocytes capable of killing tumour cells without prior sensitization [3–5]. This led to considerable enthusiasm over the possibility that they function as one of the main effector cells of immunosurveillance. Several studies in the 1980s reported a higher cancer incidence in individuals with genetic disorders such as Chediak-Higashi syndrome and X-linked lymphoproliferative syndrome, which lead to defective NK cell function [6, 7]. Subsequent mouse studies showed increased tumour growth in mice with impaired NK cell activity or mice treated with an NK cell-depleting agent [8, 9]. A long-term epidemiological study following cancer patients reported that subjects with lower NK cell activity had a higher incidence of several types of cancer [10]. Collectively, data from both mouse and human studies support the theory of cancer immunosurveillance and the concept that NK cells play a critical role in tumour control and eradication [11, 12]. The two main effector functions observed by NK cells against tumour targets are target cell elimination and cytokine secretion [13]. Until recently, these two effector functions were thought to follow similar mechanisms of activation, but now it is recognized that cytokine secretion by NK cells is distinct from cytotoxicity [14].

### 1.1. Target cell elimination

NK cells kill tumour cells through granule exocytosis or death receptor ligation. Following NK cell activation, NK cells release the contents of their granules for target cell elimination. The membrane disrupting protein perforin, and a family of serine proteases termed granzymes, are the critical effector molecules contained in their granules [15]. Perforin results in the disruption of endosomal trafficking and binds in a calcium-dependent manner to phospholipid components of the lipid bilayer to facilitate entry of granzymes into the target cell cytosol [16]. Once granzymes enter the target cell, they induce apoptosis. In addition to granule exocytosis, NK cells can directly eliminate target cells through the engagement of cell surface death receptors. NK cells express Fas ligand (FasL) and TNF-related apoptosis-inducing ligand (TRAIL), which are both members of the TNF family and are shown to induce target cell apoptosis once bound to their respective receptors on target cells [16].

### 1.2. Cytokine secretion

Resting NK cells secrete a plethora of cytokines that help eliminate target cells and amplify activation signals for a more efficient immune response. NK stimulation results in enhanced secretion of cytokines, which in turn influence the activity of other immune cells. Pro-inflammatory cytokines secreted by NK cells, which include interleukin (IL)-1, IL-6, IL-12, and the chemokine CXCL8 (also known as IL-8), can enhance the activation and proliferation of T cells, dendritic cells (DCs) and macrophages [17]. By contrast, anti-inflammatory cytokines such as IL-4 and IL-10 suppress T cell and macrophage function, but activate humoral responses. Chemokines, which are chemotactic cytokines, play an important role in directing various immune cells to target sites, such that more potent responses are achieved. Chemokines released by NK cells include, in addition to CXCL8, the macrophage inflammatory protein (MIP)-1$\alpha$ and MIP-1$\beta$; chemokine (C-C motif) ligand 5 (CCL5), also known as "regulated on activation normal T cell expressed and secreted" (RANTES); monocytes chemoattractant protein (MCP)-1; and eotaxin [18, 19]. The signalling pathways and mechanisms required for cytokine secretion also appear to be distinct from secretion of cytotoxic granules [14]. The localization and trafficking of IFN-$\gamma$ and TNF-$\alpha$ were shown to take place in compartments and vesicles that do not overlap with perforin or other late endosome granule markers. Recycling endosomes (REs) are not needed for release of perforin, but are required for cytokine secretion in NK cells. Although perforin granules are released in a polarized fashion at lytic synapses, distinct carriers transport both IFN-$\gamma$ and TNF-$\alpha$ to points all over the cell surface, including within the synapse, for non-polarized release.

## 2. NK tumour recognition

Prior to the discovery of NK cell receptors, it was unclear how NK cells could identify tumour targets for lysis. The 'missing-self' recognition model was initially proposed based on the observation that NK cells kill targets with reduced or absent expression of major histocompatibility complex class I (MHC I) molecules [20, 21]. This model explains why tumour or virally-infected cells with deficient MHC class I expression are targeted by NK cells, whereas healthy autologous cells remain protected. It also explains the hybrid resistance phenomenon, in which $F_1$ hybrid mice reject parental bone marrow cells donated by either parent, despite the fact that the transplant does not express foreign MHC molecules [22]. Early experiments supported the 'missing-self' model by demonstrating selective rejection of an MHC class I-deficient version of the tumour cell line RMA in mouse models, in which the results were reversed after treating mice with an NK-depleting agent [20]. The characterization of NK cell inhibitory receptors further supported this recognition model by explaining the molecular mechanisms by which NK cells sensed the downregulation of MHC class I expression [23–29]. NK cell-mediated killing of MHC class I-deficient cells also provides a safeguard mechanism for MHC class I-restricted elimination by cytotoxic T lymphocytes. However, the 'missing-self' hypothesis alone failed to explain why NK cells spare autologous cells with absent MHC class I expression or kill tumour cells with sufficient MHC class I expression [30, 31]. The discovery of a wide array of activating NK cell receptors that detect stress-induced ligands on damaged or stressed cells led to the proposition of the 'induced-self' model, by which NK cells kill targets with upregulated expression of activating ligands. It is now understood that NK cell functions are tightly regulated by the integration of opposing signals from activating and inhibitory receptors [32]. Together these models suggest that NK cells detect changes in self-ligands on the surface of autologous cells. NK cells can also be activated through antibody-dependent cellular cytotoxicity (ADCC) whereby the NK cells are triggered directly through ligation of CD16 to kill tumour target cells to which the antibody has bound. The anti-CD20 antibody, Rituximab mediated lysis of CD20+ve lymphoma cells through this mechanism. **Figure 1** summarizes tumour recognition strategies by NK cells.

### 2.1. NK cell inhibitory receptors

Human NK cell inhibitory receptors fall into two groups: the killer immunoglobulin-like receptors (KIRs), and the lectin-like receptor NKG2A, which forms a heterodimeric complex with CD94. KIRs bind to human leukocyte antigen (HLA)-A, -B, or -C, whereas the NKG2/CD94 complexes ligate HLA-E. Human KIRs contain either two (KIR2D) or three (KIR3D) immunoglobulin (Ig)-like domains in their extracellular domain. KIR2D receptors recognize

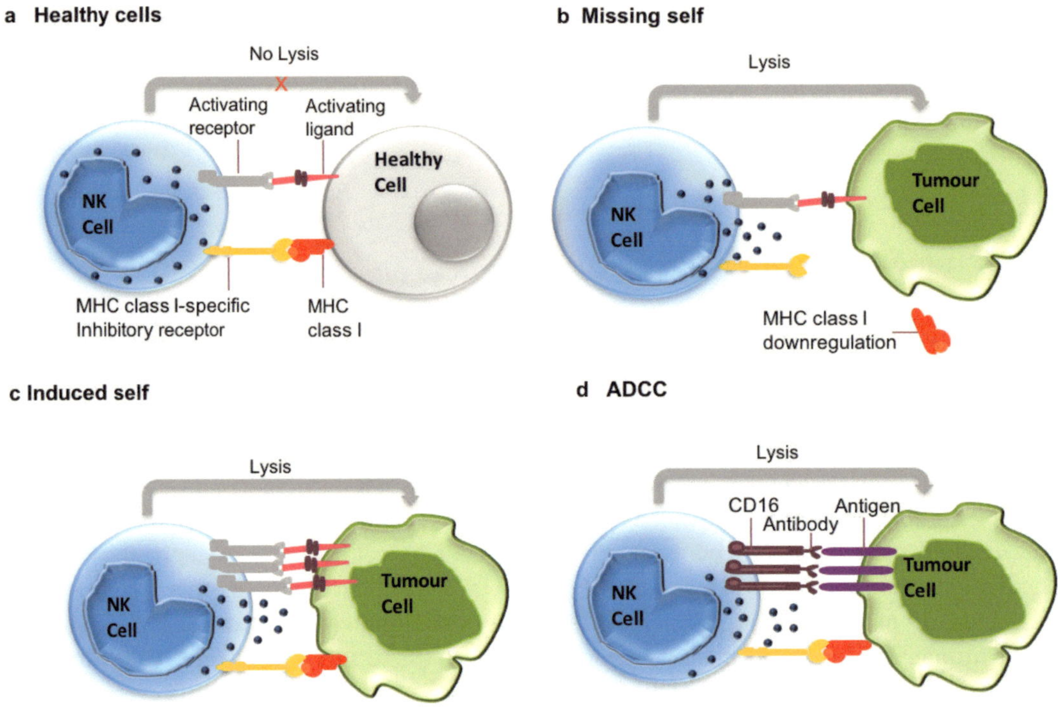


**Figure 1.** Tumour recognition strategies by NK cells. A) Balanced signals delivered by activating and inhibitory NK cells receptors are recognized as healthy and spared from NK cell-mediated lysis. B) Tumour cells downregulate MHC class I molecules, and are recognized by NK cells through 'missing self' for lysis. C) The upregulation of stress- or damage-related ligands is recognized by activating NK cell receptors and can overcome inhibitory signals to result in tumour lysis through the 'induced-self'. D) Antigen-specific antibodies can bind CD16 on NK cells to result in ADCC. ADCC: antibody-dependent cell-mediated cytotoxicity; MHC: major histocompatibility complex; NK: natural killer cell.

HLA-C alleles, whereas KIR3D receptors recognize HLA-A or HLA-B alleles. The common pathway generated by ligation of inhibitory receptors is characterized by tyrosine phosphorylation of immune tyrosine-based inhibitory motifs (ITIM) that recruit tyrosine phosphatases such as the Src homology 2 domain-containing phosphatase (SHP)-1 and SHP-2, which are responsible for the inhibition of various NK cell effector functions [33].

## 2.2. NK cell education

NK cell education refers to the mechanisms through which inhibitory input by MHC class I during development translates into functional responsiveness in mature NK cells [34]. Unlike the educational processes in T- or B-cell development, NK cell education remains a topic of intense debate, with several models proposed to explain how NK cell responsiveness relates to inhibitory signalling. NK cells that lack ITIM-bearing inhibitory receptors for self-MHC-I and NK cells from hosts that lack MHC-I ligands for ITIM-bearing inhibitory receptors have a reduced responsiveness to activation signals, such as stimulation by sensitive target cells or cross-linking of NK cell activating receptors [34–37]. These results have led to the two main models in NK cell education. The first 'disarming' model proposes that in the absence of inhibition, continuous stimulation of NK cells leads to a state of hyporesponsiveness [38]. The second model proposes that inhibitory receptors provide an ITIM-dependent signal to the NK cells that renders them responsive [39]. This model is referred to as 'arming' or 'licensing', although the latter term is now understood to include any process by which NK cells that receive signals through inhibitory receptors for self-MHC-I gain responsiveness [40]. Studies reporting that NK cell responsiveness is calibrated according to the strength of inhibitory signals received [36, 41, 42], have led to a third 'rheostat' model that aimed to reconcile the two opposing models, and account for the quantitative tuning of NK cell responsiveness [42–44]. The rheostat model postulates that NK cell responsiveness is dynamically calibrated based on the strength of inhibitory signals received. More recent data demonstrating that NK cell 'tuning' or 'licensing' may be set by transient signals and can be reversible have led to an updated model known as the 'revocable license' [45]. The revocable license model argues that NK cells can keep their license as long as they are tightly regulated by inhibitory signals, but once this inhibitory input is lost, their license is revoked. Many questions regarding the molecular basis of licensing and the effect of subsequent activation signals on licensed vs. unlicensed cells remain unanswered. In many cases, the original concept of 'missing-self' and the self-tolerance of NK cells in an MHC-I-devoid environment cannot be explained without the involvement of NK cell activating receptors.

### 2.3. NK cell activation receptors

NK cell activation receptors can be grouped into three categories: those that associate with immunoreceptor tyrosine-based activation motif (ITAM)-containing subunits, the DAP10-associated NK group 2 member D (NKG2D) receptor and a number of other receptors including DNAX accessory molecule-1 (DNAM-1), CD2 and 2B4. Receptors that associate with the ITAM-containing adapter proteins transmit signals through the recruitment of tyrosine kinases Syk or ZAP70, and include CD16, which mediates antibody-dependent cellular cytotoxicity, and the natural cytotoxicity receptors (NCRs) NKp30, NKp44, NKp46 and NKp80, which are known to play an important role in NK-mediated cytotoxicity against tumour cells [46]. NKp30 and NKp46 are constitutively expressed on all peripheral blood NK cells, whereas NKp44 is expressed only on activated NK cells. NKp30 binds the nuclear factor HLA-B-associated transcript (BAT)-3, NKp46 binds to influenza haemagglutinin and the cellular ligand for NKp80 is the activation-induced C-type lectin (AICL) [47]. NKG2D associates with the DAP10 adaptor protein and signals through a phosphoinositide 3-kinase (PI3K)-binding motif. It binds several ligands associated with stress, infection or transformation including MHC I chain-related protein A and B (MICA/B) and the UL16-binding proteins 1–4 (UBLP1-4) [48].

### 2.4. NK cell activation

NK cells require the co-engagement of multiple activating receptors in order to exhibit natural cytotoxicity against tumour target cells [49]. Upon encounter with potential target cells, an immunological synapse forms at the point of contact between the NK cell and the target cell, where NK cell receptors can interact with their respective ligands. Given sufficient activation signals, NK cell cytoskeletal rearrangements are initiated, which result in the polarization of NK cell lytic granules toward the immunological synapse, where they eventually fuse and release their cytotoxic contents on to the target cell [50]. In contrast to CTLs, NK cells have their cytotoxic granules preformed before target cell recognition, and so their release is initially constrained until sufficient signalling is achieved. NK cells have also been shown to establish cytoskeletal polarity more slowly than CTLs, and to have a unique sensitivity to minor interference with cytoskeletal dynamics [51]. This stepwise progression in activation events with specific requirements for synergistic signalling may provide a mechanistic explanation of how the spontaneous cytotoxic capacity of NK cells is regulated [52]. **Figure 2** outlines NK cell activation events at the immunological synapse with a tumour target cell.

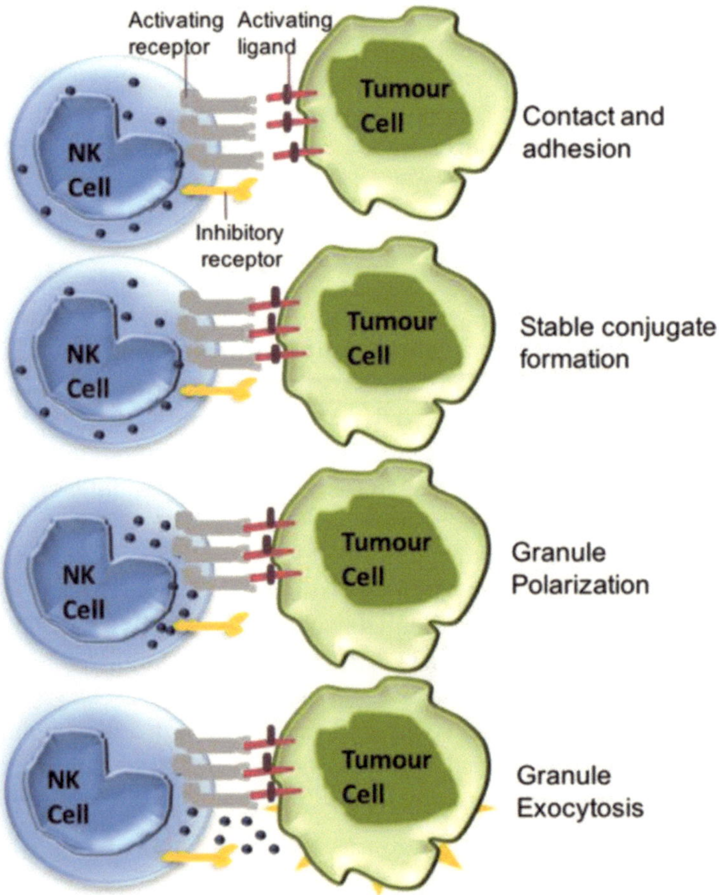


**Figure 2.** Activating immunological synapse between NK cell and tumour target. NK cell encounter with a tumour cell target generates an immunological synapse at the point of contact. If the ligand combination on the tumour target engages NK cell activating receptors sufficiently, cytoskeletal rearrangements take place resulting in granule polarization and the eventual release of cytotoxic granules on to the target cell. NK: natural killer cell.

http://dx.doi.org/10.5772/intechopen.69658

## 3. Cancer immune evasion from NK cells

Although the development of any malignancy is under surveillance by immune cells, tumour cells can still obtain means to escape from the immune system and proliferate. The recent addition of immune evasion as an emerging 'hallmark' of cancer, sheds lights on growing evidence in support of cancer evasion of immune cells [53]. Malignant cells acquire a set of biological capabilities during their development, allowing them to overcome recognition and elimination by the immune system. These capabilities are acquired with the assistance of inflammatory cells and soluble factors in the tumour microenvironment, which play an active role in the tumour development process. Kiessling et al. proposed that cancer evasion from NK cells involves an early stage of tumour formation and growth, which is associated with antigen-specific tolerance, and a later stage, which induces a state of immunodeficiency [54]. Cancer immunoediting, as proposed by Dunn et al. argues that less immunogenic variants are positively selected during tumour formation as they have a better chance of survival in a normal immunological environment [55]. This led to the formulation of the three Es of cancer immunoediting; elimination, equilibrium and escape [56]. The elimination phase involves tumour eradication by immune cells. Any tumour cells that survive the elimination phase enter the equilibrium phase. During this phase, immune cells and tumour cells are in a dynamic equilibrium, with selective pressure exerted on tumour cells, such that only the less immunogenic variants survive. In the escape phase, tumour cell variants which are positively selected in the equilibrium phase continue to grow.

Tumours can evade NK cell attack directly by insufficient expression of ligands for NK cell activation receptors, such that the activation threshold for NK cell granule exocytosis is not met. Once successful evasion from NK cell attack is achieved, the tumour cells create the microenvironment necessary for continued growth. There are several strategies for direct evasion from NK cells by tumour targets. For example, tumours have been shown to reduce expression or shed ligands for important NK cell receptors. The NKG2D ligands UBLP2, MICA and MICB are commonly shed by tumour cells to evade NK cell attack through NKG2D recognition. Alternatively, tumour cells can increase MHC class I, soluble MIC and FasL expression in order to increase NK cell inhibitory signalling [30, 57, 58]. The secretion of soluble factors such as IL-10, TGF-β and indoleamine 2, 3-dioxygense (IDO) by tumour targets suppresses the adaptive immune response to exhibit significantly less anti-tumour capacity [59–63].

Tumour cells employ numerous cell types from the immune system for indirect NK cell evasion mechanisms. Tumour cells have been reported to recruit, myeloid-derived suppressor cells (MDSCs), regulatory T cells, which release immunosuppressive Th2 cytokines and phagocytes, which release reactive oxygen species (ROS) to inhibit NK cell function [64]. Macrophages found in the tumour microenvironment can be classified as M1 or M2. The M1 subtype is associated with tumour control, through pro-inflammatory cytokine and ROS secretion, whereas the M2 subtype promotes tumour growth and invasion through the production of anti-inflammatory cytokines, upregulation of scavenging receptors and tissue remodelling [65]. Excess ROS in the tumour microenvironment can lead to tumour cell lysis. The Warburg effect, by which tumour cells rely mostly on glycolysis for energy production, enables cancer cells to resist ROS-related death and gain survival advantage for metastasis [66].

Tumour cells can also impair dendritic cell (DC) function to prevent NK cell priming, by changing their expressions of IL-6, IL-10, vascular epithelial growth factor or GM-CSF. Finally, tumour cells have also been shown to lower NK cell count by decreasing the numbers of lymphoid progenitor cells [67]. **Figure 3** describes different tumour immune evasion strategies from NK cells.

## 4. NK cell modulation for cancer therapy

The ability of NK cells to kill tumour cells has made them very attractive in immunotherapy. NK cell impairments associated with tumour development and progression have been frequently reported in cancer patients, including weakened effector functions and an altered phenotype with downregulation of activating NK cell receptors [68]. Different strategies have been employed to repair, replace or enhance the biological functions of autologous or

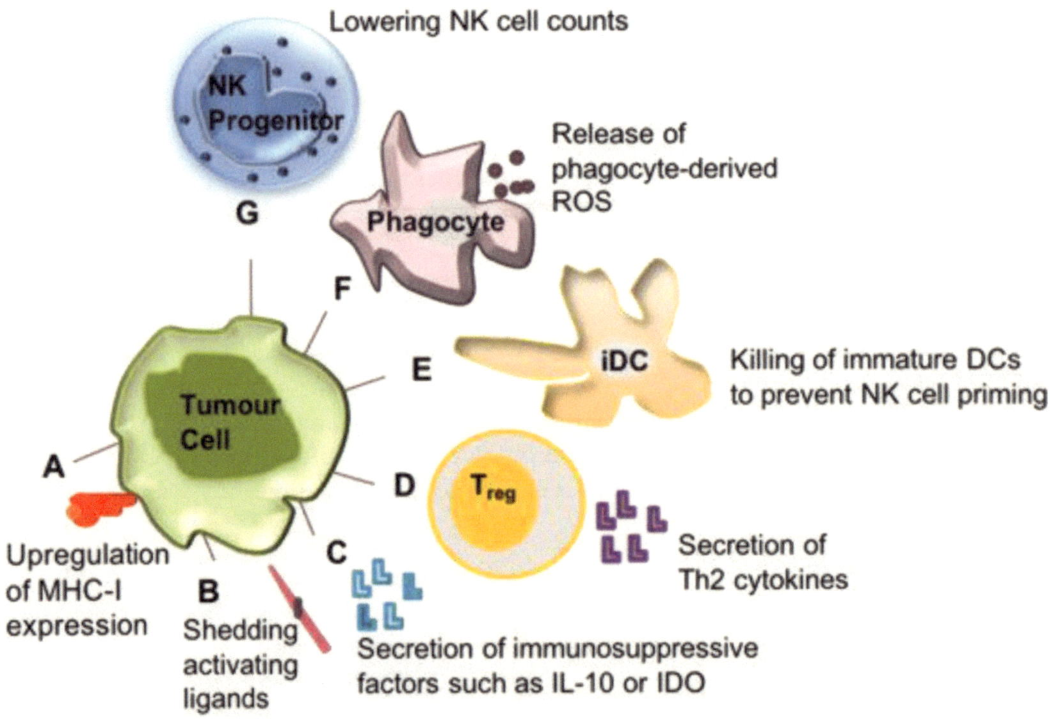


**Figure 3.** Tumour Evasion from NK cells. Tumour cells use direct and indirect mechanisms to evade NK cell attack. Direct mechanisms include A) upregulation of MHC class I expression B) shedding of soluble ligands for NK cell activation receptors and C) release of inhibitory cytokines. Indirect mechanisms include D) activation of inhibitory regulatory T cells E) killing of immature dendritic cells to prevent NK cell priming F) release of phagocyte-derived inhibitory cytokines and G) reducing the number of NK progenitor cells to lower NK cell counts. NK: natural killer cell; DC: dendritic cell, IL-10: interleukin 10; IDO: indoleamine 2,3-dioxygenase; MHC: major histocompatibility complex; ROS: reactive oxygen species; Th2: T helper cell type 2.

allogeneic NK cells *in vivo* and *ex vivo*. In a clinical setting, the key factors to be considered are the number, purity, proliferative capacity and activation state of NK cells. The most limiting of these factors is obtaining a sufficient number of NK cells, hence the extensive development of *ex vivo* expansion methods for NK cell adoptive immunotherapy applications. The impressive clinical responses seen following administration of chimeric antigen receptor T cells (CAR-T) has led to trials of CAR-NK cells at centres in the US and Europe. Reports of pre-clinical data are encouraging and suggest that the more constrained proliferation of CAR-NK cells *in vivo* and the lower release of inflammatory cytokines may provide improve the safety profile.

The delivery of IL-2, IL-12 and IL-15 genes to the human NK cell line NK-92 has also been shown to enhance proliferative and cytotoxic capabilities. These cytokines are known to play important roles in the enhancement of survival and activation of many immune cells including T cells, B cells and NK cells. Strategies to enhance endogenous NK cell function *in vivo* through cytokines were pioneered by Rosenberg et al. who demonstrated great initial potential for IL-2 administration in advanced cancer patients [69]. *In vitro* stimulation of NK cells by activating cytokines such as IL-2 is known as the lymphokine-activated killer (LAK) phenomenon [70]. In early experiments, NK cells were activated *ex vivo* and adoptively transferred to patients with advanced metastatic renal cancer and melanoma along with IL-2 infusions. However, overall data from clinical trials since then have failed to provide a convincing proof of efficacy [68]. The clinical efficacy of LAK therapy was limited by the toxicity of IL-2 and the potential expansion of T regulatory cells. Mouse NK cells stimulated *in vitro* with a combination of IL-12, IL-15 and IL-18 were recently shown to have enhanced effector functions and longer survival after adoptive cell transfer [71]. Target cell stimulation of NK cells is an alternative to *in vitro* cytokine stimulation. Recent studies reported a tumour-priming approach, in which human NK cells are activated by co-incubation with an NK-resistant leukaemia cell line in the absence of IL-2 [72]. The clinical potential of these tumour-primed NK cells has been explored in acute myeloid leukaemia and multiple myeloma with promising results in autologous and allogeneic settings [73].

The last three decades unravelled different molecular mechanisms governing NK cell-mediated anti-tumour functions. This led to the development of a variety of strategies for NK cell-based immunotherapy of cancer. However, many challenges still remain as we better our molecular and functional characterization of NK cells and their receptors, and decipher the different signalling pathways involved in NK cell recognition of targets. NK cell responses can differ according to the type, combination and intensity of signals. Thus, a better understanding of tumour-specific responses at the bench, will lead to novel therapeutic strategies with better efficacy in the clinic.

## Author details

May Sabry and Mark W. Lowdell*

*Address all correspondence to: m.lowdell@ucl.ac.uk

Department of Haematology, University College London Medical School, University College London, London, United Kingdom

## References


[1] Morvan MG, Lanier LL. NK cells and cancer: You can teach innate cells new tricks. Nature Reviews Cancer. 2016;**16**(1):7-19

[2] Burnet M. Cancer; A biological approach. I. The processes of control. British Medical Journal. 1957;**1**(5022):779-786

[3] Herberman RB, Nunn ME, Lavrin DH. Natural cytotoxic reactivity of mouse lymphoid cells against syngeneic acid allogeneic tumors. I. Distribution of reactivity and specificity. International Journal of Cancer. 1975;**16**(2):216-229

[4] Kiessling R, Klein E, Pross H, Wigzell H. "Natural" killer cells in the mouse. II. Cytotoxic cells with specificity for mouse Moloney leukemia cells. Characteristics of the killer cell. European Journal of Immunology. 1975;**5**(2):117-121

[5] Kiessling R, Klein E, Wigzell H. "Natural" killer cells in the mouse. I. Cytotoxic cells with specificity for mouse Moloney leukemia cells. Specificity and distribution according to genotype. European Journal of Immunology. 1975;**5**(2):112-117

[6] Roder JC, Haliotis T, Klein M, Korec S, Jett JR, Ortaldo J, et al. A new immunodeficiency disorder in humans involving NK cells. Nature. 1980;**284**(5756):553-555

[7] Sullivan JL, Byron KS, Brewster FE, Purtilo DT. Deficient natural killer cell activity in x-linked lymphoproliferative syndrome. Science. 1980;**210**(4469):543-545

[8] Talmadge JE, Meyers KM, Prieur DJ, Starkey JR. Role of natural killer cells in tumor growth and metastasis: C57BL/6 normal and beige mice. Journal of the National Cancer Institute. 1980;**65**(5):929-935

[9] Gorelik E, Wiltrout RH, Okumura K, Habu S, Herberman RB. Role of NK cells in the control of metastatic spread and growth of tumor cells in mice. International Journal of Cancer. 1982;**30**(1):107-112

[10] Imai K, Matsuyama S, Miyake S, Suga K, Nakachi K. Natural cytotoxic activity of peripheral-blood lymphocytes and cancer incidence: An 11-year follow-up study of a general population. Lancet. 2000;**356**(9244):1795-1799

[11] Waldhauer I, Steinle A. NK cells and cancer immunosurveillance. Oncogene. 2008;**27**(45): 5932-5943

[12] Orange JS. Natural killer cell deficiency. Journal of Allergy and Clinical Immunology. 2013;**132**(3):515-525; quiz 26

[13] Vivier E, Tomasello E, Baratin M, Walzer T, Ugolini S. Functions of natural killer cells. Nature Immunology. 2008;**9**(5):503-510

[14] Reefman E, Kay JG, Wood SM, Offenhauser C, Brown DL, Roy S, et al. Cytokine secretion is distinct from secretion of cytotoxic granules in NK cells. The Journal of Immunology. 2010;**184**(9):4852-4862

[15] Smyth MJ, Thia KY, Cretney E, Kelly JM, Snook MB, Forbes CA, et al. Perforin is a major contributor to NK cell control of tumor metastasis. The Journal of Immunology. 1999;**162**(11):6658-6662

[16] Lavrik I, Golks A, Krammer PH. Death receptor signaling. Journal of Cell Science. 2005;**118**(Pt 2):265-267

[17] Elenkov IJ, Chrousos GP. Stress hormones, proinflammatory and antiinflammatory cytokines, and autoimmunity. Annals of the New York Academy of Sciences. 2002;**966**: 290-303

[18] Cuturi MC, Anegon I, Sherman F, Loudon R, Clark SC, Perussia B. et al. Production of hematopoietic colony-stimulating factors by human natural killer cells. The Journal of Experimental Medicine. 1989;**169**(2):569-583

[19] Roda JM, Parihar R, Magro C, Nuovo GJ, Tridandapani S, Carson WE, III. Natural killer cells produce T cell-recruiting chemokines in response to antibody-coated tumor cells. Cancer Research. 2006;**66**(1):517-526

[20] Karre K, Ljunggren HG, Piontek G, Kiessling R. Selective rejection of H-2-deficient lymphoma variants suggests alternative immune defence strategy. Nature. 1986;**319**(6055): 675-678

[21] Ljunggren HG, Karre K. In search of the 'missing self': MHC molecules and NK cell recognition. Immunology Today. 1990;**11**(7):237-244

[22] Murphy WJ, Kumar V, Bennett M. Rejection of bone marrow allografts by mice with severe combined immune deficiency (SCID). Evidence that natural killer cells can mediate the specificity of marrow graft rejection. The Journal of Experimental Medicine. 1987;**165**(4):1212-1217

[23] Brooks AG, Posch PE, Scorzelli CJ, Borrego F, Coligan JE. NKG2A complexed with CD94 defines a novel inhibitory natural killer cell receptor. The Journal of Experimental Medicine. 1997;**185**(4):795-800

[24] Carretero M, Cantoni C, Bellon T, Bottino C, Biassoni R, Rodriguez A, et al. The CD94 and NKG2-A C-type lectins covalently assemble to form a natural killer cell inhibitory receptor for HLA class I molecules. European Journal of Immunology. 1997;**27**(2):563-567

[25] Colonna M, Samaridis J. Cloning of immunoglobulin-superfamily members associated with HLA-C and HLA-B recognition by human natural killer cells. Science. 1995;**268**(5209):405-408

[26] D'Andrea A, Chang C, Franz-Bacon K, McClanahan T, Phillips JH, Lanier LL. Molecular cloning of NKB1. A natural killer cell receptor for HLA-B allotypes. The Journal of Immunology. 1995;**155**(5):2306-2310

[27] Karlhofer FM, Ribaudo RK, Yokoyama WM. MHC class I alloantigen specificity of Ly-49+ IL-2-activated natural killer cells. Nature. 1992;**358**(6381):66-70

[28] Sivori S, Vitale M, Bottino C, Marcenaro E, Sanseverino L, Parolini S, et al. CD94 functions as a natural killer cell inhibitory receptor for different HLA class I alleles: Identification of the inhibitory form of CD94 by the use of novel monoclonal antibodies. European Journal of Immunology. 1996;**26**(10):2487-2492

[29] Wagtmann N, Biassoni R, Cantoni C, Verdiani S, Malnati MS, Vitale M, et al. Molecular clones of the p58 NK cell receptor reveal immunoglobulin-related molecules with diversity in both the extra- and intracellular domains. Immunity. 1995;**2**(5):439-449

[30] Costello RT, Sivori S, Marcenaro E, Lafage-Pochitaloff M, Mozziconacci MJ, Reviron D, et al. Defective expression and function of natural killer cell-triggering receptors in patients with acute myeloid leukemia. Blood. 2002;**99**(10):3661-367

[31] Ruggeri L, Capanni M, Urbani E, Perruccio K, Shlomchik WD, Tosti A, et al. Effectiveness of donor natural killer cell alloreactivity in mismatched hematopoietic transplants. Science. 2002;**295**(5562):2097-100.

[32] Brumbaugh KM, Binstadt BA, Leibson PJ. Signal transduction during NK cell activation: Balancing opposing forces. Current Topics in Microbiology and Immunology. 1998;**230**:103-122

[33] Lanier LL. NK cell recognition. Annual Review of Immunology. 2005;**23**:225-274

[34] Anfossi N, Andre P, Guia S, Falk CS, Roetynck S, Stewart CA, et al. Human NK cell education by inhibitory receptors for MHC class I. Immunity. 2006;**25**(2):331-342

[35] Fernandez NC, Treiner E, Vance RE, Jamieson AM, Lemieux S, Raulet DH. A subset of natural killer cells achieves self-tolerance without expressing inhibitory receptors specific for self-MHC molecules. Blood. 2005;**105**(11):4416-4423

[36] Johansson S, Johansson M, Rosmaraki E, Vahlne G, Mehr R, Salmon-Divon M, et al. Natural killer cell education in mice with single or multiple major histocompatibility complex class I molecules. The Journal of Experimental Medicine. 2005;**201**(7): 1145-1155

[37] Kim S, Poursine-Laurent J, Truscott SM, Lybarger L, Song YJ, Yang L, et al. Licensing of natural killer cells by host major histocompatibility complex class I molecules. Nature. 2005;**436**(7051):709-713

[38] Raulet DH, Vance RE. Self-tolerance of natural killer cells. Nature Reviews Immunology. 2006;**6**(7):520-531

[39] Yokoyama WM, Kim S. Licensing of natural killer cells by self-major histocompatibility complex class I. Immunological Reviews. 2006;**214**:143-154

[40] Elliott JM, Yokoyama WM. Unifying concepts of MHC-dependent natural killer cell education. Trends in Immunology. 2011;**32**(8):364-372

[41] Brodin P, Lakshmikanth T, Johansson S, Karre K, Hoglund P. The strength of inhibitory input during education quantitatively tunes the functional responsiveness of individual natural killer cells. Blood. 2009;**113**(11):2434-2441

[42] Joncker NT, Raulet DH. Regulation of NK cell responsiveness to achieve self-tolerance and maximal responses to diseased target cells. Immunological Reviews. 2008;**224**:85-97

[43] Hoglund P, Brodin P. Current perspectives of natural killer cell education by MHC class I molecules. Nature Reviews Immunology. 2010;**10**(10):724-734

[44] Joncker NT, Fernandez NC, Treiner E, Vivier E, Raulet DH. NK cell responsiveness is tuned commensurate with the number of inhibitory receptors for self-MHC class I: The rheostat model. The Journal of Immunology. 2009;**182**(8):4572-4580

[45] Long EO, Kim HS, Liu D, Peterson ME, Rajagopalan S. Controlling natural killer cell responses: Integration of signals for activation and inhibition. Annual Review of Immunology. 2013;**31**:227-258

[46] Moretta L, Biassoni R, Bottino C, Cantoni C, Pende D, Mingari MC, et al. Human NK cells and their receptors. Microbes & Infection. 2002;**4**(15):1539-1544

[47] Mandelboim O, Lieberman N, Lev M, Paul L, Arnon TI, Bushkin Y, et al. Recognition of haemagglutinins on virus-infected cells by NKp46 activates lysis by human NK cells. Nature. 2001;**409**(6823):1055-1060

[48] Mistry AR, O'Callaghan CA. Regulation of ligands for the activating receptor NKG2D. Immunology. 2007;**121**(4):439-447

[49] Bryceson YT, March ME, Ljunggren HG, Long EO. Synergy among receptors on resting NK cells for the activation of natural cytotoxicity and cytokine secretion. Blood. 2006;**107**(1):159-166

[50] Orange JS. Formation and function of the lytic NK-cell immunological synapse. Nature Reviews Immunology. 2008;**8**(9):713-725

[51] Wulfing C, Purtic B, Klem J, Schatzle JD. Stepwise cytoskeletal polarization as a series of checkpoints in innate but not adaptive cytolytic killing. Proceedings of the National Academy of Sciences of the United States of America. 2003;**100**(13):7767-7772

[52] Mace EM, Dongre P, Hsu HT, Sinha P, James AM, Mann SS, et al. Cell biological steps and checkpoints in accessing NK cell cytotoxicity. Immunology & Cell Biology. 2014;**92**(3):245-255

[53] Hanahan D, Weinberg RA. Hallmarks of cancer: The next generation. Cell. 2011;**144**(5): 646-674

[54] Kiessling R, Wasserman K, Horiguchi S, Kono K, Sjoberg J, Pisa P, et al. Tumor-induced immune dysfunction. Cancer Immunology, Immunotherapy Cancer Immunology, Immunotherapy. 1999;**48**(7):353-362

[55] Dunn GP, Bruce AT, Ikeda H, Old LJ, Schreiber RD. Cancer immunoediting: From immunosurveillance to tumor escape. Nature Immunology. 2002;**3**(11):991-998

[56] Dunn GP, Old LJ, Schreiber RD. The three Es of cancer immunoediting. Annual Review of Immunology. 2004;**22**:329-360

[57] Bennett MW, O'Connell J, O'Sullivan GC, Brady C, Roche D, Collins JK, et al. The Fas counterattack in vivo: Apoptotic depletion of tumor-infiltrating lymphocytes associated with Fas ligand expression by human esophageal carcinoma. The Journal of Immunology. 1998;**160**(11):5669-5675

[58] Yamauchi A, Taga K, Mostowski HS, Bloom ET. Target cell-induced apoptosis of interleukin-2-activated human natural killer cells: Roles of cell surface molecules and intracellular events. Blood. 1996;**87**(12):5127-5135

[59] Morse MA, Mosca PJ, Clay TM, Lyerly HK. Dendritic cell maturation in active immunotherapy strategies. Expert Opinion on Biological Therapy. 2002;**2**(1):35-43

[60] Orleans-Lindsay JK, Barber LD, Prentice HG, Lowdell MW. Acute myeloid leukaemia cells secrete a soluble factor that inhibits T and NK cell proliferation but not cytolytic function—implications for the adoptive immunotherapy of leukaemia. Clinical & Experimental Immunology. 2001;**126**(3):403-411

[61] Shields JD, Kourtis IC, Tomei AA, Roberts JM, Swartz MA. Induction of lymphoid-like stroma and immune escape by tumors that express the chemokine CCL21. Science. 2010;**328**(5979):749-752

[62] Yang L, Pang Y, Moses HL. TGF-beta and immune cells: An important regulatory axis in the tumor microenvironment and progression. Trends in Immunology. 2010;**31**(6): 220-227

[63] Zagury D, Gallo RC. Anti-cytokine Ab immune therapy: Present status and perspectives. Drug Discovery Today. 2004;**9**(2):72-81

[64] Romero AI, Thoren FB, Brune M, Hellstrand K. NKp46 and NKG2D receptor expression in NK cells with CD56dim and CD56bright phenotype: Regulation by histamine and reactive oxygen species. British Journal of Haematology. 2006;**132**(1):91-98

[65] Nielsen SR, Schmid MC. Macrophages as key drivers of cancer progression and metastasis. Mediators of Inflammation. 2017;**2017**:9624760

[66] Lu J, Tan M, Cai Q. The Warburg effect in tumor progression: Mitochondrial oxidative metabolism as an anti-metastasis mechanism. Cancer Letters. 2015;**356**(2 Pt A):156-164

[67] Richards J, McNally B, Fang X, Caligiuri MA, Zheng P, Liu Y. Tumor growth decreases NK and B cells as well as common lymphoid progenitor. PLoS One. 2008;**3**(9):e3180

[68] Sutlu T, Alici E. Natural killer cell-based immunotherapy in cancer: Current insights and future prospects. Journal of Internal Medicine. 2009;**266**(2):154-181

[69] Rosenberg SA, Lotze MT, Muul LM, Chang AE, Avis FP, Leitman S. et al. A progress report on the treatment of 157 patients with advanced cancer using lymphokine-activated killer cells and interleukin-2 or high-dose interleukin-2 alone. The New England Journal of Medicine. 1987;**316**(15):889-897

[70] Grimm EA, Mazumder A, Zhang HZ, Rosenberg SA. Lymphokine-activated killer cell phenomenon. Lysis of natural killer-resistant fresh solid tumor cells by interleukin 2-activated autologous human peripheral blood lymphocytes. The Journal of Experimental Medicine. 1982;**155**(6):1823-1841

[71] Cooper MA, Elliott JM, Keyel PA, Yang L, Carrero JA, Yokoyama WM. Cytokine-induced memory-like natural killer cells. Proceedings of the National Academy of Sciences of the United States of America. 2009;**106**(6):1915-1919

[72] North J, Bakhsh I, Marden C, Pittman H, Addison E, Navarrete C, et al. Tumor-primed human natural killer cells lyse NK-resistant tumor targets: Evidence of a two-stage process in resting NK cell activation. The Journal of Immunology. 2007;**178**(1):85-94

[73] Katodritou E, Terpos E, North J, Kottaridis P, Verrou E, Gastari V, et al. Tumor-primed natural killer cells from patients with multiple myeloma lyse autologous, NK-resistant, bone marrow-derived malignant plasma cells. American Journal of Hematology. 2011;**86**(12):967-973

Chapter 3

# Natural Killer Cells in the Near Future of Immuno-Oncological Therapeutic Approaches

Hend Mohamed El Tayebi

Additional information is available at the end of the chapter

http://dx.doi.org/10.5772/intechopen.70567

**Abstract**

Natural killer (NK) cells are called natural killers because they do not need to recognize a specific antigen before releasing their toxins and destroying virally infected or cancer cells. Their killing ability is mainly attributed to a large number of cytolytic granules containing proteins known as perforins and granzymes. NK cells also play a part in the adaptive immune responses through mediating antibody-dependent cell-mediated cytotoxicity (ADCC). Furthermore, NK cells play a role in the regulation and activation of other cells of the immune system. This occurs through the release of cytokines and chemokines such as interferon-gamma (IFN-$\gamma$), tumor necrosis factor-alpha (TNF-$\alpha$), and transforming growth factor-beta (TGF-$\beta$). This chapter reviews the functional highlights of NK cells through their different mechanism, in addition to discussing the potential involvement of natural killer cells in future application of immunotherapies for cancer.

**Keywords:** natural killer cells, inhibitory receptors, activating receptors, cancer, immunotherapy, epigenetics, microRNAs

## 1. Introduction

### 1.1. Natural killer cells (NK cells)

Natural killer (NK) cells are branded to be the native defenders of the innate immune system. NK cells are large granular cytolytic lymphocytes. They originate from hematopoietic stem cells (HSC) and undergo maturation primarily in the bone marrow (BM) [1, 2]. They constitute 2–18% of all circulating lymphocytes; they are also found in peripheral tissues like the liver, peritoneal cavity, and placenta [3, 4]. "Natural cytotoxicity" delineates an effectively contributing phenomenon of NK cells as the first resident invaders against viral infections and more in general against pathogens without prior sensitization [5–12]. NK cells are also involved in immune-surveillance against malignancies and prevent dissemination of metastatic tumors [13, 14]. These effector functions are mediated through cellular cytotoxicity, in addition to secretion of several chemokines and cytokines [14]. NK cells cross-talking among immune cells, as well, play a mandatory control in mediating the anti-tumor adaptive immunity of T- and B cells that contrastingly require initial priming for the expression of their activity [15, 16]. The sophisticated players of the innate immunity, NK cells exhibit distinct morphologic phenotypic and functional properties from T- and B cells [17].

### 1.2. Human natural killer cell morphology and subsets

Phenotypically, human NK cells are characterized by the expression of CD56 and lack of the surface marker of T cell CD3. In addition, co-expression of CD16 (Fc$\gamma$RIIIA, the low affinity receptor for IgG) on a majority of peripheral NK cells renders them strong mediators of antibody-dependent cellular cytotoxicity (ADCC) against IgG-coated cells [18].

Nevertheless, the non-homogenous cell compartments of NK cells divide them distinctly into two subpopulations based upon CD56 cell surface density. Accordingly, various models have been proposed regarding the phylogeny and ontogeny of these human NK cell subsets. Initially, $CD56^{bright}$ or $CD56^{dim}$ could differentiate from a common NK cell precursor, each act as separate entity. Depending on the microenvironment, inter-switching between these two subsets ranks a second possibility. Third, $CD56^{bright}$ may be precursors of $CD56^{dim}$ (or vice versa) [19, 20]. Poor understanding of their origin and the possible relationship between the subsets remains a controversy. However, each subset has distinguished functions [21, 22].

In peripheral blood, low-density expression of CD56 ($CD56^{dim}$) and high expression of CD16 ($CD16^{bright}$) makes up the majority (90%) of human NK cells, whereas $CD56^{bright}$ comprise the remaining 10% [22]. $CD56^{bright}$ NK cells termed as such as they express 5- to 10-fold higher level of CD56 and present either no, or at most, dim expression of CD16 [102]. By contrast, $CD56^{bright}$ NK cells predominate in lymph nodes and inflamed tissues [23]. Functionally, $CD56^{dim}$ cells represent "classical NK cells" with strong cytotoxic capacity involved with natural and AB-mediated cell cytotoxicity [20, 24, 25]. In contrast, $CD56^{bright}$ NK cells are characterized by enhanced cytokine production and having immune-regulatory function but poor killing properties as shown in **Figure 1** [26].

Phenotypically, $CD56^{dim}$ and $CD56^{bright}$ exhibit differential receptor profile; for example $CD56^{dim}$ NK cell exhibit much higher levels of KIR, whereas resting $CD56^{bright}$ NK cells have high expression of CD94/NKG2A. Functionally, $CD56^{dim}$ NK cells are essentially cytotoxic cells that produce low levels of cytokines in response to monokine stimulation. However, they are potent mediators of cytotoxic functions due to high levels of CD16 surface expression. On the other hand, $CD56^{bright}$ NK cells are known as immunoregulatory cells that produce high levels of cytokines such as interferon-gamma (IFN-$\gamma$), interleukin-10 (IL-10), and TGF-$\beta$ upon activation. It has low expression of CD16, thus performing reduced cytotoxic functions.

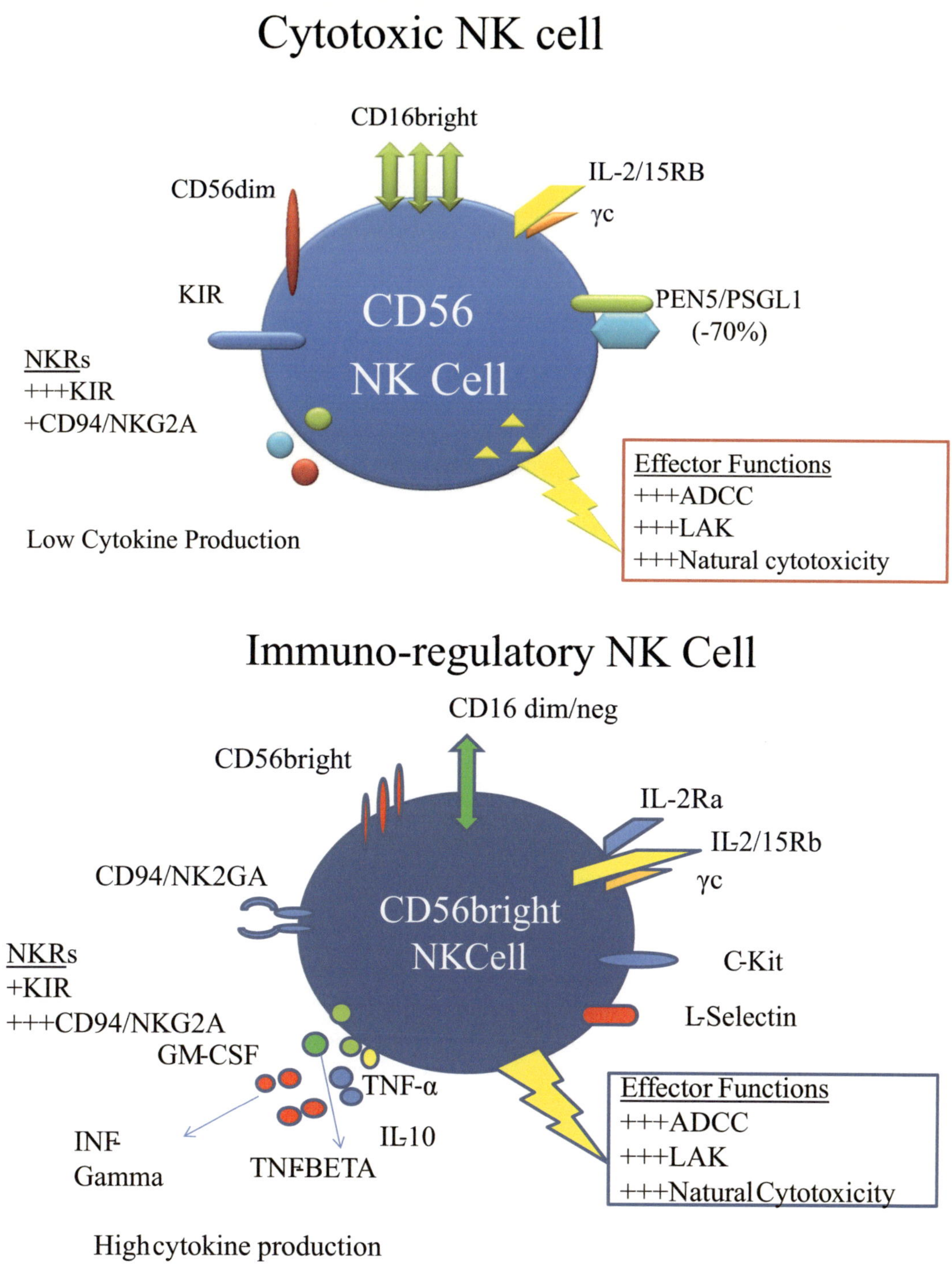


**Figure 1.** Human NK cell subsets differ both phenotypically and functionally.

## 2. Repertoire of receptors orchestrating natural killer cell signals

NK cells have a unique feature of discerning the infected or malignant cells from normal "self" cells via a complex balance between activating and inhibitory receptor-ligand interactions [27]. In addition, resting inactivated NK cell surface constitutively expresses a wide range of receptors that upon their activation by different ligands, initiation of several downstream signaling pathways take place, and finally resulting in boosting the NK cytotoxicity and cytokines production [28].

### 2.1. Activating receptors and their ligands

Upon instances of viral infection and malignant transformation, cellular stress often upregulate ligands for activating receptors and downregulate the self-marker major histocompatibility complex 1 (MHC class I) [29–31]. The interplay and cooperation of NK activating receptors creates a critical threshold of signaling that exceeds the counter balancing influence of the inhibitory receptors, in order for NK cells to mount a productive response [32]. Activating receptors embrace adaptor molecules such as DAP12 bearing immunoreceptor tyrosine-based activating motifs (ITAMs), while other receptors, such as NKG2D (natural killer group 2D), bind to non-ITAM-bearing proteins, providing NK cells with a strong stimulus [29–31]. Thoroughly, several activating receptors including NKG2D, the natural cytotoxicity receptors (NCRs), the nectin and nectin-like receptors, and NKp80 have now been characterized on NK cells [33–37]. These NCRs encompass NKp46, NKp44, and NKp30 collectively were found to play a central role in tumor cell recognition and killing [38]. Interaction of these receptors with their analogous ligands include the human leukocyte antigen-B-associated transcript 3 (BAT-3) and B7H6 for NKp30, a novel isoform of the mixed-lineage leukemia-5 protein (MLL5) for NKp44 and Nectin-2 (CD112) for DNAM-1, and MICA/B and ULBPs for NKG2D [39, 40] all depicted in **Figure 2**.

NKG2D is perhaps one of the best characterized among the activating NK cell receptors. It is a potent stimulatory, C-type lectin-like immunoreceptor that is expressed on NK cells, NKT cells, $\gamma\delta$+ T cells, and CD8+ T cells. It recognizes at least six ligands having MHC class I homology. MICA, MICB, and ULBP4 are transmembrane proteins [37, 41], while ULBP1, 2, and 3 are glycophosphatidylinositol (GPI)-anchored proteins [39]. Importantly, these NKG2D ligands are not expressed on normal tissues, but rather are induced during times of genotoxic or cellular stress as is seen with viral and malignant transformation [42]. Dissimilar to the other activating receptors, NKG2D does not utilize ITAM as a signaling peptide. However, upon receptor-ligand interaction, NKG2D phosphorylates an adaptor protein DAP-10 that recruits and activates phosphatidylinositol3 (PI-3) kinase, which in turn results in perforin-dependent cytotoxicity [43, 44]. Tumors exploit their common vulnerability and disarm NK cells and cytolytic T cell effector systems by targeting NKG2D. This draws an attention on the epithelial cancers that shed MICA/B ligands into the serum; these soluble ligands downmodulate NKG2D expression on these effector cells with consequent reduction in their cytolytic effectiveness [45–48].

http://dx.doi.org/10.5772/intechopen.70567

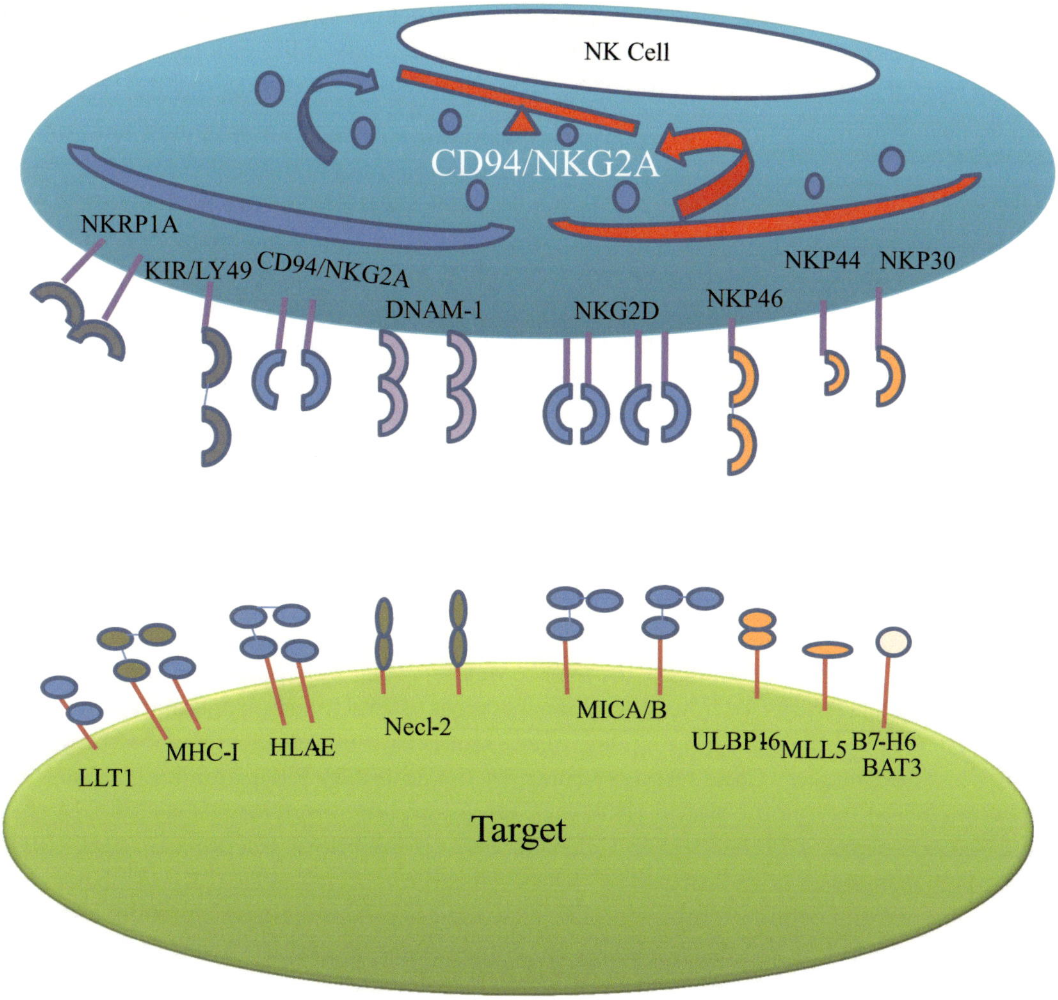


**Figure 2.** The dynamic equilibrium regulating natural killer cell activation.

### 2.2. Inhibitory receptors and their ligands

Self-immune-surveillance of NK cells activity is inhibited through the recognition of the MHC class I, which is expressed by all healthy cells; by NK cell inhibitory receptors under normal physiological conditions [49, 50]. These receptors comprise the inhibitory killer immunoglobulin-like receptors (KIRs), monomeric type 1 glycoproteins of the immunoglobulin super family that bind to classical MHC class Ia ligands (HLA-A, B, and C), and the inhibitory CD94-NKG2A heterodimeric, C-type lectin-like receptor that bind the non-classical MHC class Ib (HLA-E) as shown in **Figure 2** [29, 51, 52]. Recognition of HLA-E by NKG2A/CD94 receptors enables NK cells to monitor the expression of other HLA class I proteins on cells. CD94 dominates the interaction with HLA-E, whereas NKG2A is more peripheral to the interface [53]. Since,

HLA-E expression on the cell surface bound to peptides, depends on classical and non-classical MHC-I proteins production; from which these peptides are derived [53–55]. This double-check mechanism ensures that cells are producing MHC-I molecules in a normal manner [56].

Even in the absence of KIRs-MHC class Ia mediated self-tolerance, other inhibitory receptor-ligand systems help the NK cells to determine whether tolerance of the host tissue is appropriate. Backing up the other inhibitory NK receptors, is the C-type lectin-like receptor NKR-P1A (CD161) that interacts with a host encoded non-MHC ligand "lectin-like transcript-1 (LLT-1)" illustrated in **Figure 2** [57, 58]. Interestingly, engagement of NK inhibitory receptors including NKG2A with their ligands activates the same signaling mechanisms. Upon phosphorylation of the inhibitory receptors' cytoplasmic immunoreceptor tyrosine-based inhibition motifs (ITIMs), the downstream targets: Src homology 2 domain-containing phosphatases (SHP-1 and SHP-2) are recruited directly to antagonize the signaling pathways of the activating receptors [59–63]. In an elaboration, these tyrosine phosphatases suppress NK cell responses by dephosphorylating the protein substrates of the tyrosine kinases "ITAMs" linked to the activating receptors. Consequently, they terminate $Ca^{2+}$ influx, degranulation, cytokine production, and proliferation of NK cells. Notably, these events are transient, spatially localized, and do not interfere with the ability of the same NK cells to get activated upon encounter with subsequent viral or tumor target cells [32].

NK cells rely on a vast combinatorial array of receptors, rather than possessing one dominant receptor to initiate its effector functions. Upon instances of viral infection and malignant transformation, cellular stress often upregulate ligands for activating receptors and downregulate MHC class I expression. These receptors comprise the inhibitory killer immunoglobulin-like receptors (KIRs) that bind classical HLA-A, B, and C, and the inhibitory CD94-NKG2A that bind the non-classical MHC class Ib (HLA-E). Backup inhibitory receptors like NKR-P1A (CD161) that interacts with a non-MHC ligand "lectin-like transcript-1 (LLT-1)." Balancing off, the activating receptors comprise, NCRs (NKp30, NKp44, and NKp46) that interact with their ligands including the human leukocyte antigen-B-associated transcript 3 (BAT-3) and B7H6 for NKp30 and the mixed-lineage leukemia-5 protein (MLL5) for NKp44, and also, nectin-2 for DNAM-1, and MICA/B and ULBPs for NKG2D activating receptors [56–58].

## 3. Dictation of natural killer cell function

NK cells effector functions is a matter of convoluted balance between activating and inhibitory receptors previously explained. The unique feature of those cells to recognize their targets without prior activation has perplexed researchers along the way since early 1990s. NK cells checks for the presence of MHC class I expression that are only present on normal "self" cells just like checking for an ID, and to consider everything lacking this "self" as foreign, which is the case in transformed or virally infected cells; this was first explained by Kärre and colleagues postulating the "missing self" hypothesis [64]. Recognition of the MHC class I molecules is achieved via the inhibitory receptors of NK cells that include members of the killer cell Ig-like receptors (i.e., KIR) [65], in addition to a CD94/NKG2A heterodimer [66].

Upon activation of such inhibitory receptors recruitment of the protein tyrosine phosphatases SHP-1 or SHP-2 was reported which bring about the inhibition of the NK cell activity [67]. Presence of the MHC class I molecules on a given target cell normally will "turn off" the activity of NK cells. However, absence of these molecules was not enough to "turn on" their activity. Instead an activation signal is required, that is mediated by several activating receptors such as natural cytotoxicity receptors (NCRs) that include NKp30, NKp46, and NKp44 as well as the activating receptor NKG2D [68]. Nevertheless, it was reported that NK cell activation mediated by these receptors was tightly controlled by inhibitory receptors as well. Consequently, state of NK cell activation is reached by a balance between the turn on/ turn off signals.

In normal cells, both activating and inhibitory receptors are cross-linked to their ligands but the inhibitory signals received will be able to counteract the activating signals protecting the normal cell from the NK cell cytotoxic effect. On the other hand, this balance was reported to be disrupted in transformed cells, due to a downregulation of the inhibitory ligands and/ or an upregulation of the stress-induced activating ligands, yielding them susceptible to NK cell-mediated killing [69].

## 4. Natural killer cell signaling pathways

The integration of signal transduction pathways is modulated *in vivo* by several soluble immune cytokines, including IL-2, IL-12, IL-15, and IFN-$\alpha$/$\beta$ [4, 13, 70] as well as cell-to-cell interactions involving different cell types primarily dendritic cells (DC) [13, 71], macrophages, and mesenchymal stromal cells [72, 73] determine NK cell effector responses [74, 75].

For instance, interleukin-2 (IL-2) binds to its corresponding receptor; IL-2 receptor (IL-2R) is composed of three subunits: IL-2R$\alpha$ (CD25), IL-2R$\beta$ (CD122), and the common $\gamma$ chain ($\gamma$c, CD132). Subsequently, activating downstream intracellular signaling pathways JAK-STAT pathway, MAPK-ERK pathway, and PI3K-AKT-mTOR pathway promote NK cell proliferation, cytotoxicity, and survival [28, 76, 77]. Intricately, IL-15R is a heterotrimeric receptor consisting of a unique $\alpha$ chain, a shared $\beta$ subunit with IL-2, and a common γ subunit with several cytokines [78]. Engagement of IL-15R on NK cells causes auto-phosphorylation and activation of Janus kinases (JAK1 and JAK3), which induces at least three parallel signaling cascades: Ras-Raf-MEK, PI3K-AKT-mTOR, and STAT5 pathways [28, 78]. In addition, it was recently demonstrated that the PI3K-AKT-mTOR pathway is critically activated by the most potent interleukin-15 (IL-15) enabling NK cell homeostasis, maturation, and activation. Furthermore, this pathway is also implicated in a broad range of IL-15-induced NK cell effector functions such as proliferation, cytokine production, and cytotoxicity [79]. Co-activation of NK cells by IL-12 and IL-18 or IL-15, results in the production of IFN-$\gamma$ and deactivation of the TGF-$\beta$; the immunosuppressive signaling cascade [80]. IL-21 binds to $\gamma$c receptor shared with IL-2 and IL-15 and the IL-21R$\beta$ receptor which is similar to IL-2R$\beta$, and then activates a series of intracellular signaling pathways. Thus, it stimulates cell proliferation, survival, secretion of IFN-$\gamma$, and cytotoxicity of NK cells [81, 82].

### 4.1. Functions of natural killer cells

In the immune system, the NK cells are of crucial importance due to its important functions that can be classified into three categories: (A) cytotoxicity, (B) cytokine and chemokine release, and (C) co-stimulation of other immune cells.

### 4.2. Cytotoxicity

Through their cytotoxic activity, NK cells are capable of killing viral infected and malignant cells [83]. Different cytotoxic pathways in NK cell have been characterized. First, the Prf- and Gzm-mediated cytotoxic pathway is the most common killing pathway of NK cell. In such pathway, the well-known effector molecules (perforin-1 and granzyme B) are exocytosed from their cytoplasmic granules in NK cells to the vicinity of the target cells (immunological synapse) [70]. Prf1, which is a pore performing protein, polymerizes forming pores in the phospholipid bilayer of the target cell facilitating the delivery of granzymes into the cytosol of the target cell; whereas, the serine protease GzmB cleaves several procaspases and other intracellular substrates to initiate the classical apoptotic pathways [84]. Second, the killing process may also be mediated in a perforin-independent manner through the CD95 (Fas)-CD178 (Fas ligand) pathway. Upon binding of the NK cell to the Fas expressing stressed target cells, death inducing signaling complex is formed and subsequent activation of caspases promoting the apoptotic process of the target cell [85]. Third, the antibody-dependent cellular cytotoxicity (ADCC) which is used by leukocytes that express CD16 (Fc receptors), including NK cells to kill antibody-coated target cells [86].

### 4.3. Cytokine and chemokine release

It is thought that NK cells participate in a complex interaction network with other lymphocytes, dendritic cells, and macrophages to effectively control infection and malignancy. NK cells mediate their modulatory function on the immune cells through the production of cytokines and chemokines following either cytokine- or activating-receptor stimulation on the NK cell surface. The prototype effector cytokine produced by NK cells is IFN-$\gamma$, which has pleotropic effector actions on other immune cells, antigen-presenting cells, and virally infected or malignant target cells [7]. In viral models of infection, IFN-$\gamma$ production by NK cells has been shown to be a key event in successful resolution of infection [87]. In liver, the IFN-$\gamma$ contributes to the anti-viral [88], anti-fibrotic [89], anti-regenerative [90], and anti-tumor [91] activities of resident NK cells there. NK cells release several other cytokines including interleukin-3 (IL-3) and granulocyte-macrophage colony-stimulating factor (GM-CSF), tissue necrosis factor-$\alpha$ (TNF-$\alpha$) and transforming growth factor-$\beta$ (TGF-$\beta$) and chemokines (MIP-1$\alpha$, MIP-1$\beta$, and RANTES), which depends on the NK cell stimulation type and the time course after activation [92].

### 4.4. Co-stimulation

NK cells can also interact with other immune cells through contact-dependent cell co-stimulation, this takes place upon the expression of several co-stimulatory ligands on the NK cell including CD40L (CD154) and OX40L, thus allowing NK cells to provide a co-stimulatory signal to T cells or B cells [93, 94]. So from that, NK cells serve as a bridge in an interactive loop between innate and adaptive immunity. Dendritic cells (DC) stimulate NK cells, which then deliver a co-stimulatory signal to T- or B cells allowing for an optimal immune response. In addition to signals received from soluble mediators, activation of NK cells are also done through cell contact by their receptors that recognize ligands on other cells [95].

## 5. Trafficking of natural killer cells to the microenvironment of solid tumors

Solid tumors hinder the infiltration and activation of NK cells at the tumor microenvironment (TME) leading to a challenge to NK cell efficacy [96]. The tumor suppresses cytotoxic responses by secreting IL-10, vascular endothelial growth factor (VEGF), prostaglandin E2 (PGE2), TGFβ indoleamine 2,3-dioxygenase (IDO), proteinase inhibitor-9 (PI-9), and arginase [97–99]. In addition to downregulating class I MHC, those cytokines gives rise to immature phenotype of dendritic cells [100].

In addition, the differentiation of myeloid derived suppressor cells (MDSCs) is controlled by some cytokines, such as TGF-β and PGE2. The MDSCs are then generated as highly heterogeneous population consisting of dendritic cells, granulocytes, and macrophages arrested at various differentiation stages [101]. The hypoxic tumor microenvironment results in the upregulation of arginase activity and inducible nitric oxide synthase (iNOS) by MDSCs that in turn inhibits T cells through NO signaling [102]. Moreover, this depletes arginine intracellularly and reactive oxygen species (ROS) production leading to shedding of NKG2D ligands, thus resulting in diminished immune-surveillance [102].

## 6. Epigenetics in natural killer cells

NK cells may show adaptive characters similar to B- and T-lymphocytes expressed in improved longevity and memory responses [103–105].

NK cells function mainly by producing interferon (IFN)-γ to eliminate pathogens, and release perforin to kill activated target immune cells [74, 106].

Epigenetics is a set of genome modifications that impacts the expression of a gene without changing the nucleotide sequence. Those modifications include methylation, acetylation, or phosphorylation of the histone proteins [107].

### 6.1. Epigenetic regulation of mature natural killer cell function

The activation of NK cell has been studied for several decades; however, the mechanism of generation and maintenance of functional NK cells is only partially understood.

NK cell cytotoxicity is mediated by the effector molecule, perforin, which creates pores in the phospholipid bilayer of host target cells leading to facilitation of granzymes entry resulting in induction of apoptosis.

The expression of perforin in NK cells is only induced by the direct binding of myeloid Elf1-like factor (MEF), a transcription factor that belongs to Ets family, to perforin 1 promoter at two sites. However, in cytotoxic T lymphocytes perforin 1 is regulated differentially at the transcriptional level [108]. Perforin 1 regulatory region has two enhancers that are responsive to IL-2R-activated signal transduction and bind to Stat5 [108]. IL2Rb or Stat5b knockout NK cells of mice showed significantly lower levels of perforin transcript which highlights the importance of these enhancers for perforin transcription [109]. One of the enhancers is responsive to IL-6 and IL-12 and, upon cytokine stimulation, can bind STAT1a and STAT4, respectively [110, 111].

On the other hand, granzymes are serine proteases present in cytolytic granules of NK cells and cytotoxic T cells. Granzyme B (GZMB) is the most comprehensively studied member of the granzymes family. It acts on target cell either through cleaving caspases or damaging mitochondria thus mediating cell death [112]. Transcriptional regulation of granzyme B in CD8+ T cells is mediated by binding of transcriptional factors as CREB1, RUNX1, and AP1 to granzyme B promoter, harboring a DNase-hypersensitive region, enhancing the transcription [113–115]. Granzyme B expression is epigenetically controlled by histone H3K9 acetylation in its promoter resulting in high gene expression levels [113]. Another regulator of granzyme B expression is NF-κB, where, the activation of NF-κB signaling pathway results in binding of NF-κB to an enhancer element downstream to granzyme B transcriptional start site inducing its expression [116–118].

### 6.2. Recent approaches in fine-tuning of natural killer cell function

In a study conducted by our research group, a potential role of insulin-like growth factor-1 (IGF-1) was highlighted in modulating cytolytic potential of NK cells of HCC patients. miR-486-5p acts in a cell-specific manner, differentially modulating IGF-1 expression in NK cells and their target hepatocytes with a contemporary inhibitory impact on HCC progression [119]. Moreover, in another study, NK cells of HCC patients showed miR-182 overexpression compared to controls. NKG2D and NKG2A were upregulated and downregulated, respectively, in HCC NK cells. Upon forcing miR-182 expression in the HCC NK cells, upregulation of both receptors was observed. Finally, miR-182 was reported to induce NK cell cytotoxicity represented in perforin-1 upregulation and increase in cytolytic killing of co-cultured Huh-7 cells [120].

Our research team reported a novel role of miR-615-5p in NK cells activity of HCC patients. We have previously described miR-615-5p as potent tumor suppressor microRNA in HCC via repressing a pivotal mitogen in HCC, Insulin-like growth factor-II (IGF-II) as well as cellular proliferation, viability, and migration [121]. Recently, our team proved an opposing function for miR-615-5p in the NK cells of HCC patients. Forcing the expression of miR-615-5p repressed insulin-like growth factor-type 1 receptor (IGF-IR), attenuated NKs cytotoxicity, decreased $CD56^{dim}$, increased $CD56^{bright}$ NK subsets, and reduced the cytotoxic markers NKG2D, TNF-$\alpha$, and perforins. It also repressed NKG2D ligand (ULBP2) in Huh-7 cells [122].

## Author details

Hend Mohamed El Tayebi

Address all correspondence to: hend.saber@guc.edu.eg

Genetic Pharmacology Research Group, Department of Pharmacology and Toxicology, Faculty of Pharmacy and Biotechnology, German University in Cairo, Cairo, Egypt

## References

[1] Cooper MA, Fehniger TA, Turner SC, Chen KS, Ghaheri BA, Ghayur T, Carson WE, Caligiuri MA. Human natural killer cells: A unique innate immunoregulatory role for the CD56(bright) subset. Blood. 2001;**97**(10):3146-3151

[2] Freud AG, Becknell B, Roychowdhury S, Mao HC, Ferketich AK, Nuovo GJ, Hughes TL, Marburger TB, Sung J, Baiocchi RA, Guimond M, Caligiuri MA. A human CD34(+) subset resides in lymph nodes and differentiates into CD56bright natural killer cells. Immunity. 2005;**22**(3):295-304

[3] Gregoire C, Chasson L, Luci C, Tomasello E, Geissmann F, Vivier E, Walzer T. The trafficking of natural killer cells. Immunological Reviews. 2007;**220**:169-182

[4] Smyth MJ, Hayakawa Y, Takeda K, Yagita H. New aspects of natural-killer-cell surveillance and therapy of cancer. Nature Reviews. Cancer. 2002;**2**(11):850-861

[5] Jost S, Altfeld M. Control of human viral infections by natural killer cells. Annual Review of Immunology. 2013;**31**:163-194

[6] Watzl C, Urlaub D. Molecular mechanisms of natural killer cell regulation. Frontiers in Bioscience (Landmark Edition). 2012;**17**:1418-1432

[7] Vivier E, Tomasello E, Baratin M, Walzer T, Ugolini S. Functions of natural killer cells. Nature Immunology. 2008;**9**(5):503-510

[8] Herberman RB, Nunn ME, Holden HT, Lavrin DH. Natural cytotoxic reactivity of mouse lymphoid cells against syngeneic and allogeneic tumors. II. Characterization of effector cells. International Journal of Cancer. 1975;**16**(2):230-239

[9] Herberman RB, Nunn ME, Lavrin DH. Natural cytotoxic reactivity of mouse lymphoid cells against syngeneic acid allogeneic tumors. I. Distribution of reactivity and specificity. International Journal of Cancer. 1975;**16**(2):216-229

[10] Peter HH, Kalden JR, Seeland P, Diehl V, Eckert G. Humoral and cellular immune reactions 'in vitro' against allogeneic and autologous human melanoma cells. Clinical and Experimental Immunology. 1975;**20**(2):193-207

[11] Kiessling R, Klein E, Wigzell H. "Natural" killer cells in the mouse. I. Cytotoxic cells with specificity for mouse Moloney leukemia cells. Specificity and distribution according to genotype. European Journal of Immunology. 1975;**5**(2):112-117

[12] Kiessling R, Klein E, Pross H, Wigzell H. "Natural" killer cells in the mouse. II. Cytotoxic cells with specificity for mouse Moloney leukemia cells. Characteristics of the killer cell. European Journal of Immunology. 1975;**5**(2):117-121

[13] Agaugue S, Marcenaro E, Ferranti B, Moretta L, Moretta A. Human natural killer cells exposed to IL-2, IL-12, IL-18, or IL-4 differently modulate priming of naive T cells by monocyte-derived dendritic cells. Blood. 2008;**112**(5):1776-1783

[14] Trinchieri G. Biology of natural killer cells. Advances in Immunology. 1989;**47**:187-376

[15] Paust S, Senman B, von Andrian UH. Adaptive immune responses mediated by natural killer cells. Immunological Reviews. 2010;**235**(1):286-296

[16] Di Santo JP. Natural killer cell developmental pathways: A question of balance. Annual Review of Immunology. 2006;**24**:257-286

[17] Orange JS, Ballas ZK. Natural killer cells in human health and disease. Clinical Immunology. 2006;**118**(1):1-10

[18] Cooper MA, Fehniger TA, Caligiuri MA. The biology of human natural killer-cell subsets. Trends in Immunology. 2001;**22**(11):633-640

[19] Farag SS, Caligiuri MA. Human natural killer cell development and biology. Blood Reviews. 2006;**20**(3):123-137

[20] Nagler A, Lanier LL, Cwirla S, Phillips JH. Comparative studies of human FcRIII-positive and negative natural killer cells. Journal of Immunology. 1989;**143**(10):3183-3191

[21] Jacobs R, Weber K, Wendt K, Heiken H, Schmidt RE. Altered coexpression of lectin-like receptors CD94 and CD161 on NK and T cells in HIV patients. Journal of Clinical Immunology. 2004;**24**(3):281-286

[22] Jacobs R, Hintzen G, Kemper A, Beul K, Kempf S, Behrens G, Sykora KW, Schmidt RE. CD56bright cells differ in their KIR repertoire and cytotoxic features from CD56dim NK cells. European Journal of Immunology. 2001;**31**(10):3121-3127

[23] Carson WE, Fehniger TA, Caligiuri MA. CD56bright natural killer cell subsets: Characterization of distinct functional responses to interleukin-2 and the c-kit ligand. European Journal of Immunology. 1997;**27**(2):354-360

[24] Farag SS, Van Deusen JB, Fehniger TA, Caligiuri MA. Biology and clinical impact of human natural killer cells. International Journal of Hematology. 2003;**78**(1):7-17

[25] Jacobs R, Stoll M, Stratmann G, Leo R, Link H, Schmidt RE. CD16− CD56+ natural killer cells after bone marrow transplantation. Blood. 1992;**79**(12):3239-3244

[26] Hayakawa Y, Screpanti V, Yagita H, Grandien A, Ljunggren HG, Smyth MJ, Chambers BJ. NK cell TRAIL eliminates immature dendritic cells *in vivo* and limits dendritic cell vaccination efficacy. Journal of Immunology. 2004;**172**(1):123-129

[27] Lanier LL. NK cell recognition. Annual Review of Immunology. 2005;**23**:225-274

[28] Kovanen PE, Leonard WJ. Cytokines and immunodeficiency diseases: Critical roles of the gamma(c)-dependent cytokines interleukins 2, 4, 7, 9, 15, and 21, and their signaling pathways. Immunological Reviews. 2004;**202**:67-83

[29] Vivier E, Nunes JA, Vely F. Natural killer cell signaling pathways. Science. 2004;**306**(5701):1517-1519

[30] Gilfillan S, Ho EL, Cella M, Yokoyama WM, Colonna M. NKG2D recruits two distinct adapters to trigger NK cell activation and costimulation. Nature Immunology. 2002;**3**(12):1150-1155

[31] Campbell JL, Klueva NY, Zheng HG, Nieto-Sotelo J, Ho TD, Nguyen HT. Cloning of new members of heat shock protein HSP101 gene family in wheat (*Triticum aestivum* (L.) *Moench*) inducible by heat, dehydration, and ABA(1). Biochimica et Biophysica Acta. 2001;**1517**(2):270-277

[32] Ravetch JV, Lanier LL. Immune inhibitory receptors. Science. 2000;**290**(5489):84-89

[33] Bryceson YT, March ME, Ljunggren HG, Long EO. Activation, coactivation, and costimulation of resting human natural killer cells. Immunological Reviews. 2006;**214**:73-91

[34] Welte S, Kuttruff S, Waldhauer I, Steinle A. Mutual activation of natural killer cells and monocytes mediated by NKp80-AICL interaction. Nature Immunology. 2006;**7**(12):1334-1342

[35] Fuchs A, Colonna M. The role of NK cell recognition of nectin and nectin-like proteins in tumor immunosurveillance. Seminars in Cancer Biology. 2006;**16**(5):359-366

[36] Bottino C, Moretta L, Moretta A. NK cell activating receptors and tumor recognition in humans. Current Topics in Microbiology and Immunology. 2006;**298**:175-182

[37] Bauer S, Groh V, Wu J, Steinle A, Phillips JH, Lanier LL, Spies T. Activation of NK cells and T cells by NKG2D, a receptor for stress-inducible MICA. Science. 1999;**285**(5428):727-729

[38] Moretta A, Bottino C, Vitale M, Pende D, Cantoni C, Mingari MC, Biassoni R, Moretta L. Activating receptors and coreceptors involved in human natural killer cell-mediated cytolysis. Annual Review of Immunology. 2001;**19**:197-223

[39] Cosman D, Mullberg J, Sutherland CL, Chin W, Armitage R, Fanslow W, Kubin M, Chalupny NJ. ULBPs, novel MHC class I-related molecules, bind to CMV glycoprotein UL16 and stimulate NK cytotoxicity through the NKG2D receptor. Immunity. 2001;**14**(2):123-133

[40] Chan CJ, Smyth MJ, Martinet L. Molecular mechanisms of natural killer cell activation in response to cellular stress. Cell Death and Differentiation. 2014;**21**(1):5-14

[41] Chalupny NJ, Sutherland CL, Lawrence WA, Rein-Weston A, Cosman D. ULBP4 is a novel ligand for human NKG2D. Biochemical and Biophysical Research Communications. 2003;**305**(1):129-135

[42] Gonzalez S, Groh V, Spies T. Immunobiology of human NKG2D and its ligands. Current Topics in Microbiology and Immunology. 2006;**298**:121-138

[43] Hayakawa Y, Kelly JM, Westwood JA, Darcy PK, Diefenbach A, Raulet D, Smyth MJ. Cutting edge: Tumor rejection mediated by NKG2D receptor-ligand interaction is dependent upon perforin. Journal of Immunology. 2002;**169**(10):5377-5381

[44] Wu J, Song Y, Bakker AB, Bauer S, Spies T, Lanier LL, Phillips JH. An activating immunoreceptor complex formed by NKG2D and DAP10. Science. 1999;**285**(5428):730-732

[45] Kaiser BK, Yim D, Chow IT, Gonzalez S, Dai Z, Mann HH, Strong RK, Groh V, Spies T. Disulphide-isomerase-enabled shedding of tumour-associated NKG2D ligands. Nature. 2007;**447**(7143):482-486

[46] Doubrovina ES, Doubrovin MM, Vider E, Sisson RB, O'Reilly RJ, Dupont B, Vyas YM. Evasion from NK cell immunity by MHC class I chain-related molecules expressing colon adenocarcinoma. Journal of Immunology. 2003;**171**(12):6891-6899

[47] Salih HR, Antropius H, Gieseke F, Lutz SZ, Kanz L, Rammensee HG, Steinle A. Functional expression and release of ligands for the activating immunoreceptor NKG2D in leukemia. Blood. 2003;**102**(4):1389-1396

[48] Groh V, Wu J, Yee C, Spies T. Tumour-derived soluble MIC ligands impair expression of NKG2D and T-cell activation. Nature. 2002;**419**(6908):734-738

[49] Sivori S, Vitale M, Morelli L, Sanseverino L, Augugliaro R, Bottino C, Moretta L, Moretta A. p46, a novel natural killer cell-specific surface molecule that mediates cell activation. The Journal of Experimental Medicine. 1997;**186**(7):1129-1136

[50] Ritz J, Schmidt RE, Michon J, Hercend T, Schlossman SF. Characterization of functional surface structures on human natural killer cells. Advances in Immunology. 1988;**42**:181-211

[51] Parihar R, Dierksheide J, Hu Y, Carson WE. IL-12 enhances the natural killer cell cytokine response to Ab-coated tumor cells. The Journal of Clinical Investigation. 2002;**110**(7):983-992

[52] Lanier LL. Face off—The interplay between activating and inhibitory immune receptors. Current Opinion in Immunology. 2001;**13**(3):326-331

[53] Petrie EJ, Clements CS, Lin J, Sullivan LC, Johnson D, Huyton T, Heroux A, Hoare HL, Beddoe T, Reid HH, Wilce MC, Brooks AG, Rossjohn J. CD94-NKG2A recognition of human leukocyte antigen (HLA)-E bound to an HLA class I leader sequence. The Journal of Experimental Medicine. 2008;**205**(3):725-735

[54] Lee N, Llano M, Carretero M, Ishitani A, Navarro F, Lopez-Botet M, Geraghty DE. HLA-E is a major ligand for the natural killer inhibitory receptor CD94/NKG2A. Proceedings of the National Academy of Sciences of the United States of America. 1998;**95**(9):5199-5204

[55] Braud VM, Allan DS, O'Callaghan CA, Soderstrom K, D'Andrea A, Ogg GS, Lazetic S, Young NT, Bell JI, Phillips JH, Lanier LL, McMichael AJ. HLA-E binds to natural killer cell receptors CD94/NKG2A, B and C. Nature. 1998;**391**(6669):795-799

[56] Bryceson YT, March ME, Ljunggren HG, Long EO. Synergy among receptors on resting NK cells for the activation of natural cytotoxicity and cytokine secretion. Blood. 2006;**107**(1):159-166

[57] Flaig RM, Stark S, Watzl C. Cutting edge: NTB-A activates NK cells via homophilic interaction. Journal of Immunology. 2004;**172**(11):6524-6527

[58] Shibuya K, Lanier LL, Phillips JH, Ochs HD, Shimizu K, Nakayama E, Nakauchi H, Shibuya A. Physical and functional association of LFA-1 with DNAM-1 adhesion molecule. Immunity. 1999;**11**(5):615-623

[59] Ruggeri L, Mancusi A, Capanni M, Martelli MF, Velardi A. Exploitation of alloreactive NK cells in adoptive immunotherapy of cancer. Current Opinion in Immunology. 2005;**17**(2):211-217

[60] Parham P, McQueen KL. Alloreactive killer cells: Hindrance and help for haematopoietic transplants. Nature Reviews. Immunology. 2003;**3**(2):108-122

[61] Ruggeri L, Capanni M, Urbani E, Perruccio K, Shlomchik WD, Tosti A, Posati S, Rogaia D, Frassoni F, Aversa F, Martelli MF, Velardi A. Effectiveness of donor natural killer cell alloreactivity in mismatched hematopoietic transplants. Science. 2002;**295**(5562):2097-2100

[62] Binstadt BA, Brumbaugh KM, Dick CJ, Scharenberg AM, Williams BL, Colonna M, Lanier LL, Kinet JP, Abraham RT, Leibson PJ. Sequential involvement of Lck and SHP-1 with MHC-recognizing receptors on NK cells inhibits FcR-initiated tyrosine kinase activation. Immunity. 1996;**5**(6):629-638

[63] Burshtyn DN, Scharenberg AM, Wagtmann N, Rajagopalan S, Berrada K, Yi T, Kinet JP, Long EO. Recruitment of tyrosine phosphatase HCP by the killer cell inhibitor receptor. Immunity. 1996;**4**(1):77-85

[64] Karre K, Ljunggren HG, Piontek G, Kiessling R. Selective rejection of H-2-deficient lymphoma variants suggests alternative immune defence strategy. Nature. 1986;**319**(6055):675-678

[65] Long EO, Barber DF, Burshtyn DN, Faure M, Peterson M, Rajagopalan S, Renard V, Sandusky M, Stebbins CC, Wagtmann N, Watzl C. Inhibition of natural killer cell activation signals by killer cell immunoglobulin-like receptors (CD158). Immunological Reviews. 2001;**181**:223-233

[66] O'Callaghan CA. Natural killer cell surveillance of intracellular antigen processing pathways mediated by recognition of HLA-E and Qa-1b by CD94/NKG2 receptors. Microbes and Infection. 2000;**2**(4):371-380

[67] McVicar DW, Burshtyn DN. Intracellular signaling by the killer immunoglobulin-like receptors and Ly49. Science's STKE. 2001;**2001**(75):re1

[68] Biassoni R. Human natural killer receptors, co-receptors, and their ligands. Current Protocols in Immunology. 2009; Chapter 14: Unit 14.10

[69] Watzl C. The NKG2D receptor and its ligands-recognition beyond the "missing self"? Microbes and Infection. 2003;**5**(1):31-37

[70] Vivier E, Ugolini S, Blaise D, Chabannon C, Brossay L. Targeting natural killer cells and natural killer T cells in cancer. Nature Reviews. Immunology. 2012;**12**(4):239-252

[71] Moretta A. Natural killer cells and dendritic cells: Rendezvous in abused tissues. Nature Reviews. Immunology. 2002;**2**(12):957-964

[72] Spaggiari GM, Capobianco A, Abdelrazik H, Becchetti F, Mingari MC, Moretta L. Mesenchymal stem cells inhibit natural killer-cell proliferation, cytotoxicity, and cytokine production: Role of indoleamine 2,3-dioxygenase and prostaglandin E2. Blood. 2008;**111**(3):1327-1333

[73] Spaggiari GM, Capobianco A, Becchetti S, Mingari MC, Moretta L. Mesenchymal stem cell-natural killer cell interactions: Evidence that activated NK cells are capable of killing MSCs, whereas MSCs can inhibit IL-2-induced NK-cell proliferation. Blood. 2006;**107**(4):1484-1490

[74] Lanier LL. Up on the tightrope: Natural killer cell activation and inhibition. Nature Immunology. 2008;**9**(5):495-502

[75] Lee SH, Miyagi T, Biron CA. Keeping NK cells in highly regulated antiviral warfare. Trends in Immunology. 2007;**28**(6):252-259

[76] Grund EM, Spyropoulos DD, Watson DK, Muise-Helmericks RC. Interleukins 2 and 15 regulate Ets1 expression via ERK1/2 and MNK1 in human natural killer cells. The Journal of Biological Chemistry. 2005;**280**(6):4772-4778

[77] Yu TK, Caudell EG, Smid C, Grimm EA. IL-2 activation of NK cells: Involvement of MKK1/2/ERK but not p38 kinase pathway. Journal of Immunology. 2000;**164**(12):6244-6251

[78] Ma A, Koka R, Burkett P. Diverse functions of IL-2, IL-15, and IL-7 in lymphoid homeostasis. Annual Review of Immunology. 2006;**24**:657-679

[79] Nandagopal N, Ali AK, Komal AK, Lee SH. The critical role of IL-15-PI3K-mTOR pathway in natural killer cell effector functions. Frontiers in Immunology. 2014;**5**:187

[80] Yu J, Wei M, Becknell B, Trotta R, Liu S, Boyd Z, Jaung MS, Blaser BW, Sun J, Benson DM Jr, Mao H, Yokohama A, Bhatt D, Shen L, Davuluri R, Weinstein M, Marcucci G, Caligiuri MA. Pro- and antiinflammatory cytokine signaling: Reciprocal antagonism regulates interferon-gamma production by human natural killer cells. Immunity. 2006;**24**(5):575-590

[81] Iannello A, Boulassel MR, Samarani S, Debbeche O, Tremblay C, Toma E, Routy JP, Ahmad A. Dynamics and consequences of IL-21 production in HIV-infected individuals: A longitudinal and cross-sectional study. Journal of Immunology. 2010;**184**(1):114-126

[82] Zeng R, Spolski R, Casas E, Zhu W, Levy DE, Leonard WJ. The molecular basis of IL-21-mediated proliferation. Blood. 2007;**109**(10):4135-4142

[83] Hokland M, Kuppen PJ. Natural killer cells: From "disturbing" background to central players of immune responses. Molecular Immunology. 2005;**42**(4):381-383

[84] Vivier E, Ugolini S. Natural killer cells: From basic research to treatments. Frontiers in Immunology. 2011;**2**:18

[85] Romagne F, Vivier E. Natural killer cell-based therapies. F1000 Medicine Reports. 2011;**3**:9

[86] Narni-Mancinelli E, Ugolini S, Vivier E. Tuning the threshold of natural killer cell responses. Current Opinion in Immunology. 2013;**25**(1):53-58

[87] Lu L et al. Regulation of activated CD4+ T cells by NK cells via the Qa-1-NKG2A inhibitory pathway. Immunity. 2007;**26**(5):593-604

[88] Wang SH et al. Natural killer cells suppress full cycle HCV infection of human hepatocytes. Journal of Viral Hepatitis. 2008;**15**(12):855-864

[89] Radaeva S et al. Natural killer cells ameliorate liver fibrosis by killing activated stellate cells in NKG2D-dependent and tumor necrosis factor-related apoptosis-inducing ligand-dependent manners. Gastroenterology. 2006;**130**(2):435-452

[90] Sun R, Gao B. Negative regulation of liver regeneration by innate immunity (natural killer cells/interferon-gamma). Gastroenterology. 2004;**127**(5):1525-1539

[91] Subleski JJ et al. Enhanced antitumor response by divergent modulation of natural killer and natural killer T cells in the liver. Cancer Research. 2006;**66**(22):11005-11012

[92] Zingoni A et al. Cross-talk between activated human NK cells and CD4+ T cells via OX40-OX40 ligand interactions. Journal of Immunology. 2004;**173**(6):3716-3724

[93] Blanca IR et al. Human B cell activation by autologous NK cells is regulated by CD40-CD40 ligand interaction: Role of memory B cells and CD5+ B cells. Journal of Immunology. 2001;**167**(11):6132-6139

[94] Zimme J. Natural Killer Cells: At the Forefront of Modern Immunology. Springer; Verlag Berlin Heidelberg. 2010

[95] Cai L et al. Functional impairment in circulating and intrahepatic NK cells and relative mechanism in hepatocellular carcinoma patients. Clinical Immunology. 2008;**129**(3):428-437

[96] Chew V et al. Chemokine-driven lymphocyte infiltration: An early intratumoural event determining long-term survival in resectable hepatocellular carcinoma. Gut. 2012;**61**(3):427-438

[97] Jinushi M et al. Impairment of natural killer cell and dendritic cell functions by the soluble form of MHC class I-related chain a in advanced human hepatocellular carcinomas. Journal of Hepatology. 2005;**43**(6):1013-1020

[98] Vitale M et al. Effect of tumor cells and tumor microenvironment on NK-cell function. European Journal of Immunology. 2014;**44**(6):1582-1592

[99] Roszman T, Elliott L, Brooks W. Modulation of T-cell function by gliomas. Immunology Today. 1991;**12**(10):370-374

[100] Bodmer S et al. Human glioblastoma cell derived transforming growth factor-β2: Evidence for secretion of both high and low molecular weight biologically active forms. Journal of Neuroimmunology. 1991;**34**(1):33-42

[101] Elliott RL, Blobe GC. Role of transforming growth factor beta in human cancer. Journal of Clinical Oncology. 2005;**23**(9):2078-2093

[102] Zitvogel L, Tesniere A, Kroemer G. Cancer despite immunosurveillance: Immunoselection and immunosubversion. Nature Reviews. Immunology. 2006;**6**(10):715-727

[103] Gabrilovich DI, Ostrand-Rosenberg S, Bronte V. Coordinated regulation of myeloid cells by tumours. Nature Reviews. Immunology. 2012;**12**(4):253-268

[104] Siemens DR et al. Hypoxia increases tumor cell shedding of MHC class I chain-related molecule: Role of nitric oxide. Cancer Research. 2008;**68**(12):4746-4753

[105] Bryceson YT et al. Molecular mechanisms of natural killer cell activation. Journal of Innate Immunity. 2011;**3**(3):216-226

[106] Sun JC, Lanier LL. NK cell development, homeostasis and function: Parallels with CD8(+) T cells. Nature Reviews. Immunology. 2011;**11**(10):645-657

[107] Lodoen MB, Lanier LL. Natural killer cells as an initial defense against pathogens. Current Opinion in Immunology. 2006;**18**(4):391-398

[108] Vesely MD et al. Natural innate and adaptive immunity to cancer. Annual Review of Immunology. 2011;**29**:235-271

[109] Suganuma T, Workman JL. Signals and combinatorial functions of histone modifications. Annual Review of Biochemistry. 2011;**80**:473-499

[110] Zhang J et al. Interleukin 2 receptor signaling regulates the perforin gene through signal transducer and activator of transcription (Stat)5 activation of two enhancers. The Journal of Experimental Medicine. 1999;**190**(9):1297-1308

[111] Imada K et al. Stat5b is essential for natural killer cell-mediated proliferation and cytolytic activity. The Journal of Experimental Medicine. 1998;**188**(11):2067-2074

[112] Yu CR et al. Role of a STAT binding site in the regulation of the human perforin promoter. Journal of Immunology. 1999;**162**(5):2785-2790

[113] Yamamoto K et al. The human perforin gene is a direct target of STAT4 activated by IL-12 in NK cells. Biochemical and Biophysical Research Communications. 2002;**297**(5):1245-1252

[114] Lieberman J. The ABCs of granule-mediated cytotoxicity: New weapons in the arsenal. Nature Reviews. Immunology. 2003;**3**(5):361-370

[115] Araki Y et al. Histone acetylation facilitates rapid and robust memory CD8 T cell response through differential expression of effector molecules (eomesodermin and its targets: Perforin and granzyme B). Journal of Immunology. 2008;**180**(12):8102-8108

[116] Babichuk CK, Duggan BL, Bleackley RC. In vivo regulation of murine granzyme B gene transcription in activated primary T cells. The Journal of Biological Chemistry. 1996;**271**(28):16485-16493

[117] Wargnier A et al. Identification of human granzyme B promoter regulatory elements interacting with activated T-cell-specific proteins: Implication of Ikaros and CBF binding sites in promoter activation. Proceedings of the National Academy of Sciences of the United States of America. 1995;**92**(15):6930-6934

[118] Huang C et al. A novel NF-kappaB binding site controls human granzyme B gene transcription. Journal of Immunology. 2006;**176**(7):4173-4181

[119] Youness RA et al. Contradicting interplay between insulin-like growth factor-1 and miR-486-5p in primary NK cells and hepatoma cell lines with a contemporary inhibitory impact on HCC tumor progression. Growth Factors. 2016;**34**(3-4):128-140

[120] Abdelrahman MM et al. Enhancing NK cell cytotoxicity by miR-182 in hepatocellular carcinoma. Human Immunology. 2016;**77**(8):667-673

[121] El Tayebi HM et al. miR-615-5p is restrictedly expressed in cirrhotic and cancerous liver tissues and its overexpression alleviates the tumorigenic effects in hepatocellular carcinoma. FEBS Letters. 2012;**586**(19):3309-3316

[122] Rahmoon MA et al. MiR-615-5p depresses natural killer cells cytotoxicity through repressing IGF-1R in hepatocellular carcinoma patients. Growth Factors. 2017;1-12. DOI: 10.1080/08977194.2017.1354859

Chapter 4

# NK Cells in Cancer Immunotherapy

Lynda Addou-Klouche

Additional information is available at the end of the chapter

http://dx.doi.org/10.5772/intechopen.71217

**Abstract**

Natural killer (NK) cells are crucial components of the innate immune system and play critical roles in host immunity against viral infections and cancer. NK cells' activity is controlled by the interaction of a wide range of receptors expressed on their surfaces with cell surface ligands. Opposite signals delivered by inhibitory and activating receptors tightly regulate NK cells' cytotoxicity. Natural killer cells can discriminate between normal and cancer cells. NK cells are known to directly recognize and kill malignant cells or induce apoptosis. However, tumor cells have the ability to evade those attacks. The main mechanisms involve the lack of expression or downregulation of the expression of major histocompatibility complex (MHC) class I molecules and secretion of soluble NKG2D ligands by tumor cells. Furthermore, tumors harbor a population of cancer stem cells (CSCs), which can drive tumor progression and therapeutical resistance. This chapter highlights the roles of NK cells in tumor immunosurveillance and their applications for cancer immunotherapy. NK cell biology and function as well as the role of their receptor interactions will be described. We will discuss the therapeutic applications of NK cells in cancer and NK cells targeting CSCs as a promising strategy for cancer therapy.

**Keywords:** NK cells, cancer-immunotherapy, cancer stem cells

## 1. Introduction

Natural killer (NK) cells constitute a minor subset of lymphocytes that are crucial components of the innate immune system and play critical roles in host immunity against malignant cells and virus-infected cells but also in bacterial, fungal, and parasite immune responses [1]. NK cells represent 10% of the lymphocytes in human peripheral blood, and they comprise the third largest population of lymphocytes following B and T cells.

Natural killer cells have diverse biological functions including killing pathogen-infected cells and cancer cells as well as an immunoregulatory role [2]. Natural killer cells can discriminate between normal cells and cells that do not express adequate amounts of major histocompatibility complex (MHC) class I molecules.

NK cell cytotoxicity is regulated by a balance between activating and inhibitory signals delivered by receptors expressed at the cell surface. These cells are known to directly recognize and kill malignant cells or induce apoptosis. However, tumor cells have the ability to evade immunosurveillance by using multiple mechanisms. Furthermore, tumors harbor a population of cancer stem cells (CSC), which is responsible of tumor progression and therapeutical resistance.

Therapeutic applications of NK cells in cancer and NK cells targeting cancer stem cells (CSCs) represent a promising strategy for cancer immunotherapy.

## 2. NK cells' biology and function

NK cells originate from common lymphoid progenitor cells and further differentiate into immature/mature NK cells in bone marrow. They are then distributed in peripheral lymphoid and nonlymphoid organs and tissues [3–5], including bone marrow, spleen, peripheral blood, placenta, lung, liver, uterus [6], and peritoneal cavity while limited numbers are localized in lymph nodes [7]. Human NK cell turnover in blood is around 2 weeks [8].

NK cells were originally described as large granular lymphocytes with natural cytotoxicity against tumor cells. NK cells were later recognized as a separate lymphocyte lineage, with both cytotoxicity and immunoregulatory role, as they are involved in the production of cytokines [9]. More recently, data revealed that activated NK cells may also influence the outcome of helminth infections. CD4-NK cells increasing early following nematode infection with *Brugia pahangi* are able to produce IL-4 and then could polarize the immune response toward a Th2 profile [10]. In fact, protection against helminthic infections are usually mediated by Th2 immune response characterized by secretion of IL-4, IL-5, and IL-13, secretion of IgE antibodies, and activation of mast cells [11, 12]. Studies revealed that the clearance of these parasites is more efficient and complete in the presence of NK cells. In the case of Th2 immunity disruption, NK cells may become an important source of IL-13 during murine gastrointestinal nematode infections [13, 14]. Human NK cells can be classified into two major subsets $CD56^{dim}$ and $CD56^{bright}$ depending on their immunophenotype and functions and more recently in terms of their homing properties [15, 16]. $CD56^{dim}$ NK cells are fully mature, make up about 90% of the NK cells in peripheral blood and inflammatory sites, and they express perforin and exhibit a high cytotoxic activity after encountering target cells [17, 18]. These $CD56^{dim}$ NK cells are cytotoxic and produce interferon $\gamma$ (IFN-$\gamma$) upon interaction with tumor cells in vitro [19]. In contrast, $CD56^{bright}$ cells are more immature, make up about 5–15% of total NK cells, and have been considered primarily as cytokine producers, while playing a limited role in cytolytic responses. Approximately, 90% of NK cells in lymph nodes belong to the $CD56^{bright}$ subset and lack perforin [20]. These cells exert immunoregulatory function by producing abundant cytokines such as IFN-γ in response to stimulation with interleukins (IL)-12, IL-15, and IL-18 [21]. In response to nematode infection, $CD56^{bright}$ NK cells can bind with a secreted protein ES from the human hookworm *Necator americanus* and induce IFN-gamma production [22]. Natural killer cells have diverse biological functions, which include recognizing and killing pathogen-infected and cancer cells. Circulating NK cells are mostly in their resting phase, but after activation by cytokines and chemokines, they are capable of extravasation and recruitment into distinct inflamed or malignant tissues [9, 23]. NK cells also have an immunoregulatory role as their ligand interaction with cell-surface receptors lead to the production of several cytokines.

NK cells mediate two predominant pathways of cell death. The first pathway, a granule exocytosis pathway [24], involves the release of cytotoxic granule, perforin (a membrane-disrupting protein), and granzymes (a family of structurally related serine proteases) responsible for NK cell-mediated killing by inducing apoptosis of the target cell [25–27]. In the second pathway, a caspase-dependent apoptosis involves the association of death receptors such as first apoptosis signal (Fas) cell surface death receptor and tumor-necrosis-factor–related apoptosis inducing ligand receptor (TRAILR) on target cells with their corresponding ligands, members of the tumor necrosis factor (TNF) family of cytokines, expressed by NK cells, and regulated by IFN-γ, such as FASL, and tumor necrosis factor-related apoptosis-inducing ligand (TRAIL), resulting in caspase-dependent target cell apoptosis [28–32]. Antibody-dependent cellular cytotoxicity (ADCC) can also be a mechanism of killing of tumor cells by NK cells by triggering the NK CD16 receptor (FcγRIII), which binds to the IgG and antibody-coated targets [33].

Natural killer cells can discriminate between normal cells and those that do not express adequate amounts of MHC class I molecules. They were originally defined by their ability to spontaneously eliminate cells lacking expression of MHC class I molecules. NK cells express receptors that bind to MHC class I molecules including the killer cell immunoglobulin-like receptors (KIRs) that play major roles in regulating the activation thresholds of NK cells in humans [34].

## 3. NK cell cytotoxicity

NK cell cytotoxicity is tightly regulated by a balance between activating and inhibitory signals [35] delivered by a multitude of receptors expressed at the cell surface [36] (**Figure 1**). The inhibitory NK cell receptors interact with MHC class I molecules expressed on almost all nucleated cells, preventing NK cell activation against healthy cells (**Figure 2a**). NK cell activation is blocked through engagement of their KIR receptors [37]. This explains self-tolerance and prevention of host cell killing. NK cells can discriminate between normal host cells and infected or abnormal cells by recognition of MHC class I molecules. It was earlier discovered that NK cells are activated when they encounter cells that lack self-MHC class I molecule. For example, under stress conditions, such as cellular transformation, cells down-regulate MHC-I expression causing NK cells to lose inhibitory signaling and be activated in

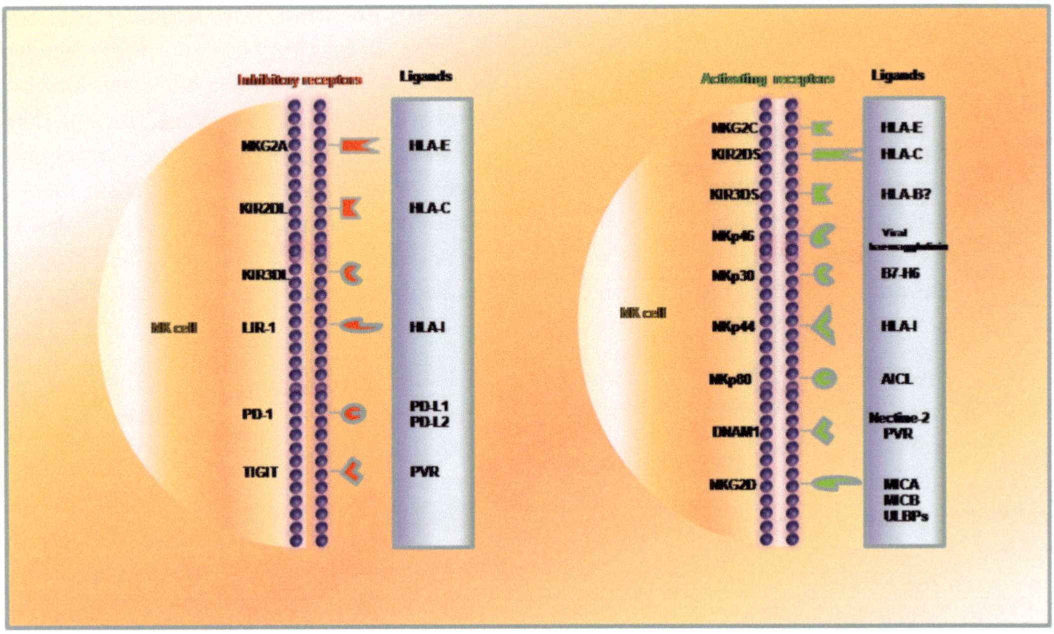


**Figure 1.** Examples of activating and inhibitory NK cell receptors and their respective ligands. AICL: activation-induced C-type lectin; B7-H6: Member of the B7 family of immunoreceptors; DNAM-1: DNAX accessory molecule 1; HLA: human leucocyte antigen; KIR2DL: killer-cell immunoglobulin-like receptor 2DL; KIR3DL: Killer-cell immunoglobulin-like receptor 3DL; KIR2D5: killer-cell immunoglobulin-like receptor 2D5; KIR3D5: killer-cell immunoglobulin-like receptor 3D5; LIR-1: leukocyte inhibitory receptor 1; MICA: MHC class I polypeptide-related sequence A; MICB: MHC class I polypeptide-related sequence B; NKG2A: natural killer group protein 2 family member A; NKG2C: natural killer group protein 2 family member C; NKp30: natural killer Cell P30-related Protein; NKp46: natural killer Cell P46-related Protein; NKp80: Natural killer Cell P80-related Protein; PD1: programmed cell death 1; PD-L1: programmed death-ligand 1; PD-L2: programmed death-ligand 2; PVR: polio virus receptor; TIGIT: T cell immunoreceptor with Ig and ITIM domains.

a process called "missing-self recognition" [38]. This model is based on the fact that NK cell activity is normally controlled by self-MHC molecules that interact with a large repertoire of inhibitory NK receptors. In this condition, activation receptors are no longer suppressed and they induce potent stimulatory signals, resulting in NK cell activation including cytokine production and granule release leading to cytotoxicity [39, 40]. Abnormal cells can also upregulate the expression of ligands to activate receptors on the NK cells that can overcome the inhibitory signals.

### 3.1. Activating NK cell receptors

NK cells require external signals to begin the process of cell activation, which usually occurs via triggering receptors. A number of receptors have been identified that allow NK cells to become activated. The major activating receptors expressed on human NK cells include the natural cytotoxicity receptors (NCRs: NKp30, NKp44, NKp46), the immunoglobulin gamma Fc-region receptor III (Fc$\gamma$RIII/CD16), activating forms of killer cell Ig-like receptors (KIR:

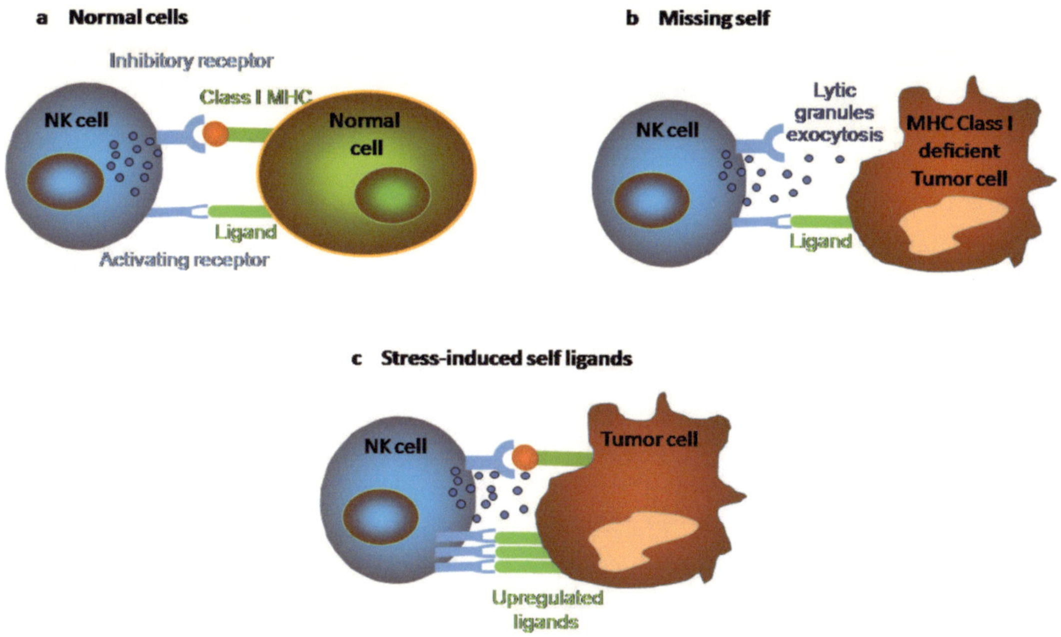


**Figure 2.** NK cell functions. (a) Inhibitory NK cell receptors interact with MHC class I molecules expressed on nucleated cells, preventing NK cell activation and lysis against normal cells. (b) NK cells can eliminate tumors cells that downregulate major histocompatibility complex (MHC) class I molecules causing NK cells to lose inhibitory signaling and be activated in a process called "missing-self recognition." (c) NK cells can kill tumor cells that retain full expression of MHC class I but overexpress induced stress ligands recognized by activating NK cell receptors, which override the inhibitory signals and elicit target cell lysis.

KIR2DS and KIR3DS), NKG2D, C-type lectin receptors (CD94/NKG2C, NKG2E/H, and NKG2F), NKp80, and 2B4 [41]. NKG2D and NCRs are particularly important receptors for triggering NK cell responses toward tumor cells [42].

A new family of receptors that recognize nectin and nectin-like molecules has recently emerged as a critical regulator of NK cell functions — DNAX accessory molecule 1 (DNAM-1, CD226) is an adhesion molecule that controls NK cell cytotoxicity and interferon-$\gamma$ production against a wide range of cancer and infected cells [43].

The B7 family member B7-H6 is a tumor cell ligand for the activating natural killer cell receptor NKp30 in humans [44]. Activating KIR receptor recognizes classical MHC-I molecules [45], whereas NKG2D recognizes the nonclassical MHC-I molecules, MICA/MICB, retinoic acid early transcript 1E protein (RAET1E), RAET1G, RAET1H, RAET1I, RAET1L, and RAET1N (also known as ULBP1–ULBP6) [46, 47]. These ligands are not present on the cell surface of most normal cells, but are upregulated at the cell surface after cellular stress, on rapidly proliferating cells, infected cells, transformed cells, and tumor cells [48], further increasing the NK cell activity [49]. CD16 binds the Fc portion of IgG antibodies to initiate antibody-dependent cellular cytotoxicity (ADCC) and provides NK cells with the ability to recognize and kill target cells coated with antibodies [50]. DNAM-1 ligands CD112 and CD155 have been described in different pathological conditions, and recent evidence indicates that their expression is regulated by cellular stress.

All of these activating receptors promote cytotoxicity and cytokine production responses through stimulating intracellular protein tyrosine kinase cascades.

### 3.2. Inhibitory NK cell receptors

Inhibitory receptors are able to prevent the activation of NK cells and have been thought of as fail-safe mechanisms to prevent attack on normal cells and tissues. In general, these receptors express one or more immunoreceptor tyrosine-based inhibition motifs (ITIM), and they recruit SH2-containing phosphatase-1 (SHP1), SH2-containing phosphatase-2 (SHP2), and/or SH2-containing inositol phosphatase (SHIP) proteins upon binding to their ligands [51]. These phosphatases prevent the activation of cellular signaling cascades by inhibiting phosphorylation of proteins.

The inhibitory receptors encompass two distinct classes: the monomeric type I glycoprotein of the immunoglobulin superfamilies KIR2DL and KIR3DL [51], leukocyte immunoglobulin-like receptors (ILT2), and the hetero-dimeric C-type lectin-like receptor (CTLR) called CD94/NKG2A (natural killer group protein 2 family member A) [52, 53].

## 4. NK cells in tumor immunosurveillance and cancer

NK cells are innate cellular components that regulate adaptive immune responses in the immune surveillance of cancer. Primary immunodeficiencies affecting NK cells were associated with higher rates of malignancy and a higher risk of developing various types of cancer [54, 55]. NK cells have been shown to control the growth and metastasis of transplantable tumors in numerous mouse models by antibody depletion of NK cells [56].

NK cells can eliminate tumors that downregulate expression of MHC class I (**Figure 2b**), possibly in response to selective pressure exerted by $CD8^+$ T cells. Furthermore, NK cells can kill tumor cells that retain full expression of MHC class I if they have upregulated ligands that engage activating NK cell receptors, thus overriding the inhibitory signals (**Figure 2c**).

For example, NKG2D ligand expression on tumor cells induces NK cell activation and is sufficient to overcome inhibitory signals delivered by MHC class I receptors, thereby enabling NK cells to eliminate tumors expressing normal levels of MHC class I [48, 57]. Mice deficient of NKG2D ($Klrk1^{-/-}$) are more susceptible to tumorigenesis [58] confirming the crucial role of NKG2D in tumor immunosurveillance.

However, tumor cells are able to evade immunosurveillance by using multiple mechanisms. Tumor cells can secrete inhibitory cytokines such as transforming growth factor-β (TGFβ) that suppresses the activity of NK cells. Furthermore, tumor cells can express inhibitory receptor-specific ligands such as glucocorticoid-induced TNFR-related protein (GITR) that can downmodulate activating receptors NKG2D on NK cells. To escape to NK cell immunosurveillance, tumor cells can also secrete immunomodulatory molecules such as prostaglandin E2 (PGE2), indoleamine 2,3-dioxygenase (IDO), adenosine, TGFβ, and interleukin-10 (IL-10). Tumor cells can proteolytically shed NKG2D ligands (NKG2DLs) leading to a decreased amount of NKG2DL and to the production of soluble ligands that downmodulate NKG2D receptor on NK cells [59, 60]. Finally, secretion of immunosuppressive molecules or expression of NKG2DLs by cells of the tumor microenvironment can downmodulate NKG2D receptor on NK cells.

Soluble NKG2DLs have been detected at high levels in the serum of cancer patients [61] and might be used as a diagnostic marker [62]. Tumor cells can escape immunosurveillance by the secretion of soluble factors such as lactate dehydrogenase, leading to NKG2DLs expression on healthy host myeloid cells [63]. NKG2D Downregulation could be the result of its chronic exposure to NKG2D ligand on tumor cells [64]. Recent work in a mouse model suggests that a shed NKG2D ligand, MULT1, stabilizes expression of NKG2D on NK cells and increase their antitumor activity [65]. Controlling NKG2DL expression level on tumors provides an attractive therapeutic strategy for immunotherapy.

In patients and animal models, impaired NK cells or NK cell deficiency have been associated not only with recurring viral infections, but also with an increased incidence of various types of cancer [55]. Tumor cells often acquire the ability to escape NK cell-mediated immune surveillance. In fact, during tumor development and progression, many malignant cells acquire the ability either to evade from NK cell recognition or to impair NK cell function.

Cells undergoing malignant transformation often downregulate their expression of MHC class I molecules, and the absence of inhibitory signaling on NK cells permits their function. A defective immunity has been well established in different types of cancer. The imbalance of immune status is inclined to immunosuppression in cancer patients, which results in tumor immune evasion. Such immunosuppression is characterized by a decrease in NK cell numbers in peripheral blood and a decreased tumor infiltrate as compared to normal tissues. Moreover, in many types of cancer, a defective expression of activating receptors and overexpression of inhibitory receptors is observed [66].

The role of NK cells against parasites that may promote or impede carcinogens is poorly understood. Chronic inflammation is a key feature in carcinogenesis associated with helminth infections. For example, *Strongyloides stercoralis* infection was associated with an increased occurrence of lymphoid cancers [67]. An association of colorectal cancer with chronic *S. stercoralis* infection has also been reported in a Columbian patient [68]. This nematode is not only a cofactor for the development of lymphoid cancers induced by HTLV-1 [69] but is also associated with the development of colon adenocarcinoma by activating the host immune response. A study reports a case of Strongyloides infection in a 72-year-old man presenting a large population of cells (NK-LGL) with a natural killer phenotype abnormally activated and diagnosed with NK-LGL leukemia [70]. The role of NK cells in the immune response to Strongyloides is not defined, but it is possible that an abnormal or clonal expansion of NK cells could suppress antihelminth immunity. Activated NK cells, perhaps producing interferon, suppressed the T-helper 2 response that previously controlled the Strongyloides infection.

# 5. NK cell in cancer immunotherapy

Cancer immunotherapy is the targeted therapy designed to induce antitumor response against malignancies by harnessing the power of the immune system [71]. The ability to recognize and lyse transformed cells without prior immunization, the ease of isolation and expansion *ex vivo,* and the shorter life span make NK cells a good alternate to immunotherapy. Furthermore, NK cell can kill cancer cells without damaging healthy tissues or risking the T cell–driven inflammatory cytokine storm that can accompany other immunotherapies. The NK cells derived from peripheral or umbilical cord cells, embryonic or induced pluripotent stem cells, and NK cell lines were being tested for treating various malignancies. Several promising clinical therapies have been used to exploit NK cell functions in treating cancer patients.

## 5.1. Adoptive NK cell transfer therapy

Adoptive NK cell transfer therapy is a strategy aimed at enhancing the biological function of the immune system by means of autologous or allogeneic NK cells. NK cells for adoptive NK cell transfer therapy (autologous or allogeneic) are usually obtained from the peripheral blood of the patient or from a donor. They can also be derived from the bone marrow, umbilical-cord blood, human embryonic stem cells, or induced pluripotent stem cells and are now considered as alternative sources of therapeutic NK cells [72].

Various approaches exist for the therapy with the adoptive transfer of NK cells. In autologous transfer, NK cells from the patient are activated and expanded in vitro in the presence of cytokines. IL-2 has been used for this purpose, but recently, the combination of IL-12, IL-15, and IL-18 might generate NK cells that are more functional and have memory properties. The expanded and activated NK cells are then transferred back into the patient. To sustain the expansion and function of the infused NK cells, patient receives IL2 cytokine administration. Although autologous NK cells might recognize activating signals such as stress molecules on cancer cells, their anti-tumor activity is limited by the inhibitory signal transmitted by self-HLA molecules.

In allogenic transfer, NK cells can be obtained from HLA-matched or haploidentical (partially matched) donors. The best responses are obtained when haploidentical donors do not express KIRs that recognize the patient's HLA molecules, because donor NK cells do not receive an inhibitory signal from the patient's cancer cells. NK cells are expanded through processes similar to those used for autologous transfer except that T cells should be removed.

### *5.1.1. CAR-engineered NK cells*

NK cells can be transduced with activating chimeric antigen receptors (CARs) that specifically bind to antigens overexpressed by tumor cells. CARs are designed by the fusion of an antigen binding with a hinge region, a transmembrane domain and one or more stimulatory molecules.

CARs can be engineered in autologous or allogeneic NK cells or in NK cell lines such as NK-92. Each CAR has the CD3ζ chain (or sometimes the FcRγ chain) as its main signaling domain. To increase persistence and superior functionality, co-stimulatory domains, usually from CD28 or CD137, can be added to the CAR construct. CARs from the first generation have no stimulatory domain, whereas CARs from the second generation and third generation have one co-stimulatory domain or two co-stimulatory domains, respectively. CAR engineering endows NK cells with antigen specificity. The binding of a CAR to the tumor antigen delivers a potent activating signal that triggers NK cell cytotoxicity, which results in the elimination of cancer cells. Several recent studies have documented a success using NK cells engineered to express activating chimeric antigen receptors (CARs) specific to tumor antigens [73]. Many B-cell acute and chronic leukemia can escape killing by natural killer cells. The introduction of chimeric antigen receptors (CAR) into T cells or NK cells could potentially overcome this resistance [74]. NK-92 leukemia cell lines were transduced to express CARs specific for CD19 [75] and CD20 [76] expressed on B cell malignancies and also for disialoganglioside GD2, a glycolipid expressed on neuroblastoma and various other cancer types [77].

In glioblastoma, the most aggressive primary brain malignancy, intracranial administration of NK-92-EGFR-CAR cells represents a promising therapy [78]. In human multiple myeloma (MM), CS1-specific (a surface protein highly expressed on MM cells) chimeric antigen receptor (CAR)-engineered natural killer cells [79] enhance responses to tumor cells in vitro and suppressed tumor growth when tested in vivo in xenograft models [65, 78, 80]. Autologous or allogeneic transplantation of CS1-specific CAR NK cells may be a promising strategy to treat multiple myeloma.

### 5.2. Cytokine-induced NK cell activation

To promote NK cell expansion, the use of IL-2 has demonstrated the effectiveness on NK cell activation and anti-tumor responses [81]. It was reported that NK cells from lung cancer patients could regain the cytotoxicity against targets after activation by IL-2 [82]. However, NK cells activation using high-dose IL-2 has some side effects because of severe capillary leaky syndrome. To improve the therapeutic efficacy and safety, a different strategy combining IL-2 with other NK cell activators was used. Hellstrand et al. [83] administered IL-2 together with histamine to 22 acute myeloid leukemia (AML) patients and showed a good clinical outcome. IL-2 diphtheria toxin (IL2DT), a recombinant cytotoxic fusion protein has been used in order to increase the depletion of regulatory T cells (Treg) and therefore improving in vivo donor NK cell expansion and remission induction [84].

### 5.3. NK cells targeting cancer stem cells

Tumor harbors a population of cancer cells with "stem-cell" like properties including self-renewal and the ability to produce differentiated progeny [85]. These cells termed cancer stem cells (CSCs) can drive tumor progression and therapeutic resistance to standard cancer therapy. In fact, cancer stem cells have been proposed as an important mechanism of tumor initiation and/or repopulation after tumor debulking by chemotherapy and/or by radiotherapy.

In addition, CSCs have been associated with tumor relapse and metastasis, even in cases of apparent complete response to systemic therapy [86]. Then, targeting CSCs is a promising strategy for cancer therapy. Natural killer cells have the ability to reject allogeneic hematopoietic stem cells, and there are increasing data demonstrating that NK cells can selectively identify and lyse CSCs. Tallerico et al. [87], for example, demonstrated that metastatic colorectal cancer, which contains a high proportion of CSCs, showed increased susceptibility to NK cytotoxicity. Similarly, Castriconi et al. [88] reported that glioblastoma-derived CSCs were susceptible to NK cell cytotoxicity. Human cancer cells with stem cell-like phenotype exhibit enhanced sensitivity to the cytotoxicity of IL-2 and IL-15 activated natural killer cells [89]. IL-2- and IL-15-activated NK cells were found to be cytotoxic against human breast cancer stem cells and CD 133+ melanoma CSCs [90]. Recently, Ames et al. [91] showed that NK cells kill CSCs from different kinds of tumors, through the interaction of the NKG2D activating receptor with its ligand (MICA/B).

## 6. Conclusions

NK cells have a crucial role in immunosurveillance against tumor development. However, when both the innate and adaptive immune systems fail and tumors develop, NK cells and their receptors can still be targeted in many therapeutic approaches. NK cells are more effective in treating hematologic malignancies than in treating solid tumors. This might result from inefficient homing of NK cells to the site of tumor. Therefore, NK cell-based immunotherapy can be successfully exploited in the hematopoietic stem cell transplantation for the treatment of hematological malignancies, but efforts have to be made to improve the homing and in vivo persistence of NK cells. Targeting CSCs with NK cell-based immunotherapy represents an attractive strategy for cancer therapy.

NK cells clearly have a role in future immunotherapies of the treatment of cancer and should continue to be evaluated in clinical trials.

## Author details

Lynda Addou-Klouche

Address all correspondence to: addouklouche.lynda@yahoo.fr

University of Sidi-Bel-Abbes, Algeria

## References

[1] Bouzani M, Ok M, McCormick A, Ebel F, Kurzai O, Morton CO, Einsele H, Loeffler J. Human NK cells display important antifungal activity against *Aspergillus fumigatus*,

which is directly mediated by IFN-gamma release. Journal of Immunology. 2011;**187**(3): 1369-1376

[2] Glas R, Franksson L, Une C, Eloranta ML, Ohlén C, Orn A, et al. Recruitment and activation of natural killer (NK) cells *in vivo* determined by the target cell phenotype. An adaptive component of NK cell-mediated responses. The Journal of Experimental Medicine. 2000;**191**(1):129-138

[3] Farag SS, Caligiuri MA. Human natural killer cell development and biology. Blood Reviews. 2006;**20**:123-137

[4] Freud AG, Caligiuri MA. Human natural killer cell development. Immunological Reviews. 2006;**214**:56-72

[5] Vacca P, Vitale C, Montaldo E, Conte R, Cantoni C, Fulcheri E, Darretta V, Moretta L, Mingari MC. CD34+ hematopoietic precursors are present in human decidua and differentiate into natural killer cells upon interaction with stromal cells. Proceedings of the National Academy of Sciences of the United States of America. 2011;**108**:2402-2407

[6] Acar N, Ustunel I, Demir R. Uterine natural killer (uNK) cells and their missions during pregnancy: A review. Acta Histochemica. 2011;**113**(2):82-91

[7] Fehniger TA, Cooper MA, Nuovo GJ, Cella M, Facchetti F, Colonna M, Caligiuri MA. CD56 bright natural killer cells are present in human lymph nodes and are activated by T cell-derived IL-2: A potential new link between adaptive and innate immunity. Blood. 2003;**101**(8):3052-3057

[8] Zhang Y et al. In vivo kinetics of human natural killer cells: The effects of ageing and acute and chronic viral infection. Immunology. 2007;**121**:258-265

[9] Campbell KS, Hasegawa J. Natural killer cell biology: An update and future directions. The Journal of Allergy and Clinical Immunology. 2013;**132**(3):536-544

[10] Balmer P, Devaney ENKT. Cells are a source of early interleukin-4 following infection with third-stage larvae of the filarial nematode *Brugia pahangi*. Infection and Immunity. 2002;**70**:2215-2219

[11] Faveeuw C, Mallevaey T, Trottein F. Role of natural killer T lymphocytes during helminthic infection. Parasite. 2008;**15**(3):384-888

[12] Allen JE, Maizels RM. Diversity and dialogue in immunity to helminths. Nature Reviews. Immunology. 2011;**11**(6):375-388

[13] McDermott JR, Humphreys NE, Forman SP, Donaldson DD, Grencis RK. Intraepithelial NK cell-derived IL-13 induces intestinal pathology associated with nematode infection. Journal of Immunology. 2005;**175**:3207-3213

[14] Hepworth MR, Grencis RK. Disruption of Th2 immunity results in a gender-specific expansion of IL-13 producing accessory NK cells during helminth infection. Journal of Immunology. 2009;**183**(6):3906-3914

[15] Caligiuri MA. Human natural killer cells. Blood. 2008;**112**(3):461-469

[16] Vivier E, Tomasello E, Baratin M, Walzer T, Ugolini S. Functions of natural killer cells. Nature Immunology. 2008;**9**(5):503-510

[17] De Maria A, Bozzano F, Cantoni C, Moretta L. Revisiting human natural killer cell subset function revealed cytolytic CD56(dim)CD16+ NK cells as rapid producers of abundant IFN-gamma on activation. Proceedings of the National Academy of Sciences of the United States of America. 2011;**108**:728-732

[18] Fauriat C, Long EO, Ljunggren HG, Bryceson YT. Regulation of human NK-cell cytokine and chemokine production by target cell recognition. Blood. 2010;**115**:2167-2176

[19] Anfossi N et al. Human NK cell education by inhibitory receptors for MHC class I. Immunity. 2006;**25**:331-342

[20] Ferlazzo G, Munz C. NK cell compartments and their activation by dendritic cells. Journal of Immunology. 2004;**172**:1333-1339

[21] Cooper MA, Fehniger TA, Caligiuri MA. The biology of human natural killercell subsets. Trends in Immunology. 2001;**22**:633-640

[22] Hsieh GC, Loukas A, Wahl AM, Bhatia M, Wang Y, Williamson AL, Kehn KW, Maruyama H, Hotez PJ, Leitenberg D, Bethony J, Constant SL. A secreted protein from the human hookworm *Necator americanus* binds selectively to NK cells and induces IFN-gamma production. Journal of Immunology. 2004;**173**(4):2699-2704

[23] Gregoire C, Chasson L, Luci C, Tomasello E, Geissmann F, Vivier E, Walzer T. The trafficking of natural killer cells. Immunological Reviews. 2007;**220**:169-182

[24] Krzewski K, Coligan JE. Human NK cell lytic granules and regulation of their exocytosis. Natural Killer Cell Biology. 2012;**3**:335

[25] Kagi D, Ledermann B, Burki K, Seiler P, Odermatt B, Olsen KJ, Podack ER, Zinkernagel RM, Hengartner H. Cytotoxicity mediated by T cells and natural killer cells is greatly impaired in perforin-deficient mice. Nature. 1994;**369**:31-37

[26] Trapani JA, Davis J, Sutton VR, Smyth MJ. Proapoptotic functions of cytotoxic lymphocyte granule constituents in vitro and in vivo. Current Opinion in Immunology. 2000;**12**:323-329

[27] Voskoboinik I, Whisstock JC, Trapani JA. Perforin and granzymes: Function, dysfunction and human pathology. Nature Reviews. Immunology. 2015;**15**:388-400

[28] Nagata S. Apoptosis by death factor. Cell. 1997;**88**:355-365

[29] Screpanti V, Wallin RP, Ljunggren HG, Grandien A. A central role for death receptor-mediated apoptosis in the rejection of tumors by NK cells. Journal of Immunology. 2001;**167**:2068-2073

[30] Takeda K, Hayakawa Y, Smyth MJ, Kayagaki N, Yamaguchi N, Kakuta S, Iwakura Y, Yagita H, Okumura K. Involvement of tumor necrosis factor-related apoptosis-inducing

ligand in surveillance of tumor metastasis by liver natural killer cells. Nature Medicine. 2001;**7**:94-100

[31] Cretney E, Takeda K, Yagita H, Glaccum M, Peschon JJ, Smyth MJ. Increased susceptibility to tumor initiation and metastasis in TNF-related apoptosis-inducing ligand-deficient mice. Journal of Immunology. 2002;**168**:1356-1361

[32] Smyth MJ et al. Activation of NK cell cytotoxicity. Molecular Immunology. 2005;**42**: 501-510

[33] Hooijberg E, Sein JJ, van den Berk PC, Hekman A. Characterization of a series of isotype switch variants of a new CD20 monoclonal antibody. Hybridoma 1996;**15**:23-31

[34] Campbell KS, Purdy AK. Structure/function of human killer cell immunoglobulin-like receptors: Lessons from polymorphisms, evolution, crystal structures and mutations. Immunology. 2011;**132**:315-325

[35] Morvan MG, Lanier LLNK. Cells and cancer: You can teach innate cells new tricks. Nature Reviews. Cancer. 2016;**16**(1):7-19

[36] Del Zotto G, Marcenaro E, Vacca P, Sivori S, Pende D, Della Chiesa M, Moretta F, Ingegnere T, Mingari MC, Moretta A, Moretta L. Markers and function of human NK cells in normal and pathological conditions. Cytometry. Part B, Clinical Cytometry. 2017;**92**(2):100-114

[37] Lanier LL. Up on the tightrope: Natural killer cell activation and inhibition. Nature Immunology. 2008;**9**:495-502

[38] Kärre K, Ljunggren HG, Piontek G, Kiessling R. Selective rejection of H-2-deficient lymphoma variants suggests alternative immune defence strategy. Nature. 1986;**319**:675-678

[39] Bauer S, Groh V, Wu J, Steinle A, Phillips JH, Lanier LL, Spies T. Activation of NK cells and T cells by NKG2D, a receptor for stress-inducible MICA. Science. 1999;**285**(5428):727-739

[40] Cassidy SA, Cheent KS, Khakoo SI. Effects of peptide on NK cell-mediated MHC I recognition. Frontiers in Immunology. 2014;**5**:133

[41] MacFarlane IVAW, Campbell KS. Signal transduction in natural killer cells. Current Topics in Microbiology and Immunology. 2006;**298**:23-57

[42] Mentlik James A, Cohen AD, Campbell KS. Combination immune therapies to enhance anti-tumor responses by NK cells. Frontiers in Immunology. 2013;**4**:481

[43] De Andrade LF, Smyth MJ, Martinet L. DNAM-1 control of natural killer cells functions through nectin and nectin-like proteins. Immunology and Cell Biology. 2014;**92**(3):237-244

[44] Brandt CS, Baratin M, Yi EC, Kennedy J, Gao Z, Fox B, et al. The B7 family member B7-H6 is a tumor cell ligand for the activating natural killer cell receptor NKp30 in humans. The Journal of Experimental Medicine. 2009;**206**:1495-1503

[45] Purdy AK, Campbell KS. Natural killer cells and cancer: Regulation by the killer cell Ig-like receptors (KIR). Cancer Biology & Therapy. 2009;**8**(23):2211-2220

[46] Steinle A, Li P, Morris DL, Groh V, Lanier LL, Strong RK, et al. Interactions of human NKG2D with its ligands MICA, MICB, and homologs of the mouse RAE-1 protein family. Immunogenetics. 2001;**53**:279-287

[47] Lanier LL. NKG2D receptor and its ligands in host defense. Cancer Immunology Research. 2015;**3**:575-582

[48] Raulet DH, Gasser S, Gowen BG, Deng W, Jung H. Regulation of ligands for the NKG2D activating receptor. Annual Review of Immunology. 2013;**31**:413-441

[49] Terszowski G, Passweg JR, Stern M. Natural killer cell immunity after transplantation. Swiss Medical Weekly. 2012;**142**:w13700

[50] Ahmad A, Menezes J. Antibody-dependent cellular cytotoxicity in HIV infections. The FASEB Journal. 1996;**10**:258-266

[51] Lanier LL. NK cell recognition. Annual Review of Immunology. 2005;**23**:225-274

[52] Lee N, Llano M, Carretero M, Ishitani A, Navarro F, Lopez-Botet M, Geraghty DE. HLA-E is a major ligand for the natural killer inhibitory receptor CD94/NKG2A. Proceedings of the National Academy of Sciences of the USA. 1998;**95**:5199-5204 malhotra/shanker2011

[53] Malhotra A, Shanker A. NK cells: Immune cross-talk and therapeutic implications. Immunotherapy. 2011;**3**(10):1143-1166

[54] Imai K, Matsuyama S, Miyake S, Suga K, Nakachi K. Natural cytotoxic activity of peripheral-blood lymphocytes and cancer incidence: An 11-year follow-up study of a general population. Lancet. 2000;**356**:1795-1799

[55] Orange JS. Natural killer cell deficiency. The Journal of Allergy and Clinical Immunology. 2013;**132**:515-525

[56] Smyth MJ, Hayakawa Y, Takeda K, Yagita H. New aspects of natural-killer-cell surveillance and therapy of cancer. Nature Reviews. Cancer. 2002;**2**(11):850-861

[57] Cerwenka A, Baro JL, Lanier LL. Ectopic expression of retinoic acid early inducible-1 gene (*RAE-1*) permits natural killer cell-mediated rejection of a MHC class I-bearing tumor *in vivo*. Proceedings of the National Academy of Sciences of the United States of America. 2001;**98**:11521-11526

[58] Guerra N et al. NKG2D-deficient mice are defective in tumor surveillance in models of spontaneous malignancy. Immunity. 2008;**28**:571-580

[59] Groh V, Wu J, Yee C, Spies T. Tumor-derived soluble MIC ligands impair expression of NKG2D and T-cell activation. Nature. 2002;**419**:734-738

[60] Kaiser BK et al. Disulphide-isomerase-enabled shedding of tumor-associated NKG2D ligands. Nature. 2007;**447**:482-486

[61] Salih HR, Holdenrieder S, Steinle A. Soluble NKG2D ligands: Prevalence, release, and functional impact. Frontiers in Bioscience. 2008;(13):3448-3456

[62] Holdenrieder S et al. Soluble MICA in malignant diseases. International Journal of Cancer. 2006;**118**:684-687

[63] Crane CA et al. Immune evasion mediated by tumor-derived lactate dehydrogenase induction of NKG2D ligands on myeloid cells in glioblastoma patients. Proceedings of the National Academy of Sciences of the United States of America. 2014;**111**:12823-12828

[64] Champsaur M, Lanier LL. Effect of NKG2D ligand expression on host immune responses. Immunological Reviews. 2010;**235**:267-285

[65] Deng W et al. A shed NKG2D ligand that promotes natural killer cell activation and tumor rejection. Science. 2015;**348**:136-139

[66] Guillerey C, Huntington ND, MJ1 S. Targeting natural killer cells in cancer immunotherapy. Nature Immunology. 2016;**17**(9):1025-1036

[67] Tanaka T, Hirata T, Parrott G, Higashiarakawa M, Kinjo T, Kinjo T, Hokama A, Fujita J. Relationship among *Strongyloides stercoralis* infection, human T-cell lymphotropic virus type 1 infection, and cancer: A 24-year cohort inpatient study in Okinawa, Japan. The American Journal of Tropical Medicine and Hygiene. 2016;**94**(2):365-370

[68] Tomaino C, Catalano C, Tiba M, Aron J, Su. A first case report of colorectal cancer associated with chronic *Strongyloides stercoralis* colitis and the complex management decisions that follow. Gastroenterology. 2015;**148**(4):Suppl.1):S575

[69] Satoh M, Toma H, Sugahara K, Etoh K, Shiroma Y, Kiyuna S, Takara M, Matsuoka M, Yamaguchi K, Nakada K, Fujita K, Kojima S, Hori E, Tanaka Y, Kamihira S, Sato Y, Watanabe T. Involvement of IL-2/IL-2R system activation by parasite antigen in polyclonal expansion of CD4(+)25(+) HTLV-1-infected T-cells in human carriers of both HTLV-1 and *S. stercoralis*. Oncogene. 2002;**21**(16):2466-2475

[70] Myers B, Speight EL, Huissoon AP, Davies JM. Natural killer-cell lymphocytosis and strongyloides infection. Clinical and Laboratory Haematology. 2000;**22**(4):237-238

[71] Cheng M, Chen Y, Xiao W, Sun R, Tian Z. NK cell-based immunotherapy for malignant diseases. Cellular & Molecular Immunology. 2013;**10**:230-252

[72] Becker PS et al. Selection and expansion of natural killer cells for NK cell-based immunotherapy. Cancer Immunology, Immunotherapy. 2016;**65**:477-484

[73] Hermanson DL, Kaufman DS. Utilizing chimeric antigen receptors to direct natural killer cell activity. Frontiers in Immunology. 2015;**6**:195

[74] Romanski A, Uherek C, Bug G, Seifried E, Klingemann H, Wels WS, Ottmann OGT. CD19-CAR engineered NK-92 cells are sufficient to overcome NK cell resistance in B-cell malignancies. Journal of Cellular and Molecular Medicine. 2016;**20**(7):1287-1294

[75] Boissel L, Betancu M, Wels WS, Tuncer H, Klingemann H. Transfection with mRNA for CD19 specific chimeric antigen receptor restores NK cell mediated killing of CLL cells. Leukemia Research. 2009;**33**:1255-1259

[76] Müller T et al. Expression of a CD20-specific chimeric antigen receptor enhances cytotoxic activity of NK cells and overcomes NK-resistance of lymphoma and leukemia cells. Cancer Immunology, Immunotherapy. 2007;**57**:411-423

[77] Ahmed M, Hu J, Cheung NK. Structure based refinement of a humanized monoclonal antibody that targets tumor antigen disialoganglioside GD2. Frontiers in Immunology. 2014;**5**:372

[78] Han J et al. CAR-engineered NK cells targeting wild-type EGFR and EGFRvIII enhance killing of glioblastoma and patient-derived glioblastoma stem cells. Scientific Reports. 2015;**5**:11483

[79] Jiang H et al. Transfection of chimeric anti-CD138 gene enhances natural killer cell activation and killing of multiple myeloma cells. Molecular Oncology. 2014;**8**:297-310

[80] Müller N, Michen S, Tietze S, Töpfer K, Schulte A, Lamszus K, Schmitz M, Schackert G, Pastan I, Temme A. Engineering NK cells modified with an EGFRvIII-specific chimeric antigen receptor to overexpress CXCR4 improves immunotherapy of CXCL12/SDF-1$\alpha$-secreting Glioblastoma. Journal of Immunotherapy. 2015;**38**(5):197-210

[81] Becknell B, Caligiuri MA. Interleukin-2, interleukin-15, and their roles in human natural killer cells. Advances in Immunology. 2005;**86**:209-239

[82] Robinson BW, Morstyn G. Natural killer (NK)-resistant human lung cancer cells are lysed by recombinant interleukin-2-activated NK cells. Cellular Immunology. 1987;**106**:215-222

[83] Hellstrand K, Mellqvist UH, Wallhult E, Carneskog J, Kimby E, Celsing F, Brune M. Histamine and interleukin-2 in acute myelogenous leukemia. Leukemia & Lymphoma. 1997;**27**:429-438

[84] Bachanova V, Cooley S, Defor TE, Verneris MR, Zhang B, McKenna DH, Curtsinger J, Panoskaltsis-Mortari A, Lewis D, Hippen K, McGlave P, Weisdorf DJ, Blazar BR, Miller JS. Clearance of acute myeloid leukemia by haploidentical natural killer cells is improved using IL-2 diphtheria toxin fusion protein. Blood. 2014;**123**:3855-3863

[85] Clarke MF. Oncogenes, self-renewal and cancer. Pathologie Biologie (Paris). 2006;**54**(2): 109-111

[86] Visvader JE, Lindeman GJ. Cancer stem cells: Current status and evolving complexities. Cell Stem Cell. 2012;**10**:717-728

[87] Tallerico R, Todaro M, Di Franco S, et al. Human NK cells selective targeting of colon cancer-initiating cells: A role for natural cytotoxicity receptors and MHC class I molecules. Journal of Immunology. 2013;**190**(5):2381-2390

[88] Castriconi R, Daga A, Dondero A, et al. NK cells recognize and kill human glioblastoma cells with stem cell-like properties. Journal of Immunology. 2009;**182**(6):3530-3519

[89] Yin T, Wang G, He S, Liu Q, Sun J, Wang Y. Human cancer cells with stem cell-like phenotype exhibit enhanced sensitivity to the cytotoxicity of IL-2 and IL-15 activated natural killer cells. Cellular Immunology. 2016;**300**:41-45

[90] Pietra G, Manzini C, Vitale M, Balsamo M, Ognio E, Boitano M, Queirolo P, Moretta L, Mingari MC. Natural killer cells kill human melanoma cells with characteristics of cancer stem cells. International Immunology. 2009;**21**(7):793-801

[91] Ames E, Canter RJ, Grossenbacher SK, Mac S, Chen M, Smith RC, Hagino T, Perez-Cunningham J, Sckisel GD, Urayama S, Monjazeb AM, Fragoso RC, Sayers TJ, Murphy WJ. NK cells preferentially target tumor cells with a cancer stem cell phenotype. Journal of Immunology. 2015;**195**(8):4010-4019

Chapter 5

# The Role of Activating and Inhibitory NK Cell Receptors in Antitumor Immune Response

Gordana Konjević, Ana Vuletić,
Katarina Mirjačić Martinović and Radan Džodić

Additional information is available at the end of the chapter

http://dx.doi.org/10.5772/intechopen.69729

**Abstract**

Natural killer (NK) cells express many newly identified activating and inhibitory receptors that upon engagement by cognate ligands on target tumor cells regulate NK cell antitumor activity. Recently, several paired NK cell receptor families that include receptors with similar binding specificities but opposite function have been defined. The expression of most important activating receptors, natural killer group 2D (NKG2D), natural cytotoxic receptors (NCR), DNAX accessory molecule-1 (DNAM1) and activating killer cell immunoglobulin-like receptors (KAR) is often decreased, while the expression of most prominent inhibitory NK cell receptors, killer cell inhibitory immunoglobulin-like receptors (KIR) and CD94/NKG2A, may occasionally be increased in malignancies. These data indicate that impaired NK cell antitumor response results from NK cell receptor alterations induced by suppressive factors in the tumor microenvironment, including cytokines, growth factors, enzymes and metabolites, as well as by chronic NK cell receptor engagement by the tumor. The established alterations in NK cell receptor expression in cancer patients represent potential disease biomarkers and may aid in choosing therapies that upregulate activating or block inhibitory receptor function. Accumulating knowledge of NK cell biology has been helpful in creating novel therapeutic approaches that by release from tumor-influenced immunosuppression potentiate NK cell activity in cancer patients.

**Keywords:** NK cells, inhibitory and activating receptors, immunosuppression, cancer, immunotherapy

## 1. Introduction

Natural killer (NK) cells are equipped with multiple activating and inhibitory cell surface receptors and play a key role in controlling tumor growth and metastasis. NK cells have originally been described to belong to the innate arm of the immune system and are able to discriminate between normal and transformed cells on the basis of major histocompatibility complex (MHC) class I molecule expression in the organism. As normal cells express major histocompatibility complex (MHC) class I molecules that engage NK cell inhibitory receptors, they are protected from NK cell-mediated lysis. Therefore, according to the "missing-self" hypothesis, activation of NK cells occurs in contact with malignantly transformed cells that have lost MHC class I molecules and that have additionally acquired stress-induced ligands for activating NK cell receptors. Maintenance of NK cell antitumor function relies on the balance between these activating and inhibitory signals mediated by NK cell receptors [1].

Considering that NK cells are defined as $CD3^{-}CD56^{+}CD16^{+/-}$ cells according to the density of expression of these receptors, these cells are divided into two subsets. The larger cytotoxic subset with high density of CD16, low density of CD56 ($CD56^{dim}CD16^{bright}$), and abundant perforin and granzyme granules, and the other, smaller regulatory subset with low density or absence of CD16, high density of CD56 ($CD56^{bright}CD16^{dim/-}$) and the ability to produce abundant cytokines including interferon-gamma (IFN-γ), tumor necrosis factor (TNF), interleukin (IL)-10, IL-13, and granulocyte-macrophage colony-stimulating factor (GM-CSF) [2]. $CD56^{bright}CD16^{dim}$subset has a greater migratory potential and is recruited into tumor tissue, although $CD56^{dim}CD16^{bright}$NK cells have also been detected in certain tumors [3]. Recent data have shown in mucosa-associated lymph tissue (MALT), the presence of a novel family of tissue-resident innate lymphoid cells (ILC), with NK-like characteristics. This novel family is classified into three groups (ILC1, ILC2, and ILC3) and contrary to classical cytotoxic NK cells, considered to belong to ILC1 group, the involvement of other ILC subsets in cancer progression or resistance is still controversial [4].

Several new families of receptors have been recently identified on NK cells and growing knowledge indicates that some families are composed of paired receptors that inspite of binding similar ligands have opposite, activating, or inhibitory function [5]. The most important activating NK cell receptors are NKp46, NKp30, and NKp44 that belong to natural cytotoxic receptors (NCR) family, natural killer group 2D (NKG2D) that belongs to NKG2 calcium-dependent lectin-like (NKG2 C-lectin) family, DNAX accessory molecule 1 (DNAM1) that belongs to the family of nectin-binding adhesion molecules and activating killer cell immunoglobulin-like receptors (KAR). On the contrary, the most important family of inhibitory NK cell receptors belongs to killer cell immunoglobulin-like (KIR) receptor family, while NKG2 C-lectin family also includes inhibitory CD94/NKG2A NK cell receptors (**Table 1**). Upon binding ligands, these activating and inhibitory NK cell receptors cooperate and determine NK cell cytotoxicity against transformed cells [6]. However, tumor-derived immunosuppressive factors play a major role in evading NK cell responses to tumors by interfering with NK cell activation pathways or the complex receptor array that regulate NK cell activation and antitumor activity [3, 7].

The objective of this chapter is to present current data based on the knowledge of many newly identified activating and inhibitory NK cell receptors whose balance regulates NK cell antitumor activity. Numerous alterations in NK cell receptor expression and signaling pathways induced by tumor-derived immunosuppressive factors that are responsible for poor

http://dx.doi.org/10.5772/intechopen.69729

| Receptor familes | | | Ligands | Signaling molecules |
|---|---|---|---|---|
| **NCR** | **Activating** | NKp46 | HSPG, heparin, vimentin | FcRγ and CD3ζ, ZAP70/Syk |
| | | NKp44 | NKp44L | DAP12, ZAP70/Syk |
| | | NKp30a, b | B7-H6, BAG-6 | CD3ζ, ZAP70/Syk |
| | **Inhibitory** | NKp44 | PCNA | ITIM, SHP1, 2 |
| | | NKp30c | ? | ? |
| **Paired receptors** | | | | |
| **NKG2** | **Activating** | NKG2D | MICA/B, ULBP1-6 | DAP10, Grb2, Vav, SOS |
| | | CD94/NKG2C | HLA-E | DAP12, ZAP70/Syk |
| | **Inhibitory** | CD94/NKG2A | | |
| | | CD94/NKG2E | HLA-E | ITIM, SHP1, 2 |
| | | CD94/NKG2F | | |
| **KIR** | **Inhibitory** | 2DL1/L2/L3 | HLA-C | ITIM, SHP1, 2 |
| | | 3DL1/L2/L3 | HLA- A, -B | |
| | **Activating** | 2DS1/S2/S4 | HLA-C/? | DAP12, ZAP70/Syk |
| | | 3DS1 | ? | |
| **Adhesion molecules** | **Activating** | DNAM-1 | PVR, nectin-2 | ITSM, Vav, PLCγ |
| | **Inhibitory** | TIGIT | PVR, nectin-2 | ITIM, SHP1, 2 |
| | | TACTILE | | |
| **FcγRIII** | **Activating** | CD16 | Fc IgG | FcRγ and CD3ζ, ZAP70/Syk |
| **NKPR1** | **Activating** | CD161 | ? | ? |
| | **Inhibitory** | | LLT1 | ITIM, SHP1, 2 |

**Table 1.** NK cell activating and inhibitory receptors.

NK cell cytotoxic function in cancer patients will be defined. Understanding of the alterations in NK cell receptors and function can contribute in the assessment of biomarkers of the state of malignant disease and may aid in the selection of immunotherapy that supports an effective NK cell antitumor response.

## 2. NK cell receptors

### 2.1. Natural cytotoxic receptors

The NCR represent a group of human NK cell activating receptors that belong to the immunoglobulin superfamily and include NKp46, NKp30, and NKp44. NKp46 and NKp30 are constitutively expressed on all activated and resting NK cells, whereas NKp44 expression on NK cells requires activation by IL-2. This makes NKp46 and NKp30 the only NK-specific markers known today, although recent evidence suggests that a very small subset of T cells expresses NKp46 [8].

Tumor-associated ligands for most NCR have only been recently described. B7-H6 was the first identified cellular ligand for an NCR expressed on the surface of cancer cells that binds to the activating receptors NKp30 [9]. Recently, a novel isoform of the mixed lineage leukemia-5 (MLL5) nuclear protein was proposed as a cancer cell-expressed ligand for NKp44 [10]. Ligands for NKp46 have been described to have viral structural motives that belong to hemagglutinin-like molecules or to be heparan sulfate proteoglycans (HSPG) [11]. The cytoplasmatic domains of NCR do not possess any signaling motives except for NKp44 that contains an immunoreceptor tyrosine-based inhibition motif (ITIM) that has been reported functional only upon binding to certain ligands. Therefore, NCR associate with CD3 ζ-chain, FcεRIγ and DAP12 adaptor proteins that undergo phosphorylation of their immunoreceptor tyrosine-based activation motives (ITAM), recruit sarcoma homology 2 (SH2) domains of spleen tyrosine kinase (Syc)/zeta-chain-associated protein kinase 70 (ZAP70) and ultimately lead to extracellular signal-regulated kinase (ERK) activation and cytotoxic granule mobilization [8].

Conversely, it has recently been shown that the constitutively inactive cytoplasmatic ITIM domain of NKp44 receptor becomes functionally active only upon binding proliferating cell nuclear antigen (PCNA) leading to the inhibition of NK cell function [12] that might be involved in tumor immune evasion. Similarly, as NKp30 is comprised of three different isoforms, NKp30a, b, and c it has been shown that binding of NKp30c induces an immunosuppressive signal by producing IL-10 that is associated with reduced NK cell effector functions. Therefore, the final outcome of NKp44 and NKp30 activation depends on the presence of ligands on target cells, as well as receptor isoforms expressed on the surface of NK cells, respectively [13].

NCR, aside from direct antitumor cytotoxicity can also mediate the production of proinflammatory cytokines by NK cells that have an immunoregulatory role and engage in orchestrating antitumor immune response. In this sense, it has been shown that cross-linking of NKp46 and NKp44 resulted in NK cell production of IFNγ and TNF that are responsible for dendritic cell (DC) maturation and regulation of adaptive response to tumors. However, binding of inhibitory NKp30c induces production of IL-10 that reduces NK cell function [14].

Downregulation of NCR expression can be induced by soluble factors such as transforming growth factor beta (TGF-β), IL-10, L-kynurenine, a product of tryptophan degradation by tumor-derived indolamin-2,3-dioxygenase (IDO). Decreased expression of some NCR has been reported in several malignancies, namely low NKp46 in melanoma, pancreatic, gastric, cervical cancer, and acute myeloid leukemia (AML) [15–17], NKp44 in numerous solid and hematological malignancies, and NKp30 in breast, hepatocellular cancer (HCC), chronic lymphocytic leukemia (CLL), and AML [15, 16, 18–20]. Moreover, ILC3 cells expressing NKp44 activating receptor in human nonsmall-cell lung cancer (NSCLC) tissue were shown to have tumor protective role [4]. However, overexpression of PCNA in certain tumors results in NKp44 receptor-mediated inhibition of NK cell activity [8].

## 2.2. Families of paired receptors in NK cells

### *2.2.1. NK group 2 calcium-dependent lectin-like receptor family*

This family of calcium-dependent lectin-like receptors includes CD94-NKG2-A/C/E/F/H heterodimer and NKG2D homodimer receptors present on NK cells. This family is composed of paired NK cells receptors with similar binding specificities to nonclassical MHC class I molecules on the surface of potential target cells but either activating or inhibitory functions [21].

#### *2.2.1.1. Natural killer group 2D*

It is an activating receptor expressed on virtually all NK cells. NKG2D recognizes a number of MHC-class-I-related molecules, major histocompatibility complex class I chain-related molecule (MIC) A/B and UL16-binding protein (ULBP) expressed on cells in stressful conditions, such as transformation [22]. Owing to their ability to trigger activation of the immune system, it has now been shown that their expression is very tightly controlled at transcriptional level [23]. NKG2D is a pivotal activating receptor that upon binding stress-induced ligands and phosphorylation of intracellular adaptor protein DNAX-activation protein 10 (DAP10) recruits various signaling pathways and induces tumor cytotoxicity [24].

Decreased expression of NKG2D in cancer patients is mediated by TGFβ and IL-10 produced by tumor cells and immunosuppressive immune cells, tumor-associated macrophages (TAM), myeloid-derived suppressor cells (MDSC), regulatory T cells (Treg) in the tumor microenvironment [25]. Also, persistent stimulation of NKG2D receptor by its tumor cell-associated ligands, as well as, soluble ligands induced by matrix metalloproteinases (MMP) proteolytic cleavage from tumor cells may lead to functional exhaustion of NK cells [26].

Downregulation of NKG2D expression together with degradation of its intracellular signal transducing adapter, DAP10 [27], by its ligand has also been shown in experimental settings of conjugate formation between NK cells, not only of healthy individuals but also of metastatic melanoma patients, with K562, an erythromyeloid cell line, or FemX, a melanoma-derived tumor cell line [28–30]. This effect is more pronounced for K562 tumor cells as they highly express MICA/B ligands specific for NKG2D receptors [31], while for FemX tumor cell line so far no data exist regarding the expression of MICA/B ligands, although it can be assumed that, as most tumor cells, this cell line expresses some level of these stress-induced ligands. The importance of NKG2D receptor in NK cell cytotoxic function underlies a significant positive correlation of its expression with NK cytotoxicity in healthy individuals, as well as in melanoma patients, in spite of different levels of expression [32–34].

These data indicate that activating NKG2D receptor has a role in NK cell tumor immunosurveillance and in immune-mediated rejection of tumor cells and that NKG2D downregulation as a consequence of tumor immunoediting favors tumor progression [13].

#### *2.2.1.2. Heterodimeric NK group 2 calcium-dependent lectin-like A/B/C/E/H receptors*

These heterodimer receptors consist of CD94 subunit that is associated with the member of the NKG2 family (A/B/C/E/H). Prototypic member of this family CD94-NKG2A has an ITIM that consequently leads to the inhibition of NK cell activity by inducing dephosphorylation of surrounding tyrosine kinases and adaptor proteins. By contrast, receptors CD94-NKG2-C, CD94-NKG2-E, and CD94-NKG2-H, associate with DAP12 and function as activating receptors that participate in NK cell antitumor response. These receptors bind to nonclassical MHC class I, human leukocyte antigen (HLA)-E molecules on the surface of malignantly transformed target cells [21].

Interestingly, the ligand for this receptor family, HLA-E molecule assembles at the endoplasmic reticulum with peptides derived from the leader peptides of HLA-A, B, C, and G molecules and as in malignant transformation, the expression of classical MHC class I molecules is downregulated, the expression of HLA-E is consequently upregulated [35]. The importance of the inhibitory activity of NKG2A receptor expression is demonstrated in breast cancer and colorectal cancer (CRC) as its increased expression is associated with poor disease prognosis [18, 36]. Conversely, decreased expression of NKG2C activating receptor resulting in NK cell dysfunction has so far been reported for AML [37].

### 2.2.2. *Killer cell immunoglobulin-like receptor family*

This is a well-known paired NK cell receptor family with either inhibitory or activating functions that interact specifically with MHC class I molecules and their tissue protective role is based on the higher binding affinity and signal transduction by inhibitory KIR receptors, compared to activating KAR receptors, for MHC class I ligands. According to KIR expression on NK cells, they are divided into KIR haplotype A and B, with A being more frequent and including inhibitory receptors compared to B that includes both types of receptors with predominance of activating receptors [38].

The most prominent inhibitory killer cell immunoglobulin-like receptors (KIR) are KIR2DL1 (CD158a), KIR2DL2/3 (CD158b), and KIR3DL1-2 and inhibit NK cell activity through an ITIM by recruiting SH2 domain protein tyrosine phosphatases (SHP)-1 and -2 and adaptor proteins, including DAP-10. Moreover, blocking actin cytoskeleton-dependent raft recruitment of different receptors may be a general mechanism by which inhibitory receptors control NK cell activation [39]. Thus, activating KAR, such as KIR2DS1, KIR2DS4,and KIR2DL4, associate with DAP12 adaptor protein that deliver activation signals through an ITAM that after phosphorylation by sarcoma (Src) family kinases recruit Syk/ZAP-70 tyrosine kinases to mediate downstream activation signaling [40]. Clinical studies have correlated KIR gene content with cancer [41]. It has recently been reported that higher expression of inhibitory CD158a and CD158b receptors, especially in patients that express their specific HLA-C ligands, is associated not only with susceptibility to tumors but also with disease progression, shown by increase in NK cells with these receptors in advanced stages of melanoma [42, 43].

Inhibitory KIR receptor upregulation on NK cells in malignant tumors has been reported to be associated with immunosuppressive, as well as immunostimulatory cytokines [44–48]. Higher expression of certain inhibitory KIR receptors has been shown in pancreatic, gastric, and CRC without association with disease progression [15]. Other studies in patients with metastatic melanoma, as well as in NSCLC and breast cancer, show an increase in the expression of CD158a and CD158b inhibitory KIR receptors on NK cells [33, 49–51] that in melanoma negatively correlates with NK cell cytotoxicity [33]. In this sense, as inhibitory KIR play prominent roles in regulating NK cell activation therapeutic strategies designed to diminish KIR function that may be able to potentiate NK cell activity in treating patients with malignancies.

#### 2.2.3. *Family of nectin-binding adhesion molecules*

It is an important family of adhesion molecules that includes CD226 (DNAM1), CD96 (T cell-activated increased late expression (TACTILE)), and T-cell immunoglobulin and ITIM domain (TIGIT). These receptors bind nectin proteins, CD112 (nectin-2), and CD155 (poliovirus receptor (PVR)) and have been recently identified as crucial regulators of NK cell function. This is another family of paired NK cell receptors with similar binding specificities on the surface of target cells but with either activating (CD226) or inhibitory (CD96 and TIGIT) functions [5].

##### 2.2.3.1. *Stimulatory nectin-binding adhesion molecule*

Costimulatory adhesion receptor DNAM1, a member of immunoglobulin-superfamily has recently been shown to have a role in the recognition of tumor cells and NK cell-mediated responses to tumors. It binds to PVR and nectin-2, and recruits the tyrosine kinase fibroblast endothelial kinase (Fyn) and serine threonine protein kinase C (PKC). Moreover, interaction of DNAM1 with target cell ligands induces actin polymerization and activation of other surface receptors, which permit stable interaction of NK cells and target cells. Furthermore, the involvement of this receptor in the NK cell-mediated responses to tumors is beginning to be elucidated and results to date suggest that DNAM1 has a role in the recognition of tumor cells, as well as migration of NK cells [35, 52].

The importance of DNAM1 has been reported in breast cancer, CRC, AML, and melanoma [17, 18, 37, 53] and in melanoma, it has been shown that tumor-associated fibroblasts (TAF) by modulating the surface expression of DNAM-1 based on cell-to-cell interactions could inhibit NK cell function [54]. Also, DNAM1 ligand CD155 upregulation on multiple myeloma (MM) cells has been reported and resulted in increased sensitivity to NK cell-mediated lysis [55].

##### 2.2.3.2. *Inhibitory nectin-binding adhesion molecules*

TIGIT and TACTILE (CD96) receptors that unlike activating DNAM1 receptor contain an ITIM motive subsequently inhibit NK cell antitumor activity and counteract DNAM-mediated activation. These receptors are important in settings in which the tumor is mainly non-immunogenic, as it does not express stress ligands or costimulatory molecules, which is a common situation for many epithelial cell malignancies. For this reason, these inhibitory molecules may be promising therapeutic targets for the treatment of malignancies [5].

### 2.3. CD16 (Fc $\gamma$ receptor IIIA)

This is one of the most important NK cell cytotoxic receptors that contains two extracellular Ig-like domains and is involved in both direct [56] and, as an Fc gamma receptor type IIIA, is involved in antibody-dependent cell-mediated cytotoxicity (ADCC) [57], as well as cytokine production, proliferation, and postactivational NK cell apoptotic death [56].

CD16, as well as NKp46, associates with two cytoplasmatic domains composed of FcεRIγ or T-cell receptor (TCR) ζ chains that comprise ITAM, which upon ligand-binding become phosphorylated and induce signal transduction by activation of nonreceptor tyrosine kinases Syk and ZAP-70 [57].

The expression CD16 as a prominent NK cell cytotoxic receptor has been found to be decreased on NK cells in breast cancer and MM patients [18, 58] not only due to postactivational receptor internalization but also following target cell induced activation of MMP, namely ADAM 17, as shown during *in vitro* NK cell cultivation with tumor cells [59, 60]. Moreover, as CD16 defines the two functionally different NK cell subsets, its decreased expression influences the ratio of these subsets, leading to the loss $CD16^{bright}$ cytotoxic subset, a finding that has been detected in numerous malignancies such as breast cancer, MM, and melanoma [6, 33].

### 2.4. Natural killer cell surface protein P1A

This is a member of the C-type lectin family that is primarily designated as an activating receptor that plays a role in NK cell-mediated cytotoxicity and it has been previously shown that natural killer cell surface protein P1A (NKR-P1A)/CD161 participates in triggering NK cell cytotoxicity against numerous human tumor cell lines [61], while more recently, it has been suggested that its activating mechanism may require interaction with costimulatory receptors [62]. On identification of its lectin-like transcript 1 (LLT1) ligand, its inhibitory potential has recently been described, but its function still remains controversial. In support of the inhibitory function of NKR-P1A, it has been shown that its cytoplasmic tail contains tyrosine residue in an atypical motive (AxYxxL) that may function as a weak ITIM [63, 64]. There are some reports of decreased expression and cytokine-mediated upregulation of NKR-P1A/CD161 in metastatic melanoma and MM [29, 33, 58].

## 3. Tumor-induced immunosuppression

It has now been well documented that tumor-induced immunosuppression affects NK cell receptor repertoire and leads to progressive local and systemic inhibition of NK cell function. In tumors, a complex composition of immunosuppressive molecules TGF-β, IL-10, IDO, prostaglandin E2 (PGE2), vascular endothelial growth factor (VEGF), nitric oxide synthase (NOS), and reactive oxygen species (ROS) are produced by regulatory immune cells such as Treg, MDSC, TAM, and by tumor cells themselves (**Figure. 1**). These factors generate a chronic inflammatory immunosuppressive milieu that leads to the suppression of the antitumor effector NK cell function that supports tumor progression [3, 7, 13, 65]. In this sense, considering that the expression of activating NK cell receptors is decreased in most malignancies, and as some studies report that the expression of inhibitory KIR and CD94/NKG2A receptors on NK cells in different tumors remains unchanged, this suggests that activating receptors are main targets of tumor-mediated suppression [13].

http://dx.doi.org/10.5772/intechopen.69729

Furthermore, NK cell dysfunction due to decreased activating NK cell receptor expression may be mediated by chronic tumor cell ligand-NK cell receptor engagement that leads to an exhausted NK cell phenotype characterized by upregulated programmed death 1 (PD-1) checkpoint immunoreceptor expression [66]. Conversely, the appearance of soluble NK cell ligands due to proteolytic cleavage from tumor cells also leads to NK cell dysfunction due to chronic NK cell receptor stimulation in the absence of target tumor cells [26].

In this sense, it has now been established that during the development of solid tumors, NK cells are frequently rendered functionally impaired as a consequence of cancer immunoediting that induces immune tolerance to tumors owing to impairment of NK cell receptor repertoire and signaling, as well as immunoselection of nonimmunogenic tumor cells.

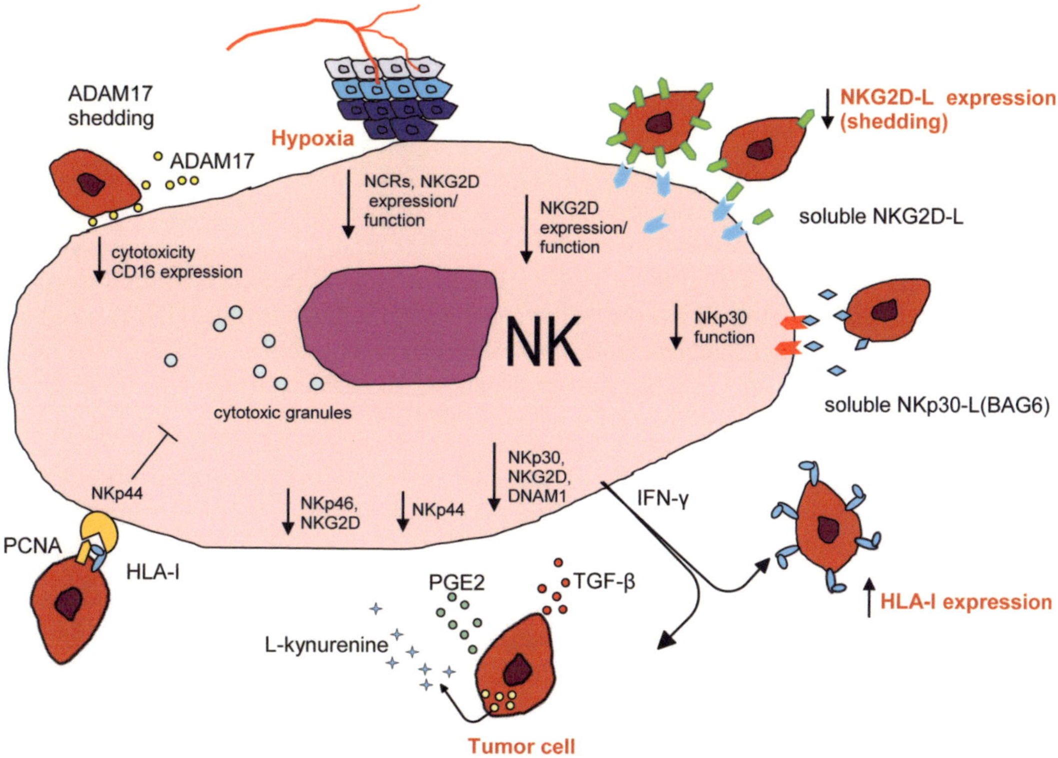


**Figure 1.** Mechanisms of NK cell receptor dysregulation in tumors. The tumor induces alterations in NK cell activating receptors by producing suppressive tumor-derived mediators including immunosuppressive cytokines (transforming growth factor beta - TGF-β), enzymes (indolamin-2,3-dioxygenase - IDO), factors (L-kynurenine, prostaglandin E2 - PGE2) that together with the presence of hypoxia can suppress NK cell antitumor activity. Chronic engagement of NK cell activating receptors with either tumor cell surface-expressed or shed NK cell ligands (NKG2D ligand - NKG2D-L) leads to progressive inhibition of NK cell antitumor response. Also, tumor-expressed proliferating cell nuclear antigen (PCNA) associated with HLA-I molecule by binding NKp44 activating receptor induces unconventional inhibitory signals in NK cells. Moreover, interferon gamma (IFN-γ) released by NK cells induces increased expression of HLA-I molecules on tumor cells, as well as tumor-produced IDO, that lead to inhibition of NK cell function.

## 4. NK cell receptors as therapeutic targets in cancer immunotherapy

As NK cell antitumor activity is regulated by numerous activating and inhibitory NK cell receptors, alterations in NK cell receptor expression and signaling underlie diminished cytotoxic NK cell function. Based on this and on predictive *in vitro* findings [6, 46–48, 67–70], cytokines, including IFNα, IL-2, IL-12, IL-15, and IL-18 have been used systemically or for *ex vivo*–activation and expansion of NK cells and have led to improved NK cells antitumor activity by increasing the expression of NK cell activating receptors and by inducing cytotoxic effector molecules [71–75]. Moreover, this cytokine-based therapy enhances NK cell proliferation and regulatory function, and it has been shown that it induces NK cells exhibiting cytokine induced memory-like properties [76] that represent a newly-defined NK cell subset with improved NK cell activity and longevity.

Considering the effect of tumor-derived immunosuppressive molecules on the decrease in the expression of activating NK cell receptors, early stage clinical trials have been introduced that use monoclonal antibodies, alone or in combination, to neutralize TGF-β, IDO, or PD-1 checkpoint inhibitor in different malignancies that led to improved antitumor NK cell function [77].

Since inhibitory KIR play prominent roles in regulating NK cell activation, therapeutic strategies in cancer to diminish KIR function have been developed. In autologous settings, anti-inhibitory KIR monoclonal antibody therapy has been introduced to support autologous NK cell administration by rendering them with higher antitumor activity, as reported in AML and MM. On the other hand, allogeneic hematopoietic stem cell transplants (HSCT) based on partially KIR/HLA mismatched alloreactive NK cell transfer that relieve donor NK cells from inhibition by recipient's MHC class I molecules, show beneficial graft-versus-tumor (GvT) effect in both pediatric and adult high-risk leukemia [78].

Moreover, it has been recognized that classical and novel pharmacological agents, such as proteasome inhibitors or histonedeacetylase inhibitors and certain chemotherapeutics [72, 74, 75], upregulate cognate ligands for activating receptors on tumor cells and provide better NK cell antitumor response.

Also, a new effective approach, in clinical trials, designed to enhance NK cell—tumor cell interaction includes genetically modified NK cells expressing cytokine transgenes, chimeric antigen receptors (CARs), or overexpressing activating receptors that recognize NK cell ligands on tumor cells are showing promising results.

As it has been shown that therapeutic antibodies that are already in use for cancer treatment also trigger NK cell-mediated ADCC activity [79, 80] have been modified to increase binding of their Fc fragment to CD16 on NK cells. These therapeutic antibodies by binding CD16 receptor induce a potent activating signal, which overcomes inhibitory signals and results in both cytotoxicity and cytokine responses [81] that enhance NK cell activation against tumor cells.

## 5. Conclusion

The knowledge of NK cells has grown to include many newly identified activating and inhibitory NK cell receptors and defined alterations in receptor expression and signaling pathways that are responsible for poor NK cell cytotoxic function in cancer patients, may be considered as biomarkers of the state of disease. These findings regarding NK cell receptors may aid in the selection of classical and newly developed therapies that favorably modulate NK cell receptor expression and function, and release them from tumor-derived immunosuppression in order to achieve an effective NK cell antitumor response.

## Acknowledgements

This work was supported by the grants of the Ministry of Education, Science and Technological Development of the Republic of Serbia, numbers III41031 and 175056.

## Author details

Gordana Konjević[1,2]*, Ana Vuletić[1], Katarina Mirjačić Martinović[1] and Radan Džodić[1,2]

*Address all correspondence to: konjevicg@ncrc.ac.rs

1 Institute of Oncology and Radiology of Serbia, Belgrade, Serbia

2 Faculty of Medicine, University of Belgrade, Belgrade, Serbia

## References

[1] Caligiuri MA. Human natural killer cells. Blood. 2008;**112**:461-469

[2] Cooper MA, Fehniger TA, Caligiuri MA. The biology of human natural killer-cell subsets. Trends in Immunology. 2001;**22**:633-640

[3] Vitalle M, Cantoni C, Pietra G, Mingari MC, Moretta L. Effect of tumor cells and tumor microenvironment on NK-cell functionEuropean Journal of Immunology. 2014;**44**: 1582-92

[4] Montaldo E, Vacca P, Vitale C, Moretta F, Locatelli F, Mingari MC, Moretta L. Human innate lymphoid cells. Immunology Letters. 2016;**179**:2-8

[5] Martinet L, Smyth MJ. Balancing natural killer cell activation through paired receptors. Nature Reviews Immunology. 2015;**15**:243-54

[6] Konjević G, Vuletić A, Mirjačić Martinović K. Natural killer cell receptors: Alterations and therapeutic targeting in malignancies. Journal of Immunology Research. 2016;**64**:25-35

[7] Pahl J, Cerwenka A. Tricking the balance: NK cells in anti-cancer immunity. Immunobiology. 2017;**222**:11-20

[8] Kruse PH, Matta J, Ugolini S, Vivier E. Natural cytotoxicity receptors and their ligands. Immunology and Cell Biology. 2014;**92**:221-229

[9] Brandt CS, Baratin M, Yi EC, Kennedy J, Gao Z, Fox B et al. The B7 family member B7-H6 is a tumor cell ligand for the activating natural killer cell receptor NKp30 in humans. Journal of Experimental Medicine. 2009;**206**:1495-1503

[10] Baychelier F, Sennepin A, Ermonval M, Dorgham K, Debré P, Vieillard V. Identification of a cellular ligand for the natural cytotoxicity receptor NKp44. Blood. 2013;**122:**2935-2942

[11] Arnon TI, Achdout H, Lieberman N, Gazit R, Gonen-Gross T, Katz G, et al. The mechanisms controlling the recognition of tumor- and virus-infected cells by NKp46. Blood. 2004;**103**:664-672

[12] Rosental B, Brusilovsky M, Hadad U, Oz D, Appel MY, Afergan F, et al. Proliferating cell nuclear antigen is a novel inhibitory ligand for the natural cytotoxicity receptor NKp44. The Journal of Immunology. 2011;**187**:5693-5702

[13] Stojanovic A, Correia MP, Cerwenka A. Shaping of NK cell responses by the tumor microenvironment. Cancer Microenvironment. 2013;**6**:135-46

[14] Hudspeth K, Silva-Santos B, Mavilio D. Natural cytotoxicity receptors: Broader expression patterns and functions in innate and adaptive immune cells. Frontiers in Immunology. 2013;**4**:69

[15] Peng YP, Zhu Y, Zhang JJ, Xu ZK, Qian ZY, Dai CC, et al. Comprehensive analysis of the percentage of surface receptors and cytotoxic granules positive natural killer cells in patients with pancreatic cancer, gastric cancer, and colorectal cancer. Journal of Translational Medicine. 2013;**11**:262.

[16] Garcia-Iglesias T, Del Toro-Arreola A, Albarran-Somoza B, Del Toro-Arreola S, Sanchez-Hernandez PE, Ramirez-Duenas MG, et al. Low NKp30, NKp46 and NKG2D expression and reduced cytotoxic activity on NK cells in cervical cancer and precursor lesions. BMC Cancer. 2009;**9**:186

[17] Mirjačić Martinović KM, Babović NLJ, Džodić RR, Jurišić VB, Tanić NT, Konjević GM. Decreased expression of NKG2D, NKp46, DNAM-1 receptors, and intracellular perforin and STAT-1 effector molecules in NK cells and their dim and bright subsets in metastatic melanoma patients. Melanoma Research. 2014;**24**:295-304

[18] Mamessier E, Sylvain A, Bertucci F, Castellano R, Finetti P, Houvenaeghel G, et al. Human breast tumor cells induce self-tolerance mechanisms to avoid NKG2D-mediated and DNAM-mediated NK cell recognition. Cancer Research. 2011;**71**:6621-6632

[19] Fiegler N, Textor S, Arnold A, Rolle A, Oehme I, Breuhahn K, et al. Downregulation of the activating NKp30 ligand B7–H6 by HDAC inhibitors impairs tumor cell recognition by NK cells. Blood. 2013;**122**:684-93

[20] Reiners KS, Topolar D, Henke A, Simhadri VR, Kessler J, Sauer M, et al. Soluble ligands for NK cell receptors promote evasion of chronic lymphocytic leukemia cells from NK cell anti-tumor activity. Blood. 2013;**121**:3658-65

[21] Braud VM, Allan DS, O'Callaghan CA, Söderström K, D'Andrea A, Ogg GS, et al. HLA-E binds to natural killer cell receptorsCD94/NKG2A, Band C. Nature. 1998;**391**:795-799

[22] Lopez-Larrea C, Suarez-Alvarez B, Lopez-Soto A, Lopez-Vazquez A, Gonzalez S. The NKG2D receptor: Sensing stressed cells. Trends in Molecular Medicine. 2008;**14**:179-89

[23] Zafirova B, Wensveen FM, Gulin M, Polić B. Regulation of immune cell function and differentiation by the NKG2D receptor. Cellular and Molecular Life Sciences. 2011;**68**:3519-3529

[24] Wu J, Song Y, Bakker AB, Bauer S, Spies T, Lanier LL, et al. An activating immunoreceptor complex formed by NKG2D and DAP10. Science. 1999;**285**:730-732

[25] Schiavoni G, Gabriele L, Mattei F. The tumor microenvironment: A pitch for multiple players. Frontiers in Oncology. 2013;**3**:90

[26] Chitadze G, Bhat J, Lettau M, Janssen O, Kabelitz D. Generation of soluble NKG2D ligands: Proteolytic cleavage, exosome secretion and functional implications. Scandinavian Journal of Immunology. 2013;**78**:120-129

[27] Gonzalez-Gugel E, Saxena M, Bhardwaj N. Modulation of innate immunity in the tumor microenvironment. Cancer Immunology, Immunotherapy. 2016;**65**:1261-1268

[28] Konjević G, Mirjacić Martinović K, Vuletić A, Jurišić V, Spužić I. Distribution of several activating and inhibitory receptors on CD3-CD16+NKcells and their correlation with NK cell function in healthy individuals. The Journal of Membrane Biology. 2009;**230**: 113-123

[29] Mirjačić Martinović K, Konjević G, Babović N, Inić M. The stage dependent changes in NK cell activity and the expression of activating and inhibitory NK cell receptors in melanoma patients. Journal of Surgical Research. 2011;**171**:637-649

[30] Konjević G, Vuletić A, Mirjacić Martinović K. Changes in NK cell effector function, subset distribution and receptor repertoire following *in vitro* NK cell and K562 tumor cell contact in melanoma patients. In: EACR Proceedings Book 5-8 June 2014; Munich. Germany: European Journal of Cancer; **50**(Suppl. 5):p 220

[31] Ito N, DeMarco RA, Mailliard RB, Han J, Rabinowich H, Kalinski P, et al. Cytolytic cells induce HMGB1 release from melanoma cell lines. Journal of Leukocyte Biology. 2007; **81**:75-83

[32] Konjević G, Mirjačić Martinović K, Vuletić A, Jović V, Jurišić V, Babović N, et al. Low expression of CD161 and NKG2D activating NK receptor is associated with impaired NK

cell cytotoxicity in metastatic melanoma patients. Clinical & Experimental Metastasis. 2007;**24**:1-11

[33] Konjević G, Mirjacić Martinović K, Jurisić V, Babović N, Spuzić I. Biomarkers of suppressed natural killer (NK) cell function in metastatic melanoma: Decreased NKG2D and increased CD158a receptors on CD3-CD16+ NK cells. Biomarkers. 2009;**14**:258-270

[34] Mirjačić Martinović K, Srdić-Rajić T, Babović N, Džodić R, Jurišić V, Konjević G. Decreased expression of pSTAT, IRF-1 and DAP10 signalling molecules in peripheral blood lymphocytes of patients with metastatic melanoma. Journal of Clinical Pathology. 2016;**69**:300-306

[35] Pegram HJ, Andrews DM, Smyth MJ, Darcy PK, Kershaw MH. Activating and inhibitory receptors of natural killer cells. Immunology and Cell Biology. 2011;**89**:216-224.

[36] Bossard C, Bezieau S, Matysiak-Budnik T, Volteau C, Laboisse CL, Jotereau F, et al. HLA-E/b2 microglobulin overexpression in colorectal cancer is associated with recruitment of inhibitory immune cells and tumor progression. International Journal of Cancer. 2012;**131**:855-863.

[37] Sanchez-Correa B, Morgado S, Gayoso I, Bergua JM, Casado JG, Arcos MJ, et al. Human NK cells in acute myeloid leukaemia patients: Analysis of NK cell-activating receptors and their ligands. Cancer Immunology, Immunotherapy. 2011;**60**:1195-1205

[38] Uhrberg M, Valiante NM, Shum BP, Shilling HG, Lienert-Weidenbach K, Corliss B, et al. Human diversity in killer cell inhibitory receptor genes. Immunity. 1997;**7**:753-763

[39] Guia S, Jaeger BN, Piatek S, Mailfert S, Trombik T, Fenis A, et al. Confinement of activating receptors at the plasma membrane controls natural killer cell tolerance. Science Signaling. 2011;**4**(167):ra21

[40] Purdy AK, Campbell KS. Natural killer cells and cancer: Regulation by the killer cell Ig-like receptors (KIR). Cancer Biology & Therapy. 2009;**8**:2211-2220

[41] Boyton RJ, Altmann DM. Natural killer cells, killer immunoglobulin-like receptors and human leucocyte antigen class I in disease. Clinical & Experimental Immunology. 2007;**149**:1-8

[42] Campillo JA, Martınez-Escribano JA, Moya-Quiles MR, Marın LA, Muro M, Guerra N, et al. Natural killer receptors on CD8 T cells and natural killer cells from different HLA-C phenotypes in melanoma patients. Clinical Cancer Research. 2006;**12**:4822-4831

[43] Naumova E, Mihaylova A, Ivanova M, Mihailova S. Impact of KIR/HLA ligand combinations on immune responses in malignant melanoma. Cancer Immunology, Immunotherapy. 2007;**56**:95-100

[44] Zwirner NW, Domaica CI. Cytokine regulation of natural killer cell effector functions. BioFactors. 2010;**36**:274-288

[45] Konjević G, Mirjačić Martinović K, Vuletić A, Radenković S. Novel aspects of in vitro IL-2 or IFN-$\alpha$ enhanced NK cytotoxicity of healthy individuals based on NKG2D and CD161 NK cell receptor induction. Biomedicine & Pharmacotherapy. 2010;**64**:663-671

[46] Mirjačić Martinović K, Babović N, Džodić R, Jurišić V, Matković S, Konjević G. Favorable in vitro effects of combined IL-12 and IL-18 treatment on NK cell cytotoxicity and CD25 receptor expression in metastatic melanoma patients. Journal of Translational Medicine. 2015;**13**:120

[47] Vuletić AM, Jovanć IP, Jurišić VB,Milovanoviić ZM, Nikolić SS, Tanić NT, et al. In-vitro activation of natural killer cells from regional lymph nodes of melanoma patients with interleukin-2 and interleukin-15. Melanoma Research. 2015;**25**:22-34

[48] Mirjačić Martinović KM, Babović NL, Džodić RR, Jurišić VB, Ninković AZ, Konjević GM. Beneficial in-vitro effects of interleukin-2, interleukin-12, and their combination on functional and receptor characteristics of natural killer cells in metastatic melanoma patients with normal serum lactate dehydrogenase levels. Melanoma Research. 2016;**26**:551-564

[49] Varker KA, Terrell CE, Welt M, Suleiman S, Thornton L, Andersen BL, et al. Impaired natural killer cell lysis in breast cancer patients with high levels of psychological stress is associated with altered expression of killer immunoglobulin like receptors. Journal of Surgical Research. 2007;**139**:36-44

[50] Al Omar SY, Marshall E, Middleton D, Christmas SE. Increased killer immunoglobulin-like receptor expression and functional defects in natural killer cells in lung cancer. Immunology. 2011;**133**:94-104

[51] Vuletić A, Jurišić V, Jovanić I, Milovanović Z, Nikolić S, Konjević G. Distribution of several activating and inhibitory receptors on CD3(-)CD56(+) NK cells in regional lymph nodes of melanoma patients. Journal of Surgical Research. 2013;**183**:860-868

[52] Lakshmikanth T, Burke S, Ali TH, Kimpfler S, Ursini F, Ruggeri L, et al. NCRs and DNAM-1 mediate NK cell recognition and lysis of human and mouse melanoma cell lines *in vitro* and *in vivo*. Journal of Clinical Investigation. 2009;**119**:1251-1263

[53] Zhang Z, Su T, He L, Wang H, Ji G, Liu X, et al. Identification and functional analysis of ligands for natural killer cell activating receptors in colon carcinoma. Tohoku Journal of Experimental Medicine. 2012;**226**:59-68

[54] Balsamo M, Scordamaglia F, Pietra G, Manzini C, Cantoni C, Boitano M, et al. Melanoma-associated fibroblasts modulate NK cell phenotype and antitumor cytotoxicity. Proceedings of the National Academy of Sciences of the United States of America. 2009;**106**:20847-20852

[55] Morisaki T, Onishi H, Katano M. Cancer immunotherapy using NKG2D and DNAM-1systems. Anticancer Research. 2012;**32**:2241-2247

[56] Warren HS, Kinnear BF. Quantitative analysis of the effect of CD16 ligation on human NK cell proliferation. Journal of Immunology. 1999;**162**:735-42

[57] Lanier LL. Natural killer cell receptor signaling. Current Opinion in Immunology. 2003; **15**:308-314

[58] Konjević G, Vuletić A, Mirjačić Martinović K, Colović N, Čolović M, Jurišić V. Decreased CD161 activating and increased CD158a inhibitory receptor expression on NK cells underlies impaired NK cell cytotoxicity in patients with multiple myeloma. Journal of Clinical Pathology. 2016;pii:jclinpath-2016-203614. DOI: 10.1136/jclinpath-2016-203614

[59] Jewett A, Tseng HC. Tumor induced inactivation of natural killer cell cytotoxic function; implication in growth, expansion and differentiation of cancer stem cells. Journal of Cancer.2011;**2**:443-457

[60] Romee R, Foley B, Lenvik T, Wang Y, Zhang B, Ankarlo D, et al. NK cell CD16 surface expression and function is regulated by a disintegrin and metalloprotease-17 (ADAM17). Blood. 2013;**121**:3599-3608

[61] Azzoni L, Zatsepina O, Abebe B, Bennett IM, Kanakaraj P, Perussia B. Differential transcriptional regulation of CD161 and a novel gene, 197/15a, by IL-2, IL-15, and IL-12 in NK and T cells. Journal of Immunology. 1998;**161**:3493-3500

[62] Lanier LL, Chang C, Phillips JH. Human NKR-P1A. A disulfide- linked homodimer of the C-type lectin superfamily expressed by a subset of NK and T lymphocytes. Journal of Immunology. 1994;**153**:2417-2428

[63] Ryan JC, Seaman WE. Divergent functions of lectin-like receptors on NK cells. Immunological Reviews. 1997;**155**:79-89

[64] Rosen DB, Bettadapura J, Alsharifi M, Mathew PA, Warren HS, Lanier LL. Cutting edge: Lectin-like transcript-1 is a ligand for the inhibitory human NKR-P1A receptor. Journal of Immunology. 2005;**175**:7796-7799

[65] Vuletić A, Jovanić I, Jurišić V, Milovanović Z, Nikolić S, Spurnić I, et al. Decreased Interferon $\gamma$ Production in CD3+ and CD3- CD56+ Lymphocyte Subsets in Metastatic Regional Lymph Nodes of Melanoma Patients. Pathology & Oncology Research. 2015;**21**:1109-1114

[66] Della Chiesa M, Pesce S, Muccio L, Carlomagno S, Sivori S, Moretta A, Marcenaro E. Features of memory-like and PD-1(+) human NK cell subsets. Frontiers in Immunology. 2016;**7**:351. DOI: 10.3389/fimmu.2016.00351

[67] Konjević G, Mirjačić Martinović K, Vuletić A, Babović N. In-vitro IL-2 or IFN-a-induced NKG2D and CD161 NK cell receptor expression indicates novel aspects of NK cell activation in metastatic melanoma patients. Melanoma Research. 2010;**20**:459-467

[68] Konjevic G, Mirjacic-Martinovic K, Vuletic A, Babovic N. In vitro increased natural killer cell activity of metastatic melanoma patients with interferon-$\alpha$ alone as opposed to its combination with 13-cis retinoic acid is associated with modulation of NKG2D and CD161 activating receptor expression. Journal of BUON. 2012;**17**:761-769

[69] Konjević G, Jurišić V, Jović V, Vuletić A, Mirjačić Martinović K, Radenković S, et al. Investigation of NK cell function and their modulation in different malignancies. Journal of Immunology Research. 2012;**52**:139-156

[70] Mirjačić Martinović KM, Vuletić AM, Lj Babović N, Džodić RR, Konjević GM, Jurišić VB. Attenuated in vitro effects of IFN-$\alpha$, IL-2 and IL-12 on functional and receptor characteristics of peripheral blood lymphocytes in metastatic melanoma patients. Cytokine. 2017;**96**:30-40

[71] Konjević G, Spužić I. Stage dependence of NK cell activity and its modulation by interleukin 2 in patients with breast cancer. Neoplasma. 1993;**40**:81-85

[72] Konjević G, Jović V, Radulović S, Jelić S, Džodić R, Spužić I. Therapeutic implications of the kinetics of immunomodulation during single or combined treatment of melanoma patients with dacarbazine and interferon-alpha. Neoplasma. 2001;**48**:175-181

[73] Konjević G, Jović V, Radomirović V, Spuzić I: [Correlation between functional capability and phenotypic characteristics of peripheral blood lymphocytes in patients with malignant melanoma]. Glas Srp Akad Nauka Med. 2002;**73**:121-36

[74] Konjević G, Jović V, Jurisić V, Radulović S, Jelić S, Spuzić I. IL-2-mediated augmentation of NK-cell activity and activation antigen expression on NK- and T-cell subsets in patients with metastatic melanoma treated with interferon-alpha and DTIC. Clinical & Experimental Metastasis. 2003;**20**:647-655

[75] Konjević G, Jović V, Vuletić A, Radulović S, Jelić S, Spužić I. CD69 on CD56+ NK cells and response to chemoimmunotherapy in metastatic melanoma. European Journal of Clinical Investigation. 2007;**37**:887-896

[76] Ni J, Miller M, Stojanovic A, Garbi N, Cerwenka A. Sustained effector function of IL-12/15/18-preactivated NK cells against established tumors. Journal of Experimental Medicine. 2012;**209**:2351-2365

[77] Adams JL, Smothers J, Srinivasan R, Hoos A. Big opportunities for small molecules in immuno-oncology. Nature Reviews Drug Discovery. 2015;**14**:603-622

[78] Pietra G, Vitale C, Pende D, Bertaina A, Moretta F, Falco M, et al. Human natural killer cells: News in the therapy of solid tumors and high-risk leukemias. Cancer Immunology, Immunotherapy. 2016;**65**:465-476

[79] Seidel UJ, Schlegel P, Lang P. Natural killer cell mediated antibody-dependent cellular cytotoxicity in tumor immunotherapy with therapeutic antibodies. Frontiers in Immunology. 2013;**4**:76

[80] Campbell KS, Hasegawa J. Natural killer cell biology: An update and future directions. Journal of Allergy and Clinical Immunology. 2013;**132**:536-544

[81] Cheng M, Chen Y, Xiao W, Sun R, Tian Z. NK cell-based immunotherapy for malignant diseases. Cellular & Molecular Immunology. 2013;**10**:230-252

Chapter 6

# Clinical Applications of Natural Killer Cells

Yui Harada, Koji Teraishi, Minori Ishii,
Hiroshi Ban and Yoshikazu Yonemitsu

Additional information is available at the end of the chapter

http://dx.doi.org/10.5772/intechopen.68991

**Abstract**

Natural killer (NK) cells are an essential component of the innate immune system, and they play a crucial role in immunity against malignancies. Recent advances in our understanding of NK cell biology have paved the way for new therapeutic strategies based on NK cells for the treatment of various cancers. In this section, we will focus on NK cell immunotherapy, including the enhancement of antibody-dependent cellular cytotoxicity, the manipulation of receptor-mediated activation, inclusion criteria based on killer cell immunoglobulin-like receptor (KIR) ligand mismatches, and adoptive immunotherapy with *ex vivo* expanded chimeric antigen receptor (CAR)-engineered or engager-modified NK cells. In contrast to T lymphocytes, donor NK cells do not attack any recipient tissues based on allogeneic human leukocyte antigens (HLAs), suggesting that NK-mediated antitumor effects may be achieved without the risk of graft-versus-host disease (GvHD). Despite reports of clinical efficacy, the application of NK cell immunotherapy is limited. Developing strategies for manipulating NK cell products, host factors, and tumor targets are thus current subjects of diligent study. Research into the biology of NK cells has indicated that NK cell immunotherapy has the potential to become the forefront of cancer immunotherapy in the coming years.

**Keywords:** NK cell, KIRs, immunotherapy, HSC transplantation, genetic modification

## 1. Introduction

Natural killer (NK) cells have been used in clinical studies in order to treat various malignancies. Missing-self is one of the mechanisms of the NK cell response that works by the detection of the loss of autologous major histocompatibility complex (MHC) class I expression.

We will mention four elements of NK cells in this chapter: (1) mechanisms of NK cells; (2) activation of NK cells; (3) inclusion criteria based on KIR ligand mismatches; and (4) genetic modifications *ex vivo*.

NK cells, which are thought to have emerged much later than B cells and T cells based on the evolutionary convergence of variable receptors, rarely cause autoimmune diseases. We will introduce the applicability of the NK cell to cancer treatment.

## 2. Activation of NK cells

NK cell-based immunotherapy has been explored for decades. Several animal experiments indicated the potential efficacy of NK cells in cancer treatment [1–3]. However, *ex vivo* NK cell expansion techniques have been insufficient regarding the numbers of cells, purity and antitumor activity to use in clinical settings. NK cells comprise only a minor population (i.e., 5–15% of peripheral lymphocytes), and only a small number of NK cells is isolated after a typical apheresis procedure. For example, approx. $77.8 \pm 14.4 \times 10^9$/L (range $62.7–95.9 \times 10^9$/L) of leukapheretic products are the result of a single apheresis of peripheral blood in a normal adult human with a mean percentage of lymphocytes of 59.8% ± 6.1 (range 53.9–66.4%), and subsequently $5–10 \times 10^8$ NK cells can be obtained [4]. On the other hand, at least $2 \times 10^7$/kg or $6 \times 10^6–6.5 \times 10^9$/body NK cells are required for each effective injection with multiple administrations [5, 6]. In addition, the reported engraftment period of NK cells was 2–189 days (median 10 days), which showed no correlation with the number of NK cells administered [7]. The NK cell infusion should thus be repeated in order to maintain a sufficient number of NK cells meeting clinical requirements, but this would be a burden on patients.

Scientists have been working to develop various methods for proliferating NK cells *ex vivo* with high cytotoxicity and high purity. Several studies used an anti-CD3 antibody (clone: OKT3) in the first few days of culture for the activation of autologous T cells to help the NK cell expansion, subsequently producing high numbers of undesirable T cells or NKT cells in the final product [8–10]. However, particularly in haploidentical NK cell transplantation, T cells must be excluded prior to the infusion in order to prevent graft versus host disease (GvHD). Other studies removed $CD3^+$ cells by magnetic beads with or without CD56-positive selection at the beginning of culture [11–13].

To acquire highly purified and expanded NK cells, an initial efficient depletion (<1%) of $CD3^+$ cells and a relatively long-term culture (over 12 days) seem to be essential [12, 13]. Because only a minor fraction of circulating NK cells is reactive to target cells (tumor cells) *in vitro*, primary NK cells show insufficient cytotoxicity [14]. Various types of stimulation have thus been reported to enable NK cells to achieve their full effector potential, such as interleukin (IL)-15 produced by dendritic cells (DCs) [15] or macrophages [16], IL-2 [17], IL-12 [18], IL-18 [19] and IL-21 [20]. Currently, the additional cytokines used in the cultivation of NK cells include IL-2, IL-15, and IL-21. IL-2, IL-15, and IL-21 share the receptor subunits IL-2/15R$\beta$ and common $\gamma$ chain [21] on the NK cell surface and have a synergetic effect. Use of IL-2 combined with IL-15 for cultivation leads to good viability and good proliferation of NK cells [22]. IL-2 is also important for NK cell infiltration and killing, and IL-15 is important for both NK cell maturation and survival [21]. IL-2 and IL-15 induce the expression of KIRs and activating receptors (NKG2D and NKp44) on NK cell surface [23]. IL-21 modifies the expression of killer cell immunoglobulin-like receptors (KIRs) and NKp44 by reducing expression of DAP-12, subsequently promote cell maturation, the ability of killing and survival [22, 23]. Several experiments used feeder cells to provide essential stimulation for NK cell cultivation through cytokine production or cell-to-cell contact [20, 23, 24]. The various cytokines and feeder cells used in some clinical trials are mentioned in a later section of this article.

### 2.1. Killer cell immunoglobulin-like receptors (KIRs)

NK cells express KIRs, most of which are inhibitory (partially activating) receptors that recognized MHC class I molecules. In the 1980s, KIRs were first described as explaining the NK cell-mediated rejection of allogeneic bone marrow transplants from a homozygous donor to a hemizygous host in lymphoma and in F1-hybrid anti-parental resistance in a rodent model [25]. In these situations, the graft fails to express at least one MHC class I allele of the host, and NK cells are highly capable of identifying the difference, thus causing rejection. This can be explained by the concept that NK cells have inhibitory receptors and begin to attack target cells if they do not express ligands that interact with the specific inhibitory receptors. This phenomenon was termed the "missing-self hypothesis", which is now accepted as one of the complex target recognition mechanisms of NK cells.

#### *2.1.1. Regulation of NK cell activity*

The activation of NK cells is regulated by various receptors including KIRs, CD94–NKG2 family, leukocyte immunoglobulin-like receptors (LILRs), natural cytotoxicity receptors (NCRs), and FcγRIIIa (CD16) [26–28]. Among these receptors, KIRs, CD94/NKG2A heterodimers, and LILRs belong to the large family of inhibitory receptors of MHC class I, mediating NK cell function by signaling through intracytoplasmic immunoreceptor tyrosine-based inhibition motifs (ITIMs) [29]. Each NK cell has a threshold of activation through a balance of total stimulation between inhibitory and activating signals [30] (**Figure 1**). In other words, NK cells selectively kill target cells that down-regulate MHC class I molecules and/or up-regulate other activating ligands [28] such as MHC class I chain (MIC)-related antigens MICA, MICB and UL-16 binding protein (ULBP). MICA, MICB, ULBPs are ligands of NKG2D homodimer, which belong to C-type lectin receptor NKG2 family expressed on the surface of NK cells and $CD8^+$ T-lymphocytes. NKG2A/CD94 and NKG2B/CD94 heterodimers transmit inhibitory signals, while NKG2C/CD94, NKG2E/CD94, NKG2H/CD94 heterodimers and NKG2D homodimer are activating receptors.

#### *2.1.2. Genetics of KIRs*

The KIR gene family includes 14 loci (KIR2DL1, KIR2DL2/3, KIR2DL4, KIR2DL5A/B, KIR2DS1, KIR2DS2, KIR2DS3, KIR2DS4, KIR2DS5, KIR3DL1/S1, KIR3DL2, KIR3DL3 and two pseudogenes, KIR2DP1 and KIR3DP1) [31]as shown in **Table 1**. These loci are located on chromosome 19q13.4, which is known as the leukocyte receptor cluster (LRC); each haplotype has 9–15 KIR genes in a row [32]. Different NK cells within individuals each express a subset of the available KIR repertoire, leading to an allelic polymorphism of KIRs. Based on studies of KIR genotype variation, two major KIR haplotype groups termed the groups 'A' and 'B' are defined [33].

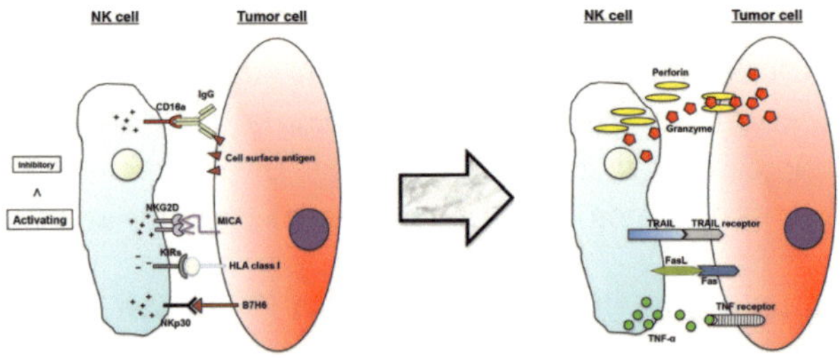


**Figure 1.** The mechanisms of cytotoxicity by NK cells.

| **Inhibitory** | **Ligands** | **Ligand missing** | **Notes** |
|---|---|---|---|
| KIR2DL1 | HLA-C2 group (Cw2, C*0307,Cw4, Cw5, Cw6, C*0707, C*0709, C*1204, C*1205, Cw15, C*1602, Cw17, Cw18) | HLA-C1/C1 | |
| KIR2DL2 | HLA-C1 group (Cw1, Cw3, Cw7, Cw8, Cw12, Cw13, Cw14, C*1507, C*1601/4)<br>HLA-B46, B73<br>HLA-C2(C*02, C*05)(weak interaction) | HLA-C2/C2(except for C*02, *05) and HLA-B46, B73 negative | |
| KIR2DL3 | HLA-C1 group (Cw1, Cw3, Cw7, Cw8, Cw12, Cw13, Cw14, C*1507, C*1601/4)<br>HLA-B46, B73 | HLA-C2/C2 and HLA-B46, B73 negative | |
| KIR3DL1 | HLA-Bw4 epitope(including HLA-A23, A24, A32) | HLA-Bw6/Bw6 and HLA-A23/24/32 negative | Expression level: *01502, *020 > *001, *007 >*004 |
| KIR3DL2 | HLA-A03, A11(+ EBNA peptide),HLA-B27 dimer | HLA-A03, A11 negative, free of EBV | *001 is homo-dimer A03/A11 could not promote NK cell Licensing |
| KIR2DL5B | Unknown | | |
| KIR2DL5T | Unknown | | |
| Activating | Ligands | Ligand missing | Notes |
| KIR2DS4 | HLA-A*1102,(A*1101, C*0304, C*0501) | HLA-A*1102 negative | |
| KIR2DS1 | HLA-C2 | HLA-C1/C1 | |
| KIR2DS2 | Unknown(HLA-C1?) | | |
| KIR3DS1 | Unknown(HLA-B*2705?) | | |
| KIR2DS3/5 | Unknown | | |
| KIR2DL4 | HLA-G | | |
| Others | Ligands | Ligand missing | Notes |
| KIR2DP1 | – | – | Pseudogene |
| KIR3DP1 | - | - | Pseudogene |

**Table 1.** Human KIRs.

Each haplotype is separated into two regions: the centromeric half (Cen) and the telomeric half (Tel). Cen and Tel motifs can be divided into Cen-A, Cen-B and Tel-A, Tel-B by the KIR genes they contain. Haplotype A is a combination of Cen-A and Tel-A, which consists of mainly inhibitory KIRs (KIR3DL3, 2DL3, 2DL1, 3DL1, 2DS4, 3DL2 and two pseudogenes). Other combinations are termed Haplotype B (such as Cen-A and Tel-B or Cen-B and Tel-B), composed of a large variation of genes characterized by the presence of more activating KIRs. All individuals can be categorized according to their haplotype: A/A, which is homozygous for group A haplotypes, or B/x, which contains either one (A/B) or two (B/B homozygotes) group B haplotypes[34]. As a consequence of this genetic variation, several studies report that donor-derived NK cells can mediate the graft-versus-leukemia (GVL) effect or even the graft-versus-tumor (GVT) effect after allogeneic hematopoietic cell transplantation (HCT) [34–36]. These are the results of a KIR-ligand mismatch, the details of which are described later in this article.

*2.1.3. KIRs subtypes*

KIRs are type I transmembrane glycoproteins expressed on the surface of NK cells, composed of two (2D) or three (3D) extracellular Ig-like domains and a cytoplasmic short (activating) or long (inhibitory) tail [31]. The length of the intracytoplasmic part determines the function; for example, receptors with long cytoplasmic tails with one or two ITIMs that bind to phosphatase SHP-1, 2 allow the transduction of inhibitory signals through its dephosphorylation. In contrast, receptors with short cytoplasmic tails possess a positively charged residue (lysine) in the transmembrane domain that enables it to associate with adaptor proteins including DAP12 and process the immunoreceptor tyrosine-based activation motifs (ITAMs) [29]. There is one exception: KIR2DL4, with a long cytoplasmic tail, binds to the activation motif of $Fc\varepsilon RI\gamma$ and thus seems to transmit the activating signal [31].

MHC class I molecules are well-known ligands for KIRs, but HLA-C molecules, in particular, are the main ligands contributing greatly to NK cell activity. Polymorphisms in amino acids at positions 77 and 80 of HLA-C show specificity for its target KIRs. Group 1 HLA-C ligands (C1) include allele-encoded molecules with serine and asparagine (Ser77 and Asn80), whereas group 2 ligands (C2) are characterized by allele-encoded molecules with asparagine and lysine (Asn77 and Lys80). C1 epitopes bind specifically to KIR2DL2/3, and C2 epitopes are ligands for KIR2DL1 [37]. However, it was shown that KIR2DL2/3 might also bind to certain HLA-C2 epitopes (C*0501, C*0202, C*0401) and some HLA-B epitopes (HLA-B*4601, B*7301) with very low affinity [38].

Among the inhibitory KIRs, KIR2DL1 results in a stronger inhibition compared to the KIR 2DL2/3 [38]. The third inhibitory KIR is KIR3DL1, which binds to HLA-Bw4 epitopes and a subset of HLA-A epitopes (A*23, A*24, and A*32). All HLA-B have either the Bw4 or Bw6 epitope, but only the Bw4 epitope is a ligand for KIRs [39]. KIR3DL2 is a framework gene, and it recognizes HLA-A*03 and HLA-A*11 with a low level of inhibition [40]. Although haplotype A includes only a single activating KIR (2DL4), at least two to five activating KIR genes (2DS1, 2DS2, 2DS3, 2DS5 and 3DS1) are subject to haplotype B. However, KIR2DS1 alone is now confirmed to have matched ligand HLA-C2 with lower avidity compared to KIR2DL1 [41].

### 2.2. Death Ligands

NK cells express members of the tumor necrosis factor (TNF) superfamily, the so-called death ligands. The cognate of the receptor on target cells by these ligands on NK cells — which include TNF-related apoptosis-inducing ligand (TRAIL), Fas ligand (FasL) and TNF-like weak inducer of apoptosis (TWEAK) — results in classical caspase-dependent apoptosis [42, 43]. In the TRAIL/TRAIL receptor system, at least five receptors have been identified and two of them, TRAIL-R1 (DR4) and TRAIL-R2 (DR5), contain cytoplasmic death domains and are able to transduce an apoptotic signal [44]. Other TRAIL receptors — TRAIL-R3 (DcR1) and TRAIL-R4 (DcR2) and a soluble receptor called osteoprotegerin (OPG: TRAIL-R5) — lack a death domain, but they are dedicated as decoy receptors to regulate TRAIL-mediated cell death [45]. In target cell expressing TRAIL receptors, the ligation of TRAIL can lead to the activation of caspase-8 and subsequently caspase-3 to induce apoptosis [46, 47]. TRAIL is up-regulated after the stimulation of interferon-gamma (IFN-$\gamma$) *in vitro* [48, 49] and also *in vivo*, which demonstrates that TRAIL is required for the IFN-$\gamma$-mediated prevention of tumors [50].

FasL is expressed on activated NK cells and cytotoxic T lymphocytes (CTLs) [42]. Although it is known that FasL is expressed on NK cells at a low level, significant amounts are stored intracellularly [51]. An activating signal of rodent NK1.1 up-regulated the expression of FasL [52]. After FasL has bound to Fas, the Fas associated with two specific proteins, Fas-associated death domain (FADD) and caspase-8, to form the death-inducing signal complex (DISC). Fas is expressed on various tissues, but the molecule is downregulated in cancers during its progression [53]. NK cells are capable of directly inducing Fas expression on tumor cells via IFN-$\gamma$ secretion, and NK cells show cytotoxicity to tumor cells expressing Fas [45].

### 2.3. Perforin and granzyme

Cytolytic killing using perforin and granzyme is a major mechanism in the elimination of infected cells and tumor cells by NK cells. NK cells contain cytoplasmic granules including perforin (a membrane-disrupting protein) and granzyme (a family of serine proteases). Once NK cells recognize target cells, they form an immunological synapse, and the secretory granules fuse with the presynaptic membrane and release perforin and granzyme into the synaptic cleft. Released perforin provides transmembrane pores on the target cell and enables granzyme to diffuse into the cell. Granzyme then initiates the apoptosis of the target cells, and the NK cells detach from the dying cells and can interact with other target cells to accomplish serial killing [54]. The release of such granules stored in the NK cells is dependent on the polarization of both microtubules and actin filaments in the cytoskeleton. The increase of intracellular calcium concentration triggered by a positive balance of activating and inhibitory signals initiate the rapid move of microtubule-organizing center (MTOC) in the cytoplasm towards the target cell, and then cytotoxic granules migrate along the MTOC [54]. Granules fuse with the presynaptic membrane, subsequently, the lytic granules can be released at the NK cell-target cell interface[55] (**Figure 2**).

http://dx.doi.org/10.5772/intechopen.68991

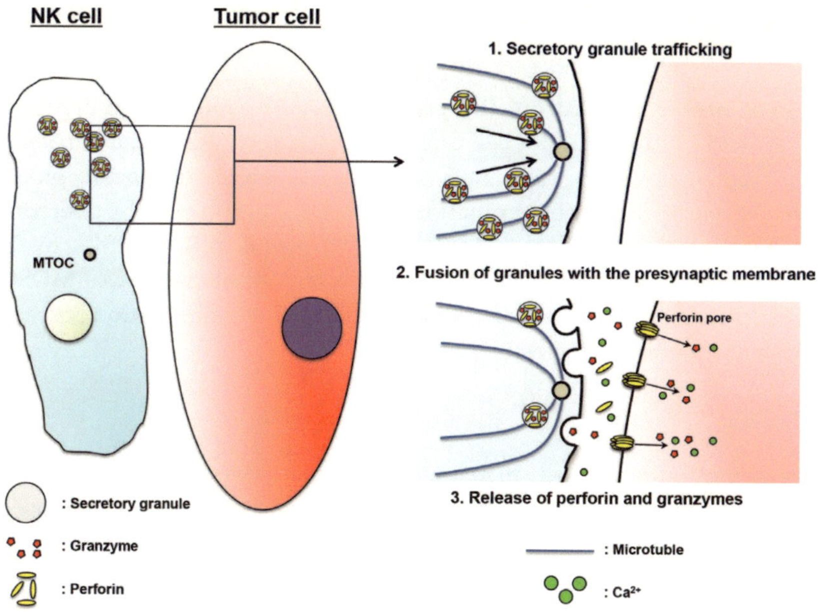


**Figure 2.** Interaction of an NK cell with a target cell.

## 3. NK cells for clinical use

### 3.1. Sources of NK cells

There are several options for sources of NK cell therapy, including peripheral blood mononuclear cells (PBMCs), umbilical cord blood (UCB), bone marrow (BM), cell lines, human embryonic stem cells (hESCs), and induced pluripotent stem cells (iPSCs).

#### *3.1.1. Peripheral blood mononuclear cells (PBMCs)*

PBMCs are the most common source of NK cells, and PBMCs can be collected by apheresis or a specific gravity centrifugal method (e.g., Ficoll separation). However, the percentage of NK cells in PBMCs is low (5–20%), and because there is a limit on the number of cells that can be recovered from a donor by lymphocyte apheresis, it is not possible that a sufficient number of NK cells for killing the target can remain in the recipient [7]. That is, in order to stay in the recipient's body until the target cells are killed, it is necessary to collect peripheral blood frequently, which is a heavy burden on the patient.

Numerous methods for amplification cultures of NK cells have been reported. Stem cell mobilization is a process whereby stem cells ($CD34^{+}$cells) are stimulated out of the bone marrow space (e.g., the hip bones and the chest bone) into the bloodstream, and granulocyte-colony stimulating factor (G-CSF) is widely used as a drug for harvesting peripheral blood stem cells from patients or healthy people. Another drug, Plerixafor [56], a CXCR4 antagonist approved in 2008, has an excellent mobilization effect in combination with G-CSF [57, 58].

An increase in a number of CD34-positive cells harvested by mobilization reduces the number of apheresis sessions required for cell therapy, which may reduce the burden on patients. When allogeneic hematopoietic stem cells are used, GVHD in the acute phase, which is thought to be caused by T-cell contamination, exists as a problem to be overcome. There is also a report that the induction of myeloid-derived suppressor cells (MDSCs) by the administration of G-CSF reduces the frequency of GVHD. It is important to note that MDSCs suppress T-cell function through an arginine depletion by arginase-1, the production of reactive oxygen species, and the induction of Treg cells [59, 60].

#### *3.1.2. Bone marrow (BM)*

Bone marrow aspiration removes a small amount of bone marrow fluid through a needle put into a bone under general anesthesia. Compared to apheresis, it is very rarely used as a starting material because of its high invasiveness to donors.

#### *3.1.3. Umbilical cord blood (CB)*

Hematopoietic reconstitution for Fanconi anemia treatment using cord blood was first performed in 1988 by Gluckman et al. [61]. Since then it has been widely accepted as a source of hematopoietic stem cells when autologous blood is not recommended or readily available. Cord blood (CB) can be donated to public CB banks for use by any patient worldwide for whom it is stored for potential autologous or family use. The majority of CB products used today are for hematopoietic stem cell transplantation and are accessed from public banks.

Cord blood presents no harm to the donor at the time of collection, and the frozen storage of collected samples is possible. In addition, cord blood of various blood types is classified and preserved in umbilical cord blood banks. When umbilical cord blood is used as the source of therapeutic NK cells, it is highly tissue-compatible according to the patient's blood type and accompanying transplantation. It is easy to select blood type-specific umbilical cord blood, with little side effects. In addition, it is possible to minimize the risk of GVHD from the absence of T cells [62–64]. As with PBMCs, a growth culture is essential because the amount of NK cells that can be obtained from a single CB sample is not an amount that can expect to provide a therapeutic effect.

#### *3.1.4. Embryonic stem cells and induced pluripotent stem cells (ES/iPS)*

Another possible source of NK cells is human embryonic stem cells (hESCs) and induced pluripotent stem cells (iPSCs). A differentiation/expansion culture from hESCs and iPSCs to NK cells is a regimen requiring more sophisticated technology compared to the PBMCs and UCB described above. The differentiation process of human iPSCs is divided into three stages of "maintenance amplification", "structure construction", and "differentiation induction". The culturing step is to generate CD34$^+$ hematopoietic progenitor cells from hESCs and iPSCs and then differentiate these cells into NK cells.

A preclinical demonstration that NK cells can be separated from the sources of these pluripotent stem cells has been described [65, 66]. However, that demonstration enabled efficient proliferation by using mouse stromal cells as feeder cells, and the involvement of heterologous cells may limit clinical application. As with UCB, advances in the development of safe, effective and standardized clinical-grade manufacturing protocols will provide opportunities to develop ready-made personalization and immunogenic cell therapy.

#### *3.1.5. Cell lines*

The cell lines that have been derived from NK cells are NK-92, NK-YS, KHYG-1, NKL, NKG, SNK-6, and IMC-1 cells [67], and several research groups are exploring the possibilities of using these cell lines for therapeutic applications. The primary advantage of an NK cell line is that it is "ready to use", and it is possible to establish comprehensive standardization and characterization of the cell source by using the master cell bank. The cell therapy product is thus considered to be an attractive merit in manufacturing. Moreover, a more homogeneous population is obtained compared to that from peripheral blood, and its homogeneous character is another advantage when performing a genetic modification operation.

NK cell line has been applied to genetic modification technology for expressing intracellular IL-2 for the forced expression of CD16, natural cytotoxicity receptor (NCR), chimeric antigen receptor (CAR) and NK cell activation [68, 69]. The most widely clinically used cell line is the NK-92 cell line, which is cytotoxic to a wide range of malignant cells [70, 71]. NK-92 cells express the receptor but hardly express KIR, NKp44 or CD16. NantKWest (Culver City, CA, USA) conducts clinical trials using NK-92 cells (Neukoplast™) and has completed a Phase 1 study (U. S. National Clinical Trial [NCT] #00900809 and NCT #00990717). Moreover, the company has begun phase 1 and phase 2 trials of haNK (high-affinity NK cells) [72] engineered to express CD16 (NCT #02465957 and NCT #03027128). In addition, as another attempt, the development of CAR-TNK expressing CD7 or CD33 has been advanced (NCT #02944162 and NCT #02742727).

### 3.2. Manufacturing method

The number of NK cells contained in a collectable amount of UCB or peripheral blood is not enough to achieve a clinical therapeutic effect. A long-term culture method is necessary to overcome this problem. For starting material, T cells and/or B cells are removed with magnetic beads to increase the purity of NK cells. This is also to prevent the proliferation of T cells caused by IL-2 during the culture period of NK cells and to avoid lower purity of the final product [8, 73].

In addition to the important cytokine IL-2, there are IL-15, which is necessary for both the maturation and survival of NK cells [21]. IL-2 and IL-15 share the same receptor component IL-2/15R$\beta$ and a common $\gamma$ chain, and they are used in a culture method without the use of feeder cells [74, 75]. IL-21 [76], a member of the IL-2 cytokine family, is a potent immunostimulatory cytokine that shows diverse regulatory effects on NK cells, T cells and B cells [77, 78] and also has the effect of enhancing rituximab-mediated antibody-dependent cell mediated cytotoxicity (ADCC) of mantle cell lymphoma [79]. In addition, there is a culture method using feeder cells to efficiently expand NK cells *ex vivo*. As feeder cells, monocytes, irradiated PBMCs, the K562 cell line and a genetically modified cell line are used.

For example, there are systems using a co-culture with NK cells and monocytes [80], with CB $CD34^+$ cells and bone marrow stromal cells [81], or K562 cells transfected with IL-21 [82]. There is also a completely closed culture using Epstein-Barr virus-transformed lymphoblastoid cell lines [83]. Thus, the use of feeder cells is an important method for securing a number of cells that can be expected to have a therapeutic effect. However, because of the problem of infectious disease risk presented by the use of an allogeneic feeder, the regulatory hurdles in the manufacture of pharmaceutical products are high [84].

To overcome this problem, Yonemitsu et al. reported a method of culturing highly activated NK cells with ≥90% purity from PBMCs in a completely closed and feeder-free system under the good manufacturing practices (GMP) [13]. As another feeder-free culture method, Spanholtz and colleagues reported a culture method that achieved amplification efficiency and high purity of 10,000 times or more in 6 weeks from UCB $CD34^+$ hematopoietic stem cell (HSCs), using a closed system process based on GMP [85]. Knorr and colleagues reported differentiation induction from $CD34^+$ hematopoietic progenitor cells produced under feeder-free conditions to cytotoxic NK cells [86].

### 3.2.1. NK cell-based immunotherapy: autologous cells

Clinical trials using autologous NK cells have been performed targeting solid tumors such as colorectal cancer, non-small cell lung cancer, melanoma, kidney cancer and esophageal cancer [87–89]. In general, autologous NK cell therapy is safe without side effects such as GvHD [87], but its therapeutic effect is limited to some cancer types [74]. An activation culture with IL-2 and OKT3 or Hsp70 has been reported to be able to efficiently induce the proliferation of NK cells [74], in particular, the retronectin culture method of Sakamoto et al. showed a high amplification efficiency (about 4720-fold) [89].

### 3.2.2. NK cell-based immunotherapy: allogeneic cells

Allogeneic NK cell products are used for the treatment of malignant tumors such as leukemia, renal cell carcinoma, colorectal cancer, and lymphoma. The major risk of allogeneic NK cell transplantation is the onset of GvHD. Measures against GvHD include the use of immunosuppressive agents, injection of high-purity NK cells by CD3 depletion, and the selection of donors consistent with the host HLA [74, 75]. In the case of haploidentical donors and recipients, to avoid GvHD, it is necessary to strictly perform T-cell depletion. In many studies, $CD56^+$ is enriched after the removal of $CD3^+$ T cells [17, 90, 91]. In cases of an allogeneic type, HLA typing and confirmation of KIR by flow cytometry are carried out, particularly in order to select the optimum donor. For details on the selection criteria, please refer to a later section of this article.

### 3.2.3. Synergistic effect: antibody drugs

An antibody drug is, in short, a medicine that functions based on the specificity with which an antibody recognizes an antigen. The characteristics of antibody drugs are high specificity (low toxicity) and high stability *in vivo*. The antibody binds only to the target antigen, and not to any other, which leads to the intended medicinal effect with only rare unexpected side effects. Antibodies are present at a stable level in the blood, and antibody medicines can also be detected at a stable level in the blood for a long period after administration, and they can exert their medicinal effects over a long term. More than 50 antibody drugs have been approved in Japan, the U.S. and Europe. Target diseases include cancer, rheumatoid arthritis and psoriasis, but most of the targets are cancers. One of the action mechanisms of antibody drugs used to treat cancer is ADCC, in which NK cell plays a central role. **Table 2** shows FDA-approved antibodies for ADCC to treat cancer.

ADCC mediated by NK cells begins with the recognition of antibodies bound to target cells. NK cells express two Fc receptors, CD16a (FcγRIIIa) [92] and CD32c (FcγRIIc) [93]. These Fc receptors recognize and bind to IgG1 and IgG3 and have a high affinity for IgG3 [94]. NK cells that recognize the antibody on the target cells transmit their signals intracellularly and kill the cells.

The signaling of human CD16 is mediated via FcεRIγ, CD3ζ, or FcεRIγ-CD3ζ heterodimer. These molecules contain an ITAM and are phosphorylated when the antibody binds to CD16 [42]. CD32c (FcγRIIc) contains an ITAM-like sequence in the cytoplasmic domain (which is

| Drug name | Trade name | Type | Target | Cancers | Approved year |
|---|---|---|---|---|---|
| Rituximab | Rituxan<br>MabThera | Chimeric IgG1κ | CD20 | Non-Hodgkin)s B-cell lymphomas Chronic lymphocytic leukemia | 1997 |
| Trastuzumab | Herceptin | Humanized IgG1κ | HER2 | Adenocarcinoma of the stomach or gastroesophageal junction<br>Breast cancer | 1998 |
| Alemtuzumab | Campath | Humanized IgG1κ | CD52 | B-cell chronic lymphocytic leukemia | 2001 |
| Cetuximab | Erbitux | Chimeric IgG1κ | EGFR | Colorectal cancer<br>Head and neck cancer | 2004 |
| Ofatumumab | Arzerra | Human IgG1κ | CD20 | Chronic lymphocytic leukemia | 2009 |
| Pertuzumab | Perjeta | Humanized IgG1κ | HER2 | Breast cancer | 2012 |
| Obinutuzumab | Gazyva | Humanized IgG1κ | CD20 | Chronic lymphocytic leukemia<br>Follicular lymphoma | 2013 |
| Dinutuximab | Unituxin | Chimeric IgG1κ | GD2 | Neuroblastoma | 2015 |
| Daratumumab | Darzalex | Humanized IgG1κ | CD38 | Multiple myeloma | 2015 |
| Elotuzumab | Empliciti | Humanized IgG1κ | SLAMF7 | Multiple myeloma | 2015 |

**Table 2.** FDA-approved antibodies for ADCC to treat cancer.

similar to that of FcγRIIa), suggesting that it transmits a signal via SRC-SYK (the SRC family of kinases and spleen tyrosine kinase [SYK]) signaling pathways [95]. However, the expression of CD32c was less than half of that of NK cells [96, 97]. Many studies focusing on CD16 have thus been conducted.

Several genetic polymorphisms of CD16 exist. Among them, the amino acid at position 158 has been shown to be important for the strength of the affinity for antibodies. The affinity depends on whether the amino acid at position 158 is phenylalanine or valine, and the valine type (158 V) has a higher affinity for the Fc of IgG. A number of reports have indicated that differences in the affinity for antibodies are correlated with therapeutic effects, and many studies have analyzed the clinical responsiveness of this gene polymorphism and antibody therapy. Cartron et al. examined the effects of rituximab treatment for non-Hodgkin's lymphoma, and they reported a higher objective response rate in CD16 (158 V) homozygous patients compared to CD16 (158F) carrier patients [98]. Wang et al. analyzed the outcomes of rituximab treatment for Follicular Lymphoma and reported significantly more likely progression-free survival at 2 years in CD16 (158 V) homozygous patients compared to CD16 (158F) carrier patients, at 45 and 14%, respectively [99].

These results suggest that the affinity of CD16 for antibodies correlates with the therapeutic effect. Thus, focusing on CD16, the modification of NK cells has been attempted. Binyamin et al. reported that introducing CD16 (158 V) into NK-92 cells not expressing CD16 improved the cytotoxicity against B-cell lymphoma with rituximab [100]. Carlsten et al. reported high ADCC activity of cultured NK cells from healthy donors with CD16 (158F/F) and transduced CD16 (158 V) mRNA by electroporation against rituximab-coated $CD20^+$ B-cell lymphoma cells [101].

As described above, since NK cells mediate antibody-dependent cytotoxic activity via Fc receptors, compatibility with antibody drugs targeting ADCC is desirable. As a strategy to further augment the antitumor effect, a plausible strategy is to enhance the affinity between the Fc receptor and the antibody. Low-molecular-weight compounds that are able to inhibit the shedding of CD16 have been reported. It is known that CD16 is cleaved by a protease such as a disintegrin and a metalloprotease 17 (ADAM17) when cells are activated [102], and thus in order to exert more sustained and enhanced ADCC activity, a method of inhibiting the cleavage of CD16 on NK cells may be important. In fact, inhibitors of ADAM17 enhanced the activity of NK cells [102, 103]. Another method to inhibit the cleavage of CD16 is a genetic modification. The substitution of the serine residue at position 197 in CD16 by a proline prevents the cleavage of CD16 on NK cells [104]. It may be possible to promote the antitumor effect by using a CD16 mutant.

## 4. Optimized selection of patients/donors

### 4.1. Clinical outcomes: on the KIR ligand mismatch model

Research reports focusing on the KIR of NK cells and the HLA of tumor cells for the purpose of treating leukemia have been drawing attention since the 2000's. In the report by Ruggeri et al.

published in *Science* in 2002, the cases in which HLA-ABC recognizable by NK cells is present in a donor but not in a recipient were defined as "KIR mismatch". It was speculated that in such cases, NK cells not receiving suppression signals from the donor HLA attack the cells of the recipient. When Ruggeri et al. started this research, it was not known that NK cells are a heterogeneous population expressing multiple inhibitory receptors, or that the specific antibodies that can be used for analysis are inadequate. Ruggeri and colleagues, therefore, examined only the HLA of donors and recipients without examining the KIR, and they analyzed patients divided into the two groups of HLA matched and mismatched transplantations. Although it may not have been an appropriate observation based on the current knowledge, at that time, the analysis was based on the following basic research data.

Ruggeri et al. examined whether CD56-positive NK cell clones collected from donors could attack leukemia cells of the recipient. They found that NK cell clones that attack leukemia cells exist, and their high frequency (≥2%) correlates well with the cases in which the donor's and recipient's KIR ligand (HLA) do not match in the GVH direction. Ruggeri et al. analyzed 35 acute lymphoblastic leukemia (ALL) and 57 acute myeloid leukemia (AML) patients who had allogeneic hematopoietic stem cell (HSC) transplantations at their institution. The result was a breakthrough result in 20 AML patients who were not KIR ligand mismatches in the GVH direction, with 0% relapse after transplantation [105]. This report was the subject of much attention, and then it was decided to conduct data analyses in medical institutions around the world seeking reproducibility of the results.

The analysis by Ruggeri et al. was by the method known as the "KIR ligand mismatch model", which examines only the donor and recipient HLA-ABC without checking the KIR. This method determines whether a KIR match or mismatch is determined. Researchers all over the world could thus easily use this method. However, most of the analysis results obtained in this way conflicted with the report by Ruggeri et al.

As an example, we will describe the analysis results obtained from the study of the Japan Marrow Donor Program (JMDP). In 2007, Morishima et al. reported the results of their analysis of 1790 patients who underwent an allogeneic bone marrow transplantation in accord with the KIR ligand mismatch model [106]. In conventional domestic allogeneic HSC transplantation, the criterion for donor selection is that the HLA-AB and -DR matched, and by this criterion 534 of the 1790 cases were HLA-C mismatched. As a result, the overall survival rate, the recurrence rate, and the incidence of GvHD were poor in the group in which the KIR ligand HLA-C was mismatched in the GVH direction.

The finding that allogeneic HSC transplantation has no merit in KIR mismatches is common in the report about cases from the U.S. National Marrow Donor Program (NMDP) and the European group for blood and marrow transplantation (EBMT) [107]. Comparing Ruggeri's 2002 report with Morishima's 2007 report, the biggest difference was the cell source for transplantations, the former being $CD34^+$ cell transplantation from haploidentical donors and the latter being conventional bone marrow transplantation. In addition, Ruggeri et al. used anti-thymocyte globulin (ATG) in all cases. A re-analysis of the registered JMDP cases reconfirmed that the transplantation performance of the HLA-C matched group was also good and that of the group with the HLA-C mismatch was poor [108].

Interestingly, the disadvantage of this HLA-C mismatch was not observed in the ATG administration group. In other words, it is suggested that not NK cell dysfunction but T cells induced by HLA-C mismatch had exacerbated the transplantation results. T cell-depleted grafting and ATG might avoid the T-cell response. There are certain reports that HLA-C mismatches are recognized by cytotoxic T lymphocytes (CTLs). There are two papers that reported a total of nine CTL clones from two patients who developed GvHD [109, 110]. Interestingly, all of the targets of the nine CTL clones were HLA-C, which was different from the HLA-C of the recipient. There is no doubt that the difference in HLA-C could be a target for CTL.

### 4.2. Receptor ligand model or missing ligand model

Although the KIR ligand mismatch model investigated only ligand (i.e., HLA) differences, eventually some researchers noted that donors' KIR should also be examined and analysed by different approaches were developed. In 2004, Leung et al. analyzed 36 children who received selective $CD34^+$ cell transplantation from haploidentical donors [111]. They first examined the presence or absence of inhibitory KIR in donor cells by flow cytometry (i.e., a phenotype assay). It was speculated that the recipient would have a KIR mismatch if the recipient did not have a ligand for KIR (suppressing type) of the donor. This is the "receptor-ligand model".

For example, when the donor has KIR2DL1 with HLA-C1/C1, when the recipient is HLA-C1/C1, it is considered a KIR match in the KIR ligand mismatch model, but it is a ligand mismatch of KIR2DL1 in the receptor-ligand model. This is a very frequent combination for Japanese (HLA-C1/C1 = 85%, $KIR2DL1^+$ = 99%). Conversely, if the donor does not have KIR2DL1 with HLA-C1/C2, if the recipient is HLA-C1/C1, it is considered a KIR mismatch in the KIR ligand mismatch model, but it is considered a KIR match in the receptor-ligand model. However, since there are few $KIR2DL1^-$ and HLA-C1/C2 among Japanese, this combination is extremely rare.

An analysis conducted to determine which model can predict recurrence more accurately revealed that the receptor-ligand model is superior [111]. Hsu et al. also reported their analysis based on the receptor-ligand model [112]. They investigated 178 cases of T cell-depleted transplantation and found that the positive rates of KIR2DL1, KIR2DL2/3, and KIR3DL1 were 93, 99, and 92%, respectively, in the donor gene, and that although there were 112 cases (63%) of the 178 patients who were expected to exhibit the GVL effect, there was a significant difference in the recurrence rate, and the disease-free survival rate/overall survival rate was also good in the AML and myelodysplastic syndrome (MDS) patients.

Hsu et al. presented a new idea in 2006 [113]. It is hard to examine the donor's KIR by genetic testing, but donors usually have genes of KIR2DL1, KIR2DL2/3, and KIR3DL1. Therefore, HLA-C1/C1 homozygous, HLA-C2/C2 homo and HLA-Bw6/Bw6 homo patients identified by examining only the recipient's HLA may experience the GVL effect from donor NK cells. This method is called the "missing ligand model". It was designed for transplantation performance analyses, not for donor selection. Hsu et al. analyzed 1770 patients who had allogeneic (unrelated) T-cell-depleted transplantation. A University of Minnesota study examined 2062 cases from the U.S. NMDP [114], and based on the idea that NK cells have a GVL effect, they excluded 568 Japanese subjects or analyzed only partial diseases with good prognosis. Nonetheless, that paper is very interesting as it shows the difference in the distribution of KIR ligand between Japanese and Westerners and the difference in the recurrence rate of disease [113]. We can see how Japanese are 'biased' toward HLA-C1.

Although few cases of GvHD in Japanese have been reported, the recurrence rate of HLA-C1/C1 patients is not much different from that of Westerners. In addition, among the Japanese, the recurrence rate is extremely small when the recipients are HLA-C2/C2 homozygous, which is a minority. However, caution is required in the interpretation of the results, as there are only three cases in which the recipient had HLA-C2/C2. Further detailed analysis is expected in the future.

### 4.3. Therapeutic effects of allogeneic transplantation of NK cells, and their limitations

In 2007, Ruggeri et al. reported the results of 122 cases of AML [115], which included 57 cases [105] and the other 55 cases. In the KIR ligand mismatch model, there were 51 cases of KIR mismatch in the GVH direction and 61 cases of matches, and the number of remission cases at the time of transplantation and the cases which were refractory to treatment were approximately 50% of the cases. The results showed that although the relapse rate was significantly lower in the cases of remission at the time of transplantation in the KIR mismatch in the GVH direction (3 vs. 47%, $p = 0.003$), in the cases in which the treatment was refractory, no treatment effect was observed (32 vs. 37%, p = NS).

Is it true that NK cells exert a GVL effect? A direct answer to that question has been reported as a KIR-mismatch NK cell transplantation in recent years. Ten children with AML [7] and 13 adults with AML [116] underwent the transplantation of CD56-positive NK cells harvested from haploidentical donors. The collected NK cells were considered KIR mismatches, and in both studies, only NK cells were transplanted after pretreatment (fludarabine and cyclophosphamide). The number of transplanted NK cells was $29 \times 10^6$/kg for the children and $2.7 \times 10^6$/kg for the adults; the numbers of transplanted T cells were $<1 \times 10^3$/kg and $< 1 \times 10^5$/kg, respectively. After transplantation, 1–10 million units of IL-2 were administered every other day, 6 times.

As a result, transient engraftment of donor NK cells was observed in all cases. Donor-derived NK cells occupied 7% (1–30%) of the peripheral blood lymphocytes at the peak of day 14 in the children's report, and at day 28, donor-derived NK cells have been detected from three of 10 patients [7]. All of the child patients had AML in complete remission, and all cases did not recur. Among the adult patients, whose leukemia was worse, one of five patients with clear recurrence showed transient remission, and two patients with genetic recurrence AML were remitted [116]. From the above results, it was demonstrated that NK cells exert a sufficient antitumor effect if the residual tumor is relatively small. However, it is not yet clear whether the therapeutic effect is proportional to the number of NK cells administered. It should be noted that even though transplanted CD3-positive cells are limited to $\leq 1 \times 10^3$/kg, there was no case of GvHD onset in either group.

## 4.4. Selection of KIR in allogeneic hematopoietic stem cell transplant donors

The target diseases in which the therapeutic effect by NK cells is confirmed in analyses of various clinical tests are mostly limited to AML. Clinical trials using conventional NK cells often do not even target other diseases. There are reports that NK cells do not show a therapeutic effect against ALL because of lymphoid cells highly MHC class I, and therefore, the inhibitory signal is strong [117]. In addition, KIR ligand mismatch can lead to GvHD by CTLs as described above. In order to avoid this, ingenuity such as umbilical cord blood transplantation or the use of ATG may be necessary.

### *4.4.1. Donor selection based on inhibitory receptors*

There is a reason to expect the GVL effect in donor NK cells not receiving a KIR signal from the recipient HLA. The main inhibitory receptors are KIR2DL1, KIR2DL2/3, KIR3DL1, and KIR3DL2. There is no evidence that the effects of these four inhibitory receptors are identical. Particularly with regard to KIR3DL2, there are reports that the KIR-positive NK cells are not even licensed, even if the recipient has HLA-A3 or A11 (KIR3DL2 ligands) [118]. Most NK cell transplantations have been expected to provide a therapeutic effect due to missing self of KIR2DL1 or KIR2DL2/3, and the number of transplantations in which a therapeutic effect by missing self of KIR3DL1 have been expected is very low. There is no transplantation in which the therapeutic effect by missing self of KIR3DL2 alone is expected.

For example, if the recipient is HLA-C1/C1 if the KIR ligand mismatch model is used, an HLA-C1/C2 or HLA-C2/C2 donor would be selected. Even if transplantation is assessed using the receptor-ligand model, the donor's KIR is often unknown. However, in Japanese, most (approx. 99%) donors KIR2DL1 can be considered positive. If so, in the receptor-ligand model, it seems that any donor could be chosen, but NK cells derived from an HLA-C1/C1 donor may show a lower GVL effect. When the recipient is HLA-Bw6/Bw6, it must first be confirmed that all of the HLA-A23, -24 and -32 are negative, and then an HLA-Bw4-positive donor should be selected. However, since 7% of Japanese are negative for KIR3DL1 gene, it must be confirmed that KIR3DL1 is positive for the donor by flow cytometry, or that the genotype is either KIR3DL1*01502 or KIR3DL1*020.

### *4.4.2. Donor selection based on haplotypes*

It was reported that donors should be chosen for haplotype B when considering the activating receptors [34]. In that study, Cooley et al. analyzed 448 AML cases of NMDP, and they observed that the 3-year overall survival rate when the donor was haplotype BX was 31%, significantly higher than the rate of 20% when it was haplotype AA ($p < 0.01$). In addition, the recurrence decreases the most in cases that the donor had Cen-B/Cen-B, and it is reported that Tel-B also leads to a reduction of recurrence and improvement of prognosis [119].

Based on the data from three groups in the United States (Memphis, Sloan Kettering, Minnesota), Leung et al. advocated a donor selection algorithm for NK cells [120]; in the transplantation of T cells containing bone marrow or peripheral blood stem cells, donors should be HLA matches, and donors with KIR ligand mismatch should be avoided. Conversely, in

T cell-depleted transplantation or umbilical cord blood transplantation, a donor for a KIR ligand mismatch should be chosen. It is also recommended that a donor with KIR that can attack the recipient's HLA (possibly KIR haplotype B) be selected. In Japan as well, if KIR haplotype testing of the donor banks becomes possible in the future, or if the NK cell preparation is put to clinical use, it will be possible to test this algorithm described by Leung et al.

#### *4.4.3. Donor selection based on activating receptor*

KIR2DS1 is activated by HLA-C2. This means that if the recipient is positive for HLA-C2 and the donor is KIR2DS1-positive (Tel-B = haplotype BX), KIR2DS1-positive NK cells will be activated and will kill the recipient's tumor cells. In actual transplantation, when NK cells were cultured *in vitro* to examine the antitumor effect on leukemic cells of patients, KIR2DS1-positive NK cells killed tumor cells of recipients with HLA-C2 [121]. An analysis of the KIR gene of AML donors and recipients (1277 cases) from the U. S. NMDP and the Center for International blood and marrow transplant research (CIBMTR) provided large-scale proof using actual transplantations, and the report was published in *The New England Journal of Medicine* [122]. The analysis revealed that recurrence was significantly reduced when the donor had KIR2DS1 (26.5 vs. 32.5% (KIR2DS1-negative), $p = 0.02$). However, this effect was canceled when the donor was HLA-C2/C2. This is thought to be a disarming phenomenon, and it can be explained as follows: the HLA-C2/C2-derived KIR2DS1-positive clone is inactivated.

In that report [122], the proportion of donors with the KIR2DS1 gene was 33%. In the report by Yabe et al. [108], the KIR2DS1 gene-positive rate was 38%. Since Yabe et al. focused only on recipients of HLA-C2/C2, they did not analyze KIR2DS1-positive donors because the number of cases was too small. In addition, it was reported that when the donors had KIR3DS1, although a decrease in the recurrence rate was not observed, the mortality rate decreased slightly [122]. Yabe et al. also analyzed leukemia patients and reported that transplantation from KIR3DS1 donors reduced the rate of acute GvHD [123]. It was also reported that the likelihood of acute GvHD increases when the donor is haplotype AA [124, 125]. The mechanisms underlying KIR/HLA interactions remain unclear, but these reports may be a reference for donor selection.

### 4.5. Immune checkpoint inhibitors

#### *4.5.1. Checkpoint of NK cells*

Checkpoint inhibitors are an extremely promising approach among immunotherapies. Treatment with anti-CTLA4 or anti-PD-1 antibody restored the T-cell activity in cancer patients and resulted in tumor regression in several patients. A combination of both of the checkpoint inhibitors anti-CTLA4 and anti-PD-1 could further enhance therapeutic benefits [126, 127]. It has been shown that NK cells from patients with multiple myeloma and renal cancer express PD-1, the signal of which reduce the cytolytic activities of NK cells [128, 129]. Treatment using patient-derived PD-1$^+$ NK cells with the anti-PD-1 antibody (pidilizumab, CT-011) increased the NK cell-mediated killing of autologous cancer cells *in vitro* [128]. The therapeutic benefit of activating PD-1$^+$ NK cells in cancer patients is currently not well understood, and the major therapeutic effect is certainly due to the re-activation of exhausted T cells.

*4.5.2. Combination with a checkpoint inhibitor: expansion of the therapeutic spectrum*

A loss or down-regulation of HLA class I antigens in tumor cells has been frequently observed in a variety of human malignancies, and this represents an important cancer-immune escape mechanism [130–134]. Using a panel of monoclonal antibodies on tumor tissue sections, these loss or down-regulation has been found in 60–90% of tumors [135–140]. Early studies using immunohistological analyses of different tumors showed a very low frequency of allelic loss. However, with the arrival of other techniques, such as studies of microsatellites to detect the loss of heterozygosity (LOH) on chromosome 6, it has been shown that LOH (haplotype loss) is the most frequent alteration of HLA class I expression [139, 141–144]. This alteration is caused by various defects in the HLA genomic region (i.e., the short arm of chromosome 6, 6p21), including chromosomal dysfunction, mitotic recombination, and genetic conversion.

The nature of the antigens that allow the immune system to distinguish cancer cells from non-cancer cells has long remained obscure. Recent technological innovations have made it possible to dissect the immune response to patient-specific neoantigens that arise as a consequence of tumor-specific mutations, and emerging data suggest that the recognition of such neoantigens is a major factor in the activity of clinical immunotherapies. These observations indicate that the neoantigen load may form a biomarker in cancer immunotherapy and provide an incentive for the development of novel therapeutic approaches that selectively enhance T-cell reactivity against this class of antigens.

If there is a neoantigen that can be a target of CTL and the patient has MHC on which the antigen is presented, and if the MHC is not lost from the tumor cells, treatments using CTL as an effector (e.g., checkpoint inhibitors) may be effective. NK cells that preferentially kill tumor cells whose expression of MHC has decreased by MHC non-restriction are expected to have a synergistic effect with a checkpoint inhibitor.

## 5. Future directions

### 5.1. Genetic modification–Gene transfer to NK cells

In order to genetically modify NK cells, efficient methods for gene transduction into NK cells are necessary. To date, such methods include viral transduction, electroporation, and nucleofection [145]. Gene transfer to not only NK cell lines such as NK-92, but also primary NK cells has been conducted. Although various gene transfer efficiencies have been described, their transduction efficiency into NK cells is generally not high. Mainly retroviral vectors and lentiviral vectors are used for gene transfer. Since a retrovirus vector cannot transduce genes into non-dividing cells, such a vector is suitable for use with NK cell lines such as NK-92 cells. When a retrovirus vector is used for primary NK cells, it is necessary to amplify the NK cells, and the transduction timing is important.

In contrast, lentiviral vectors are capable of gene transfer into both dividing and non-dividing cells. The lentiviral vectors RD114, 10A1, GALV, and VSV-G are used for the envelope of the viral vector, and RD114 and VSV-G seem to be suitable. However, it has been reported that viral vectors are recognized by antiviral mechanisms such as intracellular pattern recognition receptors, and apoptosis is induced [146]. The introduction efficiency was therefore not high.

Efforts are underway to improve the transduction efficiency. For example, by using a cytokine combination (e.g., IL-2 + IL-15 or IL-2 + IL-21), the transduction efficiency into NK cells by VSV-G pseudotyped lentiviral vector was improved by approx. fivefold compared to single cytokine-stimulated NK cells [146]. In addition, inhibitors of intracellular antiviral responses were evaluated, and the results indicated that BX795 (an inhibitor of the TBK1/IKKe complex) improved the transduction efficiency by approx. 10-fold [146]. Guven et al. reported transduction into 75.4% of NK cells after 21 days of culture by a two-round transduction with the GALV-pseudotyped retroviral vector [147]. Further improvement of the transduction efficiency into NK cells by using viral vectors is desired.

In non-viral gene transfer, mainly electroporation has been studied. Electroporation is a method of physically pulling a minute hole in a cell membrane by applying an electric pulse to a cell suspension and sending the nucleic acids into the cells. The transfer of genes into NK cells using this method has been performed. High transfection efficiency and a high survival rate have been reported in both NK cell lines and primary NK cells. Much higher transfection efficiency was achieved using mRNA compared to using DNA [148–152]. Introduction by nucleofection has also been tried, but the efficiency was not high [153, 154].

In light of these reports, the transfection of mRNA by electroporation is considered to be an efficient method from the viewpoint of gene transfer into NK cells. Shimasaki and colleagues reported that NK cells transfected with mRNA encoding CD19-specific CAR (anti-CD19-4-1BB-CD3ζ) by electroporation showed enhanced cytotoxicity for tumors in animal models [154]. On the other hand, the transfection of mRNA can obtain transient gene expression. Further research is required to determine whether a treatment effect can be expected. When persistent gene expression is the goal, gene transfer by retroviral or lentiviral vectors is suitable.

It is necessary to select a suitable gene transfer method for the purpose of treatment. In any case, it is desirable to develop more efficient, simple, highly reproducible and clinically applicable gene transfer methods for NK cells.

### 5.2. Improved persistence of NK cells *in vivo*

As a strategy for the genetic modification of NK cells to improve their survival *in vivo*, methods for transducing cytokines such as IL-2 and IL-15 into NK cells have been reported, since it was demonstrated that a local administration of IL-2 resulted in enhanced functioning of NK cells [155, 156]. IL-15 has already been used in patients with metastatic melanoma and metastatic renal cell carcinoma, and it has been reported to induce the proliferation and clinical response of NK cells. Following these findings, attempts to introduce IL-2 and IL-15 genes into NK cells were reported. Nagashima et al. showed that the NK-92 cell line transduced with IL-2 genes with a retroviral vector propagated for >5 months irrespective of IL-2 and showed higher antitumor activity than the parental cell line *in vitro* and *in vivo* [157]. Imamura et al. showed that the transfection of membrane-bound IL-15 into human PBMC-derived NK cells using a retroviral vector resulted in the cells' survival for 2 months without the addition of cytokines *in vitro*, and that the cytotoxicity of the transduced NK cells was enhanced; moreover, the antitumor activity was observed in a mouse model [158].

Sahm et al. transduced IL-15 gene into NK-92 cells and observed cell proliferation in the absence of cytokines. They also showed that the co-transduction of an EpCAM-specific chimeric antigen receptor and IL-15 into NK-92 cells enhanced the specific and efficient cytotoxic activity [159]. Jiang et al. reported high cytotoxic activity of a human NK cell line (NKL) transduced with IL-15 *in vitro* against human hepatocellular carcinoma; the transduced NKL suppressed tumor growth and prolonged survival in human hepatocellular carcinoma-transplanted model mice [160]. These reports suggested that NK cells transduced IL-2 or IL-15 can proliferate sustainably *in vitro* and *in vivo*, which resulted in improved antitumor activity.

### 5.3. Improvement of homing

It was reported that NK cells expressed different chemokine receptors depending on the activating state [161, 162]. Proper homing to the tumor tissue is an important factor in eliciting the antitumor activity of NK cells. Carlsten et al. showed that *ex vivo* expanded NK cells derived from PBMCs transfected with CCR7 mRNA using electroporation migrated significantly to CCL19, a ligand of CCR7 [163]. Sonamshi et al. reported that NK cells transferred CCR7 protein from feeder cells using trogocytosis, but not genetic manipulation, promoted the migration to CCL19 and CCL21 *in vitro*, and that the NK cells were transferred to lymph nodes in a mouse model [101]. There are few reports of genetic modification targeting homing receptors, but further progress in this field is expected.

### 5.4. Improvement of tumor-specific cytotoxic activity

As an approach to enhance specificity to tumor cells, a technique using a chimeric antigen receptor (CAR) should be mentioned. CAR is a chimeric protein composed of a single-chain antibody (the antigen-specific binding site) in which a light chain and a heavy chain derived from a monoclonal antibody recognize a tumor cell surface antigen, a transmembrane domain, and an intracellular signal domain.

In the first-generation CARs, the intracytoplasmic signal domain is composed of only the CD3ζchain. In addition to CD3ζ, the second-generation CARs have another T cell costimulatory signal domain (CD28, 4–1BB, OX40, etc.), and the activation signal is efficiently transmitted. In the third-generation CARs, two or more costimulatory signal domains are inserted. CAR-introduced T cells have already been used clinically, and excellent results have been obtained in some cases [164–167]. One of the problems with CAR-T cell therapy is a serious side effect. CAR-T cells attack not only target cells but also non-target normal cells. For example, CD-19 CAR-T cells kill not only tumor cells but also normal B cells, which cause B-cell deficiency [168]. In HER2-specific CAR therapy for colorectal cancer with lung metastasis, death due to a pulmonary complication accompanied by high cytokinemia has been reported [169].

NK cells are an attractive alternative to T cells, as NK cells have the following advantages. HLA matching is not necessary, and NK cells are used as allogenic cells. Their lifespan is limited, and they can be expected to be excluded from the body before severe side effects occur, after they kill cancer cells. The reported CAR-NK cells are summarized in **Table 3**. NK cells transduced with CD19-CAR or CD20-CAR have been used when targeting B-cell malignancies. Bossel et al. showed that NK-92 cells transfected with anti-CD19-CAR by using electroporation had high cytotoxic activity against a $CD19^+$ cell line and primary chronic lymphocytic leukemia (CLL) [150]. They also showed that tumor cells can be eliminated in xenograft mouse models by using NK-92 cells transduced with anti-CD19 CAR with lentiviral vectors [170]. Imai et al. also showed that primary NK cells transduced with anti-CD19–CD3ζ with a retroviral vector killed $CD19^+$ cells and that the cytotoxicity was improved by adding a signaling domain of 4–1BB to anti-CD19–CD3ζ [171].

| NK cell type | Target antigen | Cancer | Co-stimulatory domain | Gene transfer method | Ref |
|---|---|---|---|---|---|
| NK-92 cell line | ErbB2 (HER-2) | Breast, ovarian carcinoma | CD3ζ | Retrovirus | [175] |
| NK-92 cell line | CD20 | B-ALL, CLL | CD3ζ | Retrovirus | [170] |
| NK-92 cell line | CD19 | B-ALL, CLL | CD3ζ | Electroporation (mRNA) | [151] |
| NK-92 cell line | EpCAM | Breast carcinoma | CD28/CD3ζ | Lentivirus | [160] |
| NK-92 cell line | HLA-A2 EBNA3C | EBV+ T-cell Lymphoma | CD28/CD3ζ | Retrovirus | [178] |
| NK-92 cell line | GD2 | Neuroblastoma | CD3ζ | Retrovirus | [179] |
| NK-92 cell line | CD19/CD20 | B-ALL, CLL | CD3ζ | Electroporation (plasmid DNA)<br>Lentivirus | [180] |
| NK-92 cell line | CD19/CD20 | B-ALL, CLL | CD3ζ | Lentivirus | [68] |
| NK-92 cell line | CS1 | Multiple myeloma. | CD28/CD3ζ | Lentivirus | [181] |
| NK-92 cell line | CD138 | Multiple myeloma | CD3ζ | Lentivirus | [182] |
| NK-92 cell line | ErbB2 (HER-2) | Breast carcinoma | CD28/CD3 | Electroporation (plasmid DNA) | [176] |
| NK-92 cell line | ErbB2 (HER-2) | Breast, ovarian and renal cell carcinoma | CD3ζ<br>CD28/CD3ζ<br>CD137/CD3ζ | Lentivirus | [183] |
| YTS cell line | PSCA | Prostate cancer | CD3ζ<br>DAP12 TM and signaling | Lentivirus | [184] |
| YT cell line | CD33 | AML | CD3ζ | Electroporation (plasmid DNA) | [150] |

| NK cell type | Target antigen | Cancer | Co-stimulatory domain | Gene transfer method | Ref |
|---|---|---|---|---|---|
| YT cell line | CEA | Colon carcinoma | CD3ζ | Electroporation (plasmid DNA) | [148] |
| PBMC-NK | CD19 | B-ALL, CLL | CD3ζ | Retrovirus | [171] |
| | | | DAP10 | | |
| | | | CD137/CD3ζ | | |
| PBMC-NK | ErbB2 (HER-2) | Breast, ovarian and renal cell carcinoma | CD28/CD3ζ | Retrovirus | [174] |
| PBMC-NK | CD19/GD2 | | CD3ζ or 2B4 alone | Retrovirus | [185] |
| | | | 2B4/CD3ζ | | |
| | | | CD137/CD3ζ | | |
| PBMC-NK | CD19 | B-ALL, CLL | CD137/CD3ζ | Electroporation(mRNA) | [152] |
| PBMC-NK | CD20 | B-ALL, CLL | CD137/CD3ζ | Electroporation(mRNA) | [186] |
| PBMC-NK | NKG2D ligands | wide range | CD3ζ (with DAP10) | Retrovirus<br>Electroporation(mRNA) | [177] |

**Table 3.** CAR-NK cells.

The gene human epidermal growth factor receptor 2 (HER2) is overexpressed in many breast cancers and is correlated with disease progression [172, 173]. It is therefore considered one of the suitable targets of CAR. Kruschinski et al. transduced anti-HER2–CD28-CD3ζ into human primary NK cells using a retroviral vector, and the results demonstrated cytotoxicity to an HER2⁺ cell line. This cytotoxicity was correlated with the HER2 expression level on target cells [174]. Uherek et al. reported that anti-HER2–CD3ζ-CAR retrovirally transduced NK-92 cells efficiently killed cell lines derived from ErbB2-positive breast carcinoma, ovarian carcinoma, and squamous cell carcinoma *in vitro* and *in vivo* [175]. In a study by Liu et al., the plasmid coding anti-HER2–CD28-CD3ζCAR was transfected into NK-92 cells by electroporation, and the cells specifically killed the ErbB2-expressing human breast cancer cell lines MDA-MB-453 and SKBr3. The adoptive transfer of NK-92 cells specifically reduced the tumor size and lung metastasis of nude mice transplanted with MDA-MB-453 cells and significantly prolonged the survival of these mice [176].

As shown in **Table 3**, CAR against various tumor-associated antigens (TAA) has also been evaluated in NK cells. Chang et al. reported a modification by CAR using NKG2D, one of the human NK cell activating receptors, instead of the antigen-binding site of the antibody. Since NKG2D can bind to eight types of ligands expressed in solid tumors and blood tumors, it can be applied to a broader range of tumor cells. Primary human NK cells were transduced with a retroviral vector, using constructs designed to combine the extracellular domain of NKG2D with CD3ζ and further to express DAP10 simultaneously. This approach showed strong cytotoxic activity against various tumor cell lines and showed no damage to normal cells. It also showed strong tumor growth suppression in a mouse model of osteosarcoma [177].

## 6. Conclusions

Because NK cells are difficult to culture and it is a challenge to transduce foreign genes into NK cells, research concerning NK cells has been delayed compared to research involving T cells. However, culture and gene transfer technologies for NK cells are now developing. As introduced here, genetically modified NK cells acquired enhanced antitumor functions. These NK cells are very intriguing and are expected to be revolutionary cellular medicines for the treatment of malignancies.

NK cells are heterogeneous populations that exhibit various maturation stages and different KIR expression patterns. Since this heterogeneity has not been completely elucidated, it is not easy to choose the appropriate subset of NK cells for cancer treatment. Although allogeneic NK cell therapy using a KIR mismatch shows a strong antitumor effect against several blood cancers, the mechanisms underlying the activation and maintenance of NK cells in cancer patients are not completely understood. Cancer patients usually undergo a variety

| | Gamida Cell Lth. | Nant Kwest Inc. | Glycostem Therapeutics | GreenCross LabCell | Fate Therapeutics Inc. | GAIA BioMedicine Inc. |
|---|---|---|---|---|---|---|
| **H.Q.** | Israel | USA | Netherlands | Korea | USA | Japan |
| **Auto/Allo** | ??? | Allogeneic (Cell line) | Allogeneic | Allogeneic (Health donor) | Allogeneic | Allogeneic (Haploidentical) |
| **Materials** | PBMC/BM/ CB | NK-92 | CB CD34+ (CliniMACS) | PBMC | PBMC (CMV+ donnor)/iPS | PBMC(CliniMACS Prodigy) |
| **Feeder cell** | – | – | – | Irradiated (2000 rad) PBMC | – | – |
| **Irradiation** | – | Before administration | – | – | – | – |
| **Purity** | >97% (CD3–/ CD56+) | – | >98.1 ± 0.88% (CD3–/CD56+) | >98.1 ± 0.88% (CD3–/CD56+) | >90.9 ± 2.2% (CD3–/ CD56+) | >98.0% (CD3-/ CD56+) |
| **K562 killing** | E:T=1:1, 40–50% | E:T=5:1 (4 hr), 50% | E:T=2:1 (4 hr), 40% | E:T=10:1 (4 hr), 70–80% | – | E:T=1:1 (2 hr), >80% |
| **Handling** | CPC | Wash, Irradiation, CPC | CPC | CPC | CPC | Completely closed system |
| **Companion diagnosis** | – | – | – | – | – | HLA/KIR selection |
| **R & D Phase** | Non-clinical(Phase I/II in 2017) | Phase II | Phase I | Phase II | Non-clinical(Phase I in 2017) | Non-clinical(Phase I in 2017) |
| **Target disease** | - | Merkel cell carcinoma | AML | Hepatocellular carcinoma | AML | NSCLC, Neuroblastoma |

**Table 4.** Products of NK cells for clinical use.

of standard treatments before receiving immunotherapy, and it is important to understand the factors that influence NK cell activity in order to select the correct clinical setting for NK cell therapy. In this review, we have explained the combination with antibodies, the genetic modification technique, and the KIR mismatch pattern (which is the basis of patient selection) that has been tested to maximize the use of NK cells as a treatment for cancer. Products of NK cells for clinical use that have been developed worldwide are shown in **Table 4**.

Advances in the understanding of NK cells may also lead to the development of small-molecule inhibitors targeting intracellular signals. Because NK cells are difficult to handle, their development is delayed compared to several other immunotherapies, but it is highly likely that they will be established as innovative cell therapy in the near future.

## Conflicts of interest

Y. Harada is a member of the Scientific Advisory Boards of GAIA BioMedicine Inc. K. Teraishi is a researcher from Ono Pharmaceutical Co., Ltd. H Ban is a researcher from GAIA BioMedicine Inc. Y. Yonemitsu is a member of the Board of Directors on Science and Medicine at GAIA BioMedicine Inc.

## Author details

Yui Harada[1,2]*, Koji Teraishi[1,3], Minori Ishii[1,4], Hiroshi Ban[1,2] and Yoshikazu Yonemitsu[1,2]

*Address all correspondence to: rkfraile@med.kyushu-u.ac.jp

1 R&D Laboratory for Innovative Biotherapeutics, Graduate School of Pharmaceutical Sciences, Kyushu University, Fukuoka, Japan

2 GAIA BioMedicine, Inc., Tokyo, Japan

3 Ono Pharmaceutical Co., Ltd., Osaka, Japan

4 Department of Pediatric Surgery, Faculty of Medical Sciences, Kyushu University, Fukuoka, Japan

## References

[1] Alici E, Konstantinidis KV, Sutlu T et al. Anti-myeloma activity of endogenous and adoptively transferred activated natural killer cells in experimental multiple myeloma model. Experimental Hematology. 2007;**35**(12):1839-1846. DOI: 10.1016/j.exphem.2007.08.006

[2] Basse PH, Whiteside TL, Herberman RB. Cancer immunotherapy with interleukin-2-activated natural killer cells. Molecular Biotechnology. 2002;**21**(2):161-170. DOI: 10.1385/MB:21:2:161

[3] Siegler U, Kalberer CP, Nowbakht P, Sendelov S, Meyer-Monard S, Wodnar-Filipowicz A. Activated natural killer cells from patients with acute myeloid leukemia are cytotoxic against autologous leukemic blasts in NOD/SCID mice. Leukemia. 2005;**19**(12):2215-2222. DOI: 10.1038/sj.leu.2403985

[4] Torelli GF, Rozera C, Santodonato L et al. A good manufacturing practice method to ex vivo expand natural killer cells for clinical use. Blood Transfusion. 2015;**13**(3):464-471. DOI: 10.2450/2015.0231-14

[5] Miller JS, Soignier Y, Panoskaltsis-mortari A, et al. Successful adoptive transfer and in vivo expansion of human haploidentical NK cells in patients with cancer. Cancer. 2005;**105**(8):3051-3057. DOI: 10.1182/blood-2004-07-2974.Supported

[6] Ishikawa E, Tsuboi K, Saijo K, et al. Autologous natural killer cell therapy for human recurrent malignant glioma. Anticancer Research. 2004;**24**(3 B):1861-1871

[7] Rubnitz JE, Inaba H, Ribeiro RC et al. NKAML: A pilot study to determine the safety and feasibility of haploidentical natural killer cell transplantation in childhood acute myeloid leukemia. Journal of Clinical Oncology. 2010;**28**(6):955-959. DOI: 10.1200/JCO.2009.24.4590

[8] Carlens S, Gilljam M, Chambers BJ, et al. A new method for in vitro expansion of cytotoxic human CD3–CD56+ natural killer cells. Human Immunology. 2001;**62**(10):1092-1098. DOI: 10.1016/S0198-8859(01)00313-5

[9] Alici E, Sutlu T, Bjo B. et al. Autologous antitumor activity by NK cells expanded from myeloma patients using GMP-compliant components. Blood. 2008;**111**(6):3155-3163. DOI: 10.1182/blood-2007-09-110312

[10] Sutlu T, Stellan B, Gilljam M. et al. Clinical-grade, large-scale, feeder-free expansion of highly active human natural killer cells for adoptive immunotherapy using an automated bioreactor. Cytotherapy. 2010;**12**(8):1044-1055. DOI: 10.3109/14653249.2010.504770

[11] Bachanova V, Linda J. Burns DHM. Allogeneic natural killer cells for refractory. Cancer Immunology, Immunotherapy. 2010;**59**(11):1739-1744. DOI: 10.1007/s00262-010-0896-z. ALLOGENEIC

[12] Koehl U, Brehm C, Huenecke S. et al. Clinical grade purification and expansion of NK cell products for an optimized manufacturing protocol. Frontiers in Oncology. 2013;**3**. DOI: 10.3389/fonc.2013.00118

[13] Saito S, Harada Y, Morodomi Y. et al. Ex vivo generation of highly purified and activated natural killer cells from human peripheral blood. Human Gene Therapy Methods. 2013;**24**(4):241-252. DOI: 10.1089/hgtb.2012.183

[14] Anfossi N, André P, Guia S, et al. Human NK cell education by inhibitory receptors for MHC class I. Immunity. 2006;**25**(2):331-342. DOI: 10.1016/j.immuni.2006.06.013

[15] Lucas M, Schachterle W, Oberle K, Aichele P, Andreas D. Natural killer cell-mediated control of infections requires production of interleukin 15 by Type I IFN-triggered dendritic cells. Immunity. 2007;**26**:503-517. DOI: 10.1016/j.biotechadv.2011.08.021.Secreted

[16] Mortier E, Advincula R, Kim L, et al. Macrophage- and dendritic-cell-derived interleukin-15 receptor alpha supports homeostasis of distinct CD8+ T cell subsets. Immunity. 2009;**31**(5):811-822. DOI: 10.1016/j.immuni.2009.09.017

[17] Brehm C, Huenecke S, Quaiser A, et al. IL-2 stimulated but not unstimulated NK cells induce selective disappearance of peripheral blood cells: Concomitant results to a phase I/II study. PLoS One. 2011;**6**(11). DOI: 10.1371/journal.pone.0027351

[18] Guia S, Cognet C, de Beaucoudrey L, et al. A role for interleukin-12/23 in the maturation of human natural killer and CD56+ T cells in vivo. Blood. 2008;**111**(10):5008-5016. DOI: 10.1182/blood-2007-11-122259

[19] Chaix J, Tessmer MS, Hoebe K, et al. Priming of natural killer cells by Interleukin-18. J Immunol. 2008;**181**(3):1627-1631

[20] Lapteva N, Durett AG, Sun J, et al. Large-scale ex vivo expansion and characterization of natural killer cells for clinical applications. Cytotherapy. 2012;**14**(9):1131-1143. DOI: 10.3109/14653249.2012.700767

[21] Cooper MA, Bush JE, Fehniger TA. et al. In vivo evidence for a dependence on interleukin 15 for survival of natural killer cells. Blood. 2002;**100**(10):3633-3638. DOI: 10.1182/blood-2001-12-0293

[22] Dahlberg CIM, Sarhan D, Chrobok M, Duru AD, Alici E. Natural killer cell-based therapies targeting cancer: Possible strategies to gain and sustain anti-tumor activity. Frontiers in Immunology. 2015;**6**(NOV). DOI: 10.3389/fimmu.2015.00605

[23] Rham de C, Ferrari-Lacraz S, Jendly S, Schneiter G, et al. The proinflammatory cytokines IL-2, IL-15 and IL-21 modulate the repertoire of mature human natural killer cell receptors. Arthritis Research & Therapy. 2007;**9**:R125. DOI: 10.1186/ar2336

[24] Berg M, Lundqvist A, McCoy P, et al. Clinical-grade ex vivo-expanded human natural killer cells up-regulate activating receptors and death receptor ligands and have enhanced cytolytic activity against tumor cells. Cytotherapy. 2009;**11**(3):341-355. DOI: 10.1080/14653240902807034

[25] Ljunggren HG, Kärre K. In search of the "missing self": MHC molecules and NK cell recognition. Immunology Today. 1990;**11**(C):237-244. DOI: 10.1016/0167-5699(90)90097-S

[26] Hudson LE, Allen RL. Leukocyte Ig-like receptors—A model for MHC class I disease associations. Frontiers in Immunology. 2016;**7**(JUL):1-8. DOI: 10.3389/fimmu.2016.00281

[27] Chester C, Fritsch K, Kohrt HE. Natural killer cell immunomodulation: Targeting activating, inhibitory, and co-stimulatory receptor signaling for cancer immunotherapy. Frontiers in Immunology. 2015;**6**(DEC):1-9. DOI: 10.3389/fimmu.2015.00601

[28] Vivier E, Raulet D, Moretta A, Caligiuri M. Innate or adaptive immunity? The example of natural killer cells. Science (80). 2011;**331**(6013):44-49. DOI: 10.1126/science.1198687.Innate

[29] Vivier E, Nunes JA, Vely F. Natural killer cell signaling pathways. Science. 2004;**306**(5701): 1517-1519. DOI: 306/5701/1517 [pii]\n10.1126/science.1103478

[30] Holmes TD, El-Sherbiny YM, Davison A, Clough SL, Blair GE, Cook GP. A human NK cell activation/inhibition threshold allows small changes in the target cell surface phenotype to dramatically alter susceptibility to NK cells. The Journal of Immunology. 2011;**186**(3):1538-1545. DOI: 10.4049/jimmunol.1000951

[31] Varbanova V, Naumova E, Mihaylova A. Killer-cell immunoglobulin-like receptor genes and ligands and their role in hematologic malignancies. Cancer Immunology, Immunotherapy. 2016;**65**(4):427-440. DOI: 10.1007/s00262-016-1806-9

[32] Wilson MJ, Torkar M, Haude A et al. Plasticity in the organization and sequences of human KIR/ILT gene families. Proceedings of the National Academy of Sciences USA. 2000;**97**(9):4778-4783. DOI: 10.1073/pnas.080588597

[33] Hsu KC, Chida S, Geraghty DE, Dupont B. The killer cell immunoglobulin-like receptor (KIR) genomic region: Gene-order, haplotypes and allelic polymorphism. Immunological Reviews. 2002;**190**:40-52. DOI: imr19004 [pii]

[34] Cooley S, Trachtenberg E, Bergemann TL, et al. Donors with group B KIR haplotypes improve relapse-free survival after unrelated hematopoietic cell transplantation for acute myelogenous leukemia. Blood. 2009;**113**(3):726-732. DOI: 10.1182/blood-2008-07-171926

[35] Symons HJ, Leffell MS, Rossiter ND, Zahurak M, Jones RJ, Fuchs EJ. Transplantation. Blood. 2011;**16**(4):533-542. DOI: 10.1016/j.bbmt.2009.11.022.Improved

[36] Leung W, Handgretinger R, Iyengar R, Turner V, Holladay MS, Hale Ga. Inhibitory KIR-HLA receptor-ligand mismatch in autologous haematopoietic stem cell transplantation for solid tumour and lymphoma. British Journal of Cancer. 2007;**97**(4):539-542. DOI: 10.1038/sj.bjc.6603913

[37] Colonna M, Borsellino G, Falco M, Ferrara GB, Strominger JL. HLA-C is the inhibitory ligand that determines dominant resistance to lysis by NK1- and NK2-specific natural killer cells. Proceedings of the National Academy of Sciences USA. 1993;**90**(24):12000-12004. DOI: 10.1073/pnas.90.24.12000

[38] Moesta AK, Norman PJ, Yawata M, Yawata N, Gleimer M, Parham P. Synergistic polymorphism at two positions distal to the ligand-binding site makes KIR2DL2 a stronger receptor for HLA-C than KIR2DL3. The Journal of Immunology. 2008;**180**(6):3969-3979. DOI: 10.4049/JIMMUNOL.180.6.3969

[39] Yawata M, Yawata N, Draghi M, Little A-M, Partheniou F, Parham P. Roles for HLA and KIR polymorphisms in natural killer cell repertoire selection and modulation of effector function. The Journal of Experimental Medicine. 2006;**203**(3):633-645. DOI: 10.1084/jem.20051884

[40] Dohring C, Scheidegger D, Samaridis J, Cella M, Colonna M. A human killer inhibitory receptor specific for HLA-A1, 2. The Journal of Immunology. 1996;**156**(9):3098-3101. http://www.ncbi.nlm.nih.gov/entrez/query.fcgi?cmd=Retrieve&db=PubMed&dopt=Citation&list_uids=8617928

[41] Hilton HG, Guethlein LA, Goyos A, et al. Polymorphic HLA-C receptors balance the functional characteristics of KIR haplotypes. The Journal of Immunology. 2015;**195**:3160-3170. DOI: 10.4049/jimmunol.1501358

[42] Smyth MJ, Cretney E, Kelly JM, et al. Activation of NK cell cytotoxicity. Molecular Immunology. 2005;**42**(4 SPEC. ISS.):501-510. DOI: 10.1016/j.molimm.2004.07.034

[43] Ikner A, Ashkenazi A. TWEAK induces apoptosis through a death-signaling complex comprising receptor-interacting protein 1 (RIP1), Fas-associated death domain (FADD), and caspase-8. The Journal of Biological Chemistry. 2011;**286**(24):21546-21554. DOI: 10.1074/jbc.M110.203745

[44] Degli-Esposti M. To die or not to die—the quest of the TRAIL receptors. Journal of Leukocyte Biology. 1999;**65**(5):535-542. http://www.ncbi.nlm.nih.gov/pubmed/10331480

[45] Smyth MJ, Takeda K, Hayakawa Y, Peschon JJ, van den Brink MR., Yagita H. Nature's TRAIL—On a Path to Cancer Immunotherapy. Immunity. 2003;**18**(1):1-6. DOI: 10.1016/S1074-7613(02)00502-2

[46] Wajant H, Moosmayer D, Wüest T, et al. Differential activation of TRAIL-R1 and -2 by soluble and membrane TRAIL allows selective surface antigen-directed activation of TRAIL-R2 by a soluble TRAIL derivative. Oncogene. 2001;**20**(30):4101-4106. DOI: 10.1038/sj.onc.1204558

[47] Guicciardi ME, Gores GJ. Life and death by death receptors. The FASEB Journal. 2009;**23**(6):1625-1637. DOI: 10.1096/fj.08-111005

[48] Griffith BTS, Wiley SR, Kubin MZ, Sedger LM, Maliszewski CR, Fanger N. A necrosis factor- related cytokine, TRAIL. Cell. 1999;**189**(8)

[49] Fanger NA, Maliszewski CR, Schooley K, Griffith TS. Human dendritic cells mediate cellular apoptosis via tumor necrosis factor-related apoptosis-inducing ligand (TRAIL). The Journal of Experimental Medicine. 1999;**190**(8):1155-1164. DOI: 10.1084/jem.190.8.1155

[50] Smyth MJ, Cretney E, Takeda K. et al. Tumor necrosis factor-related apoptosis-inducing ligand (TRAIL) contributes to interferon gamma-dependent natural killer cell protection from tumor metastasis. The Journal of Experimental Medicine. 2001;**193**(6):661-670. DOI: 10.1084/jem.193.6.661

[51] Screpanti V, Wallin RPA, Grandien A, Ljunggren HG. Impact of FASL-induced apoptosis in the elimination of tumor cells by NK cells. Molecular Immunology. 2005;**42**(4 SPEC. ISS.):495-499. DOI: 10.1016/j.molimm.2004.07.033

[52] Wallin RPA, Screpanti V, Michaëlsson J, Grandien A, Ljunggren HG. Regulation of perforin-independent NK cell-mediated cytotoxicity. European Journal of Immunology. 2003;**33**(10):2727-2735. DOI: 10.1002/eji.200324070

[53] Reichmann E. The biological role of the Fas/FasL system during tumor formation and progression. Seminars in Cancer Biology. 2002;**12**:309-315

[54] Voskoboinik I, Whisstock JC, Trapani Ja. Perforin and granzymes: function, dysfunction and human pathology. Nature Reviews Immunology. 2015;**15**(6):388-400. DOI: 10.1038/nri3839

[55] Wulfing C, Purtic B, Klem J, Schatzle JD. Stepwise cytoskeletal polarization as a series of checkpoints in innate but not adaptive cytolytic killing. Proceedings of the National Academy of Sciences USA. 2003;**100**(13):7767-7772. DOI: 10.1073/pnas.1336920100

[56] DiPersio JF, Uy GL, Yasothan U. et al. Plerixafor. Nature Reviews Drug Discovery. 2009;**8**(2):105-106. DOI: 10.1038/nrd2819

[57] DiPersio JF, Micallef IN, Stiff PJ, et al. Phase III prospective randomized double-blind placebo-controlled trial of plerixafor plus granulocyte colony-stimulating factor compared with placebo plus granulocyte colony-stimulating factor for autologous stem-cell mobilization and transplantation for patients with non-Hodgkin's lymphoma. Journal of Clinical Oncology. 2009;**27**(28):4767-73. DOI: 10.1200/JCO.2008.20.7209

[58] Nademanee AP, DiPersio JF, Maziarz RT, et al. Plerixafor plus granulocyte colony-stimulating factor versus placebo plus granulocyte colony-stimulating factor for mobilization of CD34(+) hematopoietic stem cells in patients with multiple myeloma and low peripheral blood CD34(+) cell count: results of a subset analysis of a randomized trial. Biology of Blood and Marrow Transplantation. 2012;**18**(10):1564-1572. DOI: 10.1016/j.bbmt.2012.05.017

[59] Gabrilovich DI, Nagaraj S. Myeloid-derived suppressor cells as regulators of the immune system. Nature Reviews Immunology. 2009;**9**(3):162-174. DOI: 10.1038/nri2506

[60] Luyckx A, Schouppe E, Rutgeerts O, et al. G-CSF stem cell mobilization in human donors induces polymorphonuclear and mononuclear myeloid-derived suppressor cells. Clinical Immunology. 2012;**143**(1):83-87. DOI: 10.1016/j.clim.2012.01.011

[61] Gluckman E, Broxmeyer HA, Auerbach AD. et al. Hematopoietic reconstitution in a patient with Fanconi's anemia by means of umbilical-cord blood from an HLA-identical sibling. The New England Journal of Medicine. 1989;**321**(17):1174-1178. DOI: 10.1056/NEJM198910263211707

[62] Eapen M, Rubinstein P, Zhang MJ. et al. Outcomes of transplantation of unrelated donor umbilical cord blood and bone marrow in children with acute leukaemia: a comparison study. Lancet. 2007;**369**(9577):1947-1954. DOI: 10.1016/S0140-6736(07)60915-5

[63] Atsuta Y, Suzuki R, Nagamura-Inoue T, et al. Disease-specific analyses of unrelated cord blood transplantation compared with unrelated bone marrow transplantation in adult patients with acute leukemia. Blood. 2009;**113**(8):1631-1638. DOI: 10.1182/blood-2008-03-147041

[64] Takahashi S, Ooi J, Tomonari A, et al. Comparative single-institute analysis of cord blood transplantation from unrelated donors with bone marrow or peripheral blood stem-cell transplants from related donors in adult patients with hematologic malignancies after myeloablative conditioning regimen. Blood. 2007;**109**(3):1322-1330. DOI: 10.1182/blood-2006-04-020172

[65] Woll PS, Martin CH, Miller JS. et al. Human embryonic stem cell-derived NK cells acquire functional receptors and cytolytic activity. The Journal of Immunology. 2005;**175**(8):5095-5103

[66] Woll PS, Grzywacz B, Tian X. et al. Human embryonic stem cells differentiate into a homogeneous population of natural killer cells with potent in vivo antitumor activity. Blood. 2009;**113**(24):6094-6101. DOI: 10.1182/blood-2008-06-165225

[67] Rezvani K, Rouce RH. The application of natural killer cell immunotherapy for the treatment of cancer. Frontiers in Immunology. 2015;**6**:578. DOI: 10.3389/fimmu.2015.00578

[68] Boissel L, Betancur-Boissel M, Lu W. et al. Retargeting NK-92 cells by means of CD19- and CD20-specific chimeric antigen receptors compares favorably with antibody-dependent cellular cytotoxicity. Oncoimmunology. 2013;**2**(10): e26527. DOI: 10.4161/onci.26527

[69] Hermanson DL, Kaufman DS. Utilizing chimeric antigen receptors to direct natural killer cell activity. Frontiers in Immunology. 2015;**6**:195. DOI: 10.3389/fimmu.2015.00195

[70] Gong JH, Maki G, Klingemann HG. Characterization of a human cell line (NK-92) with phenotypical and functional characteristics of activated natural killer cells. Leukemia. 1994;**8**(4):652-658

[71] Yan Y, Steinherz P, Klingemann HG. et al. Antileukemia activity of a natural killer cell line against human leukemias. Clinical Cancer Research. 1998;**4**(11):2859-2868

[72] Jochems C, Hodge JW, Fantini M. et al. An NK cell line (haNK) expressing high levels of granzyme and engineered to express the high affinity CD16 allele. Oncotarget. 2016;**7**(52):86359-86373. DOI: 10.18632/oncotarget.13411

[73] Klingemann HG, Martinson J. Ex vivo expansion of natural killer cells for clinical applications. Cytotherapy. 2004;**6**(1):15-22. DOI: 10.1080/14653240310004548

[74] Iliopoulou EG, Kountourakis P, Karamouzis MV. et al. A phase I trial of adoptive transfer of allogeneic natural killer cells in patients with advanced non-small cell lung cancer. Cancer Immunology, Immunotherapy. 2010;**59**(12):1781-1789. DOI: 10.1007/s00262-010-0904-3

[75] Yoon SR, Lee YS, Yang SH. et al. Generation of donor natural killer cells from CD34(+) progenitor cells and subsequent infusion after HLA-mismatched allogeneic hematopoietic cell transplantation: a feasibility study. Bone Marrow Transplant Centre. 2010;**45**(6):1038-1046. DOI: 10.1038/bmt.2009.304

[76] Ozaki K, Kikly K, Michalovich D. et al. Cloning of a type I cytokine receptor most related to the IL-2 receptor beta chain. Proceedings of the National Academy of Sciences U S A. 2000;**97**(21):11439-11444. DOI: 10.1073/pnas.200360997

[77] Parrish-Novak J, Dillon SR, Nelson A. et al. Interleukin 21 and its receptor are involved in NK cell expansion and regulation of lymphocyte function. Nature. 2000;**408**(6808):57-63. DOI: 10.1038/35040504

[78] Leonard WJ, Spolski R. Interleukin-21: a modulator of lymphoid proliferation, apoptosis and differentiation. Nature Reviews Immunology. 2005;**5**(9):688-698. DOI: 10.1038/nri1688

[79] Shruti Bhatt, Julie Matthews, Salma Parvin. et al. Direct and immune-mediated cytotoxicity of interleukin-21 contributes to antitumor effects in mantle cell lymphoma. Blood. 2015;**126**(13):1555-1564. DOI: 10.1182/blood-2015-01-624585

[80] Miller JS, Oelkers S, Verfaillie C. et al. Role of monocytes in the expansion of human activated natural killer cells. Blood. 1992;**80**(9):2221-2229

[81] Boissel L, Tuncer HH, Betancur M. et al. Umbilical cord mesenchymal stem cells increase expansion of cord blood natural killer cells. Biology of Blood and Marrow Transplantation. 2008;**14**(9):1031-1038. DOI: 10.1016/j.bbmt.2008.06.016

[82] Shah N, Martin-Antonio B, Yang H. et al. Antigen presenting cell-mediated expansion of human umbilical cord blood yields log-scale expansion of natural killer cells with anti-myeloma activity. PLoS One. 2013;**8**(10):e76781. DOI: 10.1371/journal.pone.0076781

[83] Granzin M, Soltenborn S, Müller S. et al. Fully automated expansion and activation of clinical-grade natural killer cells for adoptive immunotherapy. Cytotherapy. 2015;**17**(5):621-632. DOI: 10.1016/j.jcyt.2015.03.611

[84] Geraghty RJ, Capes-Davis A, Davis JM. et al. Guidelines for the use of cell lines in biomedical research. British Journal of Cancer. 2014;**111**(6):1021-1046. DOI: 10.1038/bjc.2014.166

[85] Spanholtz J, Preijers F, Tordoir M. et al. Clinical-grade generation of active NK cells from cord blood hematopoietic progenitor cells for immunotherapy using a closed-system culture process. PLoS One. 2011;**6**(6):e20740. DOI: 10.1016/j.msard.2012.01.001

[86] Knorr DA, Ni Z, Hermanson D. et al. Clinical-scale derivation of natural killer cells from human pluripotent stem cells for cancer therapy. Stem Cells Translational Medicine. 2013;**2**(4):274-283. DOI: 10.5966/sctm.2012-0084

[87] Krause SW, Gastpar R, Andreesen R. et al. Treatment of colon and lung cancer patients with ex vivo heat shock protein 70-peptide-activated, autologous natural killer cells: A clinical phase 1 trial. Clinical Cancer Research. 2004;**10**(11):3699-3707. DOI: 10.1158/1078-0432.CCR-03-0683

[88] Parkhurst MR, Riley JP, Dudley ME. et al. Adoptive transfer of autologous natural killer cells leads to high levels of circulating natural killer cells but does not mediate tumor regression. Clinical Cancer Research. 2011;**17**(19):6287-6297. DOI: 10.1158/1078-0432.CCR-11-1347

[89] Sakamoto N, Ishikawa T, Kokura S. et al. Phase I clinical trial of autologous NK cell therapy using novel expansion method in patients with advanced digestive cancer. Journal of Translational Medicine. 2015;**13**:277. DOI: 10.1186/s12967-015-0632-8

[90] Koehl U, Sörensen J, Esser R. et al. IL-2 activated NK cell immunotherapy of three children after haploidentical stem cell transplantation. Blood Cells, Molecules and Diseases. 2004;**33**(3):261-266. DOI: 10.1016/j.bcmd.2004.08.013

[91] Shah NN, Baird K, Delbrook CP. et al. Acute GVHD in patients receiving IL-15/4-1BBL activated NK cells following T-cell-depleted stem cell transplantation. Blood. 2015;**125**(5):784-792. DOI: 10.1182/blood-2014-07-592881

[92] Lanier LL, Ruitenberg JJ, Phillips JH. Functional and biochemical-analysis of Cd16 antigen on natural-killer cells and granulocytes. The Journal of Immunology. 1988;**141**(10):3478-3485

[93] Morel PA, Ernst LK, Metes D. Functional CD32 molecules on human NK cells. Leukemia & Lymphoma. 1999;**35**(1-2):47-56. DOI: 10.3109/10428199909145704

[94] Bruhns P, Iannascoli B, England P. et al. Specificity and affinity of human Fc gamma receptors and their polymorphic variants for human IgG subclasses. Blood. 2009;**113**(16):3716-3725. DOI: 10.1182/Blood-2008-09-179754

[95] Hogarth PM, Pietersz GA. Fc receptor-targeted therapies for the treatment of inflammation, cancer and beyond. Nature Reviews Drug Discovery. 2012;**11**(4):311-331. DOI: 10.1038/nrd2909

[96] Breunis WB, Van Mirre E, Geissler J. et al. Copy number variation at the FCGR locus includes FCGR3A, FCGR2C and FCGR3B but not FCGR2A and FCGR2B. Human Mutation. 2009;**30**(5):E640-E650. DOI: 10.1002/humu.20997

[97] Wang W, Erbe AK, Hank JA. et al. NK cell-mediated antibody-dependent cellular cytotoxicity in cancer immunotherapy. Frontiers in Immunology. 2015;**6**:368. DOI: 10.3389/fimmu.2015.00368

[98] Cartron G, Dacheux L, Salles G. et al. Therapeutic activity of humanized anti-CD20 monoclonal antibody and polymorphism in IgG Fc receptor FcgammaRIIIa gene. Blood. 2002;**99**(3):754-758

[99] Weng WK, Levy R. Two immunoglobulin G fragment C receptor polymorphisms independently predict response to rituximab in patients with follicular lymphoma. Journal of Clinical Oncology. 2003;**21**(21):3940-3947. DOI: 10.1200/JCO.2003.05.013

[100] Binyamin L, Alpaugh RK, Hughes TL. et al. Blocking NK cell inhibitory self-recognition promotes antibody-dependent cellular cytotoxicity in a model of anti-lymphoma therapy. The Journal of Immunology. 2008;**180**(9):6392-6401. DOI: 10.4049/jimmunol.180.9.6392

[101] Carlsten M, Levy E, Karambelkar A. et al. Efficient mRNA-Based genetic engineering of human NK cells with high-affinity CD16 and CCR7 augments rituximab-induced ADCC against lymphoma and targets NK Cell migration toward the lymph node-associated chemokine CCL19. Frontiers in Immunology. 2016;**7**:105. DOI: 10.3389/fimmu.2016.00105

[102] Romee R, Foley B, Lenvik T. et al. NK cell CD16 surface expression and function is regulated by a disintegrin and metalloprotease-17 (ADAM17). Blood. 2013;**121**(18):3599-3608. DOI: 10.1182/blood-2012-04-425397

[103] Wiernik A, Foley B, Zhang B. et al. Targeting natural killer cells to acute myeloid leukemia in vitro with a CD16 x 33 bispecific killer cell engager and ADAM17 inhibition. Clinical Cancer Research. 2013;**19**(14):3844-3855. DOI: 10.1158/1078-0432.CCR-13-0505

[104] Jing Y, Ni Z, Wu J. et al. Identification of an ADAM17 cleavage region in human CD16 (FcγRIII) and the engineering of a non-cleavable version of the receptor in NK cells. PLoS One. 2015;**10**(3):e0121788. DOI: 10.1371/journal.pone.0121788

[105] Ruggeri L, Mancusi A, Burchielli E. et al. NK cell alloreactivity and allogeneic hematopoietic stem cell transplantation. Blood Cells, Molecules and Diseases. 2008;**40**(1):84-90. DOI: 10.1016/j.bcmd.2007.06.029

[106] Morishima Y, Yabe T, Matsuo K. et al. Effects of HLA allele and killer immunoglobulin-like receptor ligand matching on clinical outcome in leukemia patients undergoing transplantation with T-cell-replete marrow from an unrelated donor. Biology of Blood and Marrow Transplantation. 2007;**13**(3):315-328. DOI: 10.1016/j.bbmt.2006.10.027

[107] Farag SS, Bacigalupo A, Eapen M. et al. The effect of KIR ligand incompatibility on the outcome of unrelated donor transplantation: A report from the center for international blood and marrow transplant research, the European blood and marrow transplant registry, and the Dutch registry. Biology of Blood and Marrow Transplantation. 2006;**12**(8):876-884. DOI: 10.1016/j.bbmt.2006.05.007

[108] Yabe T, Matsuo K, Hirayasu K, et al. Donor killer immunoglobulin-like receptor (KIR) genotype-patient cognate KIR ligand combination and antithymocyte globulin preadministration are critical factors in outcome of HLA-C-KIR ligand-mismatched T cell-replete unrelated bone marrow transplantation. Biology of Blood and Marrow Transplantation. 2008;**14**(1):75-87. DOI: 10.1016/j.bbmt.2007.09.012

[109] Yazaki M, Takahashi T, Mizutani K. et al. Human leucocyte antigen-Cw-specific cytotoxic T lymphocytes generated from naive cord blood used for cord blood stem cell transplantation. Biology of Blood and Marrow Transplantation. 2002;**117**(4):893-898

[110] Sugimoto K, Murata M, Terakura S. et al. CTL clones isolated from an HLA-Cw-mismatched bone marrow transplant recipient with acute graft-versus-host disease. The Journal of Immunology. 2009;**183**(9):5991-5998. DOI: 10.4049/jimmunol.0804310

[111] Leung W, Iyengar R, Turner V. et al. Determinants of antileukemia effects of allogeneic NK cells. The Journal of Immunology. 2004;**172**(1):644-650

[112] Hsu KC, Keever-Taylor CA, Wilton A. et al. Improved outcome in HLA-identical sibling hematopoietic stem-cell transplantation for acute myelogenous leukemia predicted by KIR and HLA genotypes. Blood. 2005;**105**(12):4878-4884. DOI: 10.1182/blood-2004-12-4825

[113] Hsu KC, Gooley T, Malkki M. et al. KIR ligands and prediction of relapse after unrelated donor hematopoietic cell transplantation for hematologic malignancy. Biology of Blood and Marrow Transplantation. 2006;**12**(8):828-836. DOI: 10.1016/j.bbmt.2006.04.008

[114] Miller JS, Cooley S, Parham P. et al. Missing KIR ligands are associated with less relapse and increased graft-versus-host disease (GVHD) following unrelated donor allogeneic HCT. Blood. 2007;**109**(11):5058-5061. DOI: 10.1182/blood-2007-01-065383

[115] Ruggeri L, Mancusi A, Capanni M. et al. Donor natural killer cell allorecognition of missing self in haploidentical hematopoietic transplantation for acute myeloid leukemia: Challenging its predictive value. Blood. 2007;**110**(1):433-440. DOI: 10.1182/blood-2006-07-038687

[116] Curti A, Ruggeri L, D'Addio A. et al. Successful transfer of alloreactive haploidentical KIR ligand-mismatched natural killer cells after infusion in elderly high risk acute myeloid leukemia patients. Blood. 2011;**118**(12):3273-3279. DOI: 10.1182/blood-2011-01-329508

[117] Farnault L, Sanchez C, Baier C. et al. Hematological malignancies escape from NK cell innate immune surveillance: Mechanisms and therapeutic implications. Clinical and Developmental Immunology. 2012;**2012**:421702. DOI: 10.1155/2012/421702

[118] Fauriat C, Andersson S, Björklund AT. et al. Estimation of the size of the alloreactive NK cell repertoire: studies in individuals homozygous for the group A KIR haplotype. The Journal of Immunology. 2008;**181**(9):6010-6019

[119] Cooley S, Weisdorf DJ, Guethlein LA. et al. Donor selection for natural killer cell receptor genes leads to superior survival after unrelated transplantation for acute myelogenous leukemia. Blood. 2010;**116**(14):2411-2419. DOI: 10.1182/blood-2010-05-283051

[120] Leung W, Use of NK cell activity in cure by transplant. British Journal of Haematology. 2011;**155**(1):14-29. DOI: 10.1111/j.1365-2141.2011

[121] Pende D, Marcenaro S, Falco M. et al. Anti-leukemia activity of alloreactive NK cells in KIR ligand-mismatched haploidentical HSCT for pediatric patients: evaluation of the functional role of activating KIR and redefinition of inhibitory KIR specificity. Blood. 2009;**113**(13):3119-3329. DOI: 10.1182/blood-2008-06-164103

[122] Venstrom JM, Pittari G, Gooley TA. et al. HLA-C-dependent prevention of leukemia relapse by donor activating KIR2DS1. The New England Journal of Medicine. 2012;**367**(9):805-816. DOI: 10.1056/NEJMoa1200503

[123] Venstrom JM, Gooley TA, Spellman S. et al. Donor activating KIR3DS1 is associated with decreased acute GVHD in unrelated allogeneic hematopoietic stem cell transplantation. Blood. 2010;**115**(15):3162-3165. DOI: 10.1182/blood-2009-08-236943

[124] Ludajic K, Balavarca Y, Bickeböller H. et al. KIR genes and KIR ligands affect occurrence of acute GVHD after unrelated, 12/12 HLA matched, hematopoietic stem cell transplantation. Bone Marrow Transplant Centre. 2009;**44**(2):97-103. DOI: 10.1038/bmt.2008.432

[125] Littera R, Orrù N, Vacca A. et al. The role of killer immunoglobulin-like receptor haplotypes on the outcome of unrelated donor haematopoietic SCT for thalassaemia. Bone Marrow Transplant Centre. 2010;**45**(11):1618-1624. DOI: 10.1038/bmt.2010.24

[126] Callahan MK, Postow MA, Wolchok JD. CTLA-4 and PD-1 Pathway Blockade: Combinations in the Clinic. Frontiers in Oncology. 2015;**4**:385. DOI: 10.3389/fonc.2014.00385

[127] Valsecchi ME. Combined Nivolumab and Ipilimumab or Monotherapy in Untreated Melanoma. The New England Journal of Medicine. 2015;**373**(13):1270. DOI: 10.1056/NEJMc1509660#SA1

[128] Benson DM Jr, Bakan CE, Mishra A. et al. The PD-1/PD-L1 axis modulates the natural killer cell versus multiple myeloma effect: A therapeutic target for CT-011, a novel monoclonal anti-PD-1 antibody. Blood. 2010;**116**(13):2286-2294. DOI: 10.1182/blood-2010-02-271874

[129] Campbell KS, Hasegawa J. Natural killer cell biology: an update and future directions. Journal of Allergy and Clinical Immunology. 2013;**132**(3):536-544. DOI: 10.1016/j.jaci.2013.07.006

[130] Garrido F, Cabrera T, Accolla RS. et al. Functional and medical implications. vol. I. In: Charron D, EDK (eds). 1997. pp 445-452

[131] Marincola FM, Jaffee EM, Hicklin DJ. et al. Escape of human solid tumors from T-cell recognition: molecular mechanisms and functional significance. Advances in Immunology. 2000;**74**:181-273

[132] Campoli M, Chang CC, Ferrone S. HLA class I antigen loss, tumor immune escape and immune selection. Vaccine. 2002;**20** Suppl 4: A40-A45

[133] Chang CC, Campoli M, Ferrone S. Classical and nonclassical HLA class I antigen and NK Cell-activating ligand changes in malignant cells: current challenges and future directions. Advances in Cancer Research. 2005;**93**:189-234. DOI: 10.1016/S0065-230X(05)93006-6

[134] Aptsiauri N, Cabrera T, Mendez R. et al. Role of altered expression of HLA class I molecules in cancer progression. Advances in Experimental Medicine and Biology. 2007;**601**:123-31

[135] Blades RA, Keating PJ, McWilliam LJ. et al. Loss of HLA class I expression in prostate cancer: implications for immunotherapy. Urology. 1995;**46**(5):681-686; discussion 686-687. DOI: 10.1016/S0090-4295(99)80301-X

[136] Cabrera T, Angustias Fernandez M. et al. High frequency of altered HLA class I phenotypes in invasive breast carcinomas. Human Immunology. 1996 **50**(2):127-134

[137] Cabrera T, Collado A, Fernandez MA. et al. High frequency of altered HLA class I phenotypes in invasive colorectal carcinomas. Tissue Antigens. 1998;**52**(2):114-123

[138] Cabrera T, Salinero J, Fernandez MA. et al. High frequency of altered HLA class I phenotypes in laryngeal carcinomas. Human Immunology. 2000;**61**(5):499-506

[139] Koopman LA, Corver WE, van der Slik AR, et al. Multiple genetic alterations cause frequent and heterogeneous human histocompatibility leukocyte antigen class I loss in cervical cancer. The Journal of Experimental Medicine. 2000;**191**(6):961-976

[140] Kageshita T, Ishihara T, Campoli M, et al. Selective monomorphic and polymorphic HLA class I antigenic determinant loss in surgically removed melanoma lesions. Tissue Antigens. 2005;**65**(5):419-428

[141] Feenstra M, Verdaasdonk M, van der Zwan AW, et al. Microsatellite analysis of microdissected tumor cells and 6p high density microsatellite analysis in head and neck squamous cell carcinomas with down-regulated human leukocyte antigen class I expression. Laboratory Investigation. 2000;**80**(3):405-414

[142] Maleno I, López-Nevot MA, Cabrera T, et al. Multiple mechanisms generate HLA class I altered phenotypes in laryngeal carcinomas: High frequency of HLA haplotype loss associated with loss of heterozygosity in chromosome region 6p21. Cancer Immunology and Immunotherapy. 2002;**51**(7):389-396. DOI: 10.1007/s00262-002-0296-0

[143] Maleno I, Cabrera CM, Cabrera T, et al. Distribution of HLA class I altered phenotypes in colorectal carcinomas: High frequency of HLA haplotype loss associated with loss of heterozygosity in chromosome region 6p21. Immunogenetics. 2004;**56**(4):244-53. DOI: 10.1007/s00251-004-0692-z

[144] Maleno I, Romero JM, Cabrera T, et al. LOH at 6p21.3 region and HLA class I altered phenotypes in bladder carcinomas. Immunogenetics. 2006;**58**(7):503-510. DOI: 10.1007/s00251-006-0111-8

[145] Carlsten M, Childs RW. Genetic manipulation of NK cells for cancer immunotherapy: techniques and clinical implications. Frontiers in Immunology. 2015;**6**:266. DOI: 10.3389/fimmu.2015.00266

[146] Sutlu T, Nyström S, Gilljam M. et al. Inhibition of intracellular antiviral defense mechanisms augments lentiviral transduction of human natural killer cells: Implications for gene therapy. Human Gene Therapy. 2012;**23**(10):1090-1100. DOI: 10.1089/hum.2012.080

[147] Guven H, Konstantinidis KV, Alici E. et al. Efficient gene transfer into primary human natural killer cells by retroviral transduction. Experimental Hematology. 2005;**33**(11):1320-1328. DOI: 10.1016/j.exphem.2005.07.006

[148] Schirrmann T, Pecher G. Human natural killer cell line modified with a chimeric immunoglobulin T-cell receptor gene leads to tumor growth inhibition in vivo. Cancer Gene Therapy. 2002r;**9**(4):390-398. DOI: 10.1038/sj.cgt.7700453

[149] Grund EM, Muise-Helmericks RC. Cost efficient and effective gene transfer into the human natural killer cell line, NK92. Journal of Immunological Methods. 2005;**296**(1-2):31-36. DOI: 10.1016/j.jim.2004.10.008

[150] Schirrmann T, Pecher G. Specific targeting of CD33(+) leukemia cells by a natural killer cell line modified with a chimeric receptor. Leukemia Research. 2005;**29**(3):301-316. DOI: 10.1016/j.leukres.2004.07.005

[151] Boissel L, Betancur M, Wels WS. et al. Transfection with mRNA for CD19 specific chimeric antigen receptor restores NK cell mediated killing of CLL cells. Leukemia Research. 2009;**33**(9):1255-1259. DOI: 10.1016/j.leukres.2008.11.024

[152] Li L, Liu LN, Feller S. et al. Expression of chimeric antigen receptors in natural killer cells with a regulatory-compliant non-viral method. Cancer Gene Therapy. 2010;**17**(3):147-154. DOI: 10.1038/cgt.2009.61

[153] Shimasaki N, Fujisaki H, Cho D, et al. A clinically adaptable method to enhance the cytotoxicity of natural killer cells against B-cell malignancies. Cytotherapy. 2012;**14**(7):830-840. DOI: 10.3109/14653249.2012.671519

[154] Maasho K, Marusina A, Reynolds NM. et al. Efficient gene transfer into the human natural killer cell line, NKL, using the amaxa nucleofection system. Journal of Immunological Methods. 2004;**284**(1-2):133-140. DOI: 10.1016/j.jim.2003.10.010

[155] Schoenberg K, Trompeter HI, Uhrberg M. Delivery of DNA into natural killer cells for immunotherapy. Methods in Molecular Biology. 2008;**423**:165-172. DOI: 10.1007/978-1-59745-194-9_11

[156] Astoul P, Viallat JR, Laurent JC, et al. Intrapleural recombinant IL-2 in passive immunotherapy for malignant pleural effusion. Chest. 1993;**103**(1):209-213

[157] Goey SH, Eggermont AM, Punt CJ, et al. Intrapleural administration of interleukin 2 in pleural mesothelioma: A phase I–II study. British Journal of Cancer. 1995;**72**(5):1283-1288

[158] Nagashima S, Mailliard R, Kashii Y. et al. Stable transduction of the interleukin-2 gene into human natural killer cell lines and their phenotypic and functional characterization in vitro and in vivo. Blood. 1998;**91**(10):3850-6381

[159] Imamura M, Shook D, Kamiya T. et al. Autonomous growth and increased cytotoxicity of natural killer cells expressing membrane-bound interleukin-15. Blood. 2014;**124**(7):1081-1088. DOI: 10.1182/blood-2014-02-556837

[160] Sahm C, Schönfeld K, Wels WS. Expression of IL-15 in NK cells results in rapid enrichment and selective cytotoxicity of gene-modified effectors that carry a tumor-specific antigen receptor. Cancer Immunology, Immunotherapy. 2012;**61**(9):1451-1461. DOI: 10.1007/s00262-012-1212-x

[161] Jiang W, Zhang C, Tian Z, et al. hIL-15 gene-modified human natural killer cells (NKL-IL15) augments the anti-human hepatocellular carcinoma effect in vivo. Immunobiology. 2014;**219**(7):547-553. DOI: 10.1016/j.imbio.2014.03.007

[162] Inngjerdingen M, Damaj B, Maghazachi AA. Expression and regulation of chemokine receptors in human natural killer cells. Blood. 2001;**97**(2):367-375

[163] Miller JS, Rooney CM, Curtsinger J. et al. Expansion and homing of adoptively transferred human natural killer cells in immunodeficient mice varies with product preparation and in vivo cytokine administration: Implications for clinical therapy. Biology of Blood and Marrow Transplantation. 2014;**20**(8):1252-1257. DOI: 10.1016/j.bbmt.2014.05.004

[164] Somanchi SS, Somanchi A, Cooper LJ, et al. Engineering lymph node homing of ex vivo-expanded human natural killer cells via trogocytosis of the chemokine receptor CCR7. Blood. 2012;**119**(22):5164-5172. DOI: 10.1182/blood-2011-11-389924

[165] Kochenderfer JN, Wilson WH, Janik JE, et al. Eradication of B-lineage cells and regression of lymphoma on patient treated with autologous T cells genetically engineered to recognize CD19. Blood. 2010;**116**(20):4099-4102. DOI: 10.1182/blood-2010-04-281931

[166] Brentjens RJ, Rivière I, Park JH, et al. Safety and persistence of adoptively transferred autologous CD19-targeted T cells in patients with relapsed or chemotherapy refractory B-cell leukemias. Blood. 2001;**118**(18):4817-4828

[167] Pule MA, Savoldo B, Myers GD, Rossig C, Russell HV, Dotti G, Huls MH, Liu E, Gee AP, Mei Z, Yvon E, Weiss HL, Liu H, Rooney CM, Heslop HE, Brenner MK: Virus-specificT cells engineered to coexpress tumor-specific receptors:persistence and antitumor activityin individuals with neuroblastoma. Nature Medicine. 2008;**14**(11):1264-1270. DOI: 10.1038/nm.1882

[168] Maude SL, Frey N, Shaw PA, et al. Chimeric antigen receptor T cells for sustained remissions in leukemia. The New England Journal of Medicine. 2014;**371**(16):1507-1517. DOI: 10.1056/NEJMoa1407222

[169] Morgan RA, Yang JC, Kitano M, et al. Case report of a serious adverse eventfollowing theadministration of T cells transduced with a chimeric antigen receptor recognizing ERBB2. Molecular Therapy. 2010;**18**:843-851. DOI: 10.1038/mt.2010.24

[170] Müller T, Uherek C, Maki G, et al. Expression of a CD20-specific chimeric antigen receptor enhances cytotoxic activity of NK cells and overcomes NK-resistance of lymphoma and leukemia cells. Cancer Immunology, Immunotherapy. 2008;**57**(3):411-423. DOI: 10.1007/s00262-007-0383-3

[171] Imai C, Iwamoto S, Campana D. Genetic modification of primary natural killer cells overcomes inhibitory signals and induces specific killing of leukemic cells. Blood. 2005;**106**(1):376-383. DOI: 10.1182/blood-2004-12-4797

[172] Menard S, Pupa SM, Campiglio M, et al. Biologic and therapeutic role of HER2 in cancer. Oncogene. 2003;**22**(42):6570-6578. DOI: 10.1038/sj.onc.1206779

[173] Meric-Bernstam F, Hung MC. Advances in targeting human epidermal growth factor receptor-2 signaling for cancer therapy. Clinical Cancer Research. 2006;**12**(21):6326-6330. DOI: 10.1158/1078-0432.CCR-06-1732

[174] Kruschinski A, Moosmann A, Poschke I, et al. Engineering antigen-specific primary human NK cells against HER-2 positive carcinomas. Proceedings of the National Academy of Sciences USA. 2008;**105**(45):17481-174816. DOI: 10.1073/pnas.0804788105

[175] Uherek C, Tonn T, Uherek B, et al. Retargeting of natural killer-cell cytolytic activity to ErbB2-expressing cancer cells results in efficient and selective tumor cell destruction. Blood. 2002;**100**(4):1265-1273

[176] Liu H, Yang B, Sun T, et al. Specific growth inhibition of ErbB2-expressing human breast cancer cells by genetically modified NK-92 cells. Oncology Reports. 2015;**33**(1):95-102. DOI: 10.3892/or.2014.3548

[177] Chang YH, Connolly J, Shimasaki N, et al. A chimeric receptor with NKG2D specificity enhances natural killer cell activation and killing of tumor cells. Cancer Research. 2013;**73**(6):1777-1786. DOI: 10.1158/0008-5472.CAN-12-3558

[178] Tassev DV, Cheng M, Cheung NK. Retargeting NK92 cells using an HLA-A2-restricted, EBNA3C-specific chimeric antigen receptor. Cancer Gene Therapy. 2012;**19**(2):84-100. DOI: 10.1038/cgt.2011.66

[179] Esser R, Müller T, Stefes D, et al. NK cells engineered to express a GD2-specific antigen receptor display built-in ADCC-like activity against tumour cells of neuroectodermal origin. Journal of Cellular and Molecular Medicine. 2012;**16**(3):569-581. DOI: 10.1111/j.1582-4934.2011.01343.x

[180] Boissel L, Betancur M, Lu W, et al. Comparison of mRNA and lentiviral based transfection of natural killer cells with chimeric antigen receptors recognizing lymphoid antigens. Leukemia and Lymphoma. 2012;**53**(5):958-965. DOI: 10.3109/10428194.2011.634048

[181] Chu J, Deng Y, Benson DM, et al. CS1-specific chimeric antigen receptor (CAR)-engineered natural killer cells enhance in vitro and in vivo antitumor activity against human multiple myeloma. Leukemia. 2014;**28**(4):917-927. DOI: 10.1038/leu.2013.279

[182] Jiang H, Zhang W, Shang P, Zhang H, Fu W, Ye F, et al. Transfection of chimeric anti-CD138 gene enhances natural killer cell activation and killing of multiple myeloma cells. Molecular Oncology. 2014;**8**(2):297-310. DOI: 10.1016/j.molonc.2013.12.001

[183] Schönfeld K, Sahm C, Zhang C et al. Selective inhibition of tumor growth by clonal NK cells expressing an ErbB2/HER2-specific chimeric antigen receptor. Molecular Therapy. 2015;**23**(2):330-338. DOI: 10.1038/mt.2014.219

[184] Töpfer K, Cartellieri M, Michen S, et al. DAP12-based activating chimeric antigen receptor for NK cell tumor immunotherapy. The Journal of Immunology2015;**194**(7):3201-3212. DOI: 10.4049/jimmunol.1400330

[185] Altvater B, Landmeier S, Pscherer S, et al. 2B4 (CD244) signaling by recombinant antigen-specific chimeric receptors costimulates natural killer cell activation to leukemia and neuroblastoma cells. Clinical Cancer Research. 2009;**15**(15):4857-4866. DOI: 10.1158/1078-0432.CCR-08-2810

[186] Chu Y, Hochberg J, Yahr A, et al. Targeting CD20+ aggressive B-cell Non-Hodgkin lymphoma by anti-CD20 CAR mRNA-modified expanded natural killer cells in vitro and in NSG mice. Cancer Immunology Research. 2015;**3**(4):333-344. DOI: 10.1158/2326-6066.CIR-14-0114

Chapter 7

# Donor Natural Killer Cells and Their Therapeutic Potential in Allogeneic Hematopoietic Stem Cell Transplantation

Bo Hu and Haiyan Liu

Additional information is available at the end of the chapter

http://dx.doi.org/10.5772/intechopen.69684

**Abstract**

Natural killer (NK) cells were first identified and named for their "natural" cytotoxicity to reject bone-marrow allografts in lethally irradiated mice. Different from T cells, NK cells require no prior sensitization or immunization to lyse transformed or virally infected target cells and are non-major histocompatibility complex (MHC)–restricted. However, recent progress in understanding of NK cells biology has proved that NK cells share some similar characteristics with T cells. During development, NK cells also undergo "education" according to "missing self" principle, thereby become mature and acquire effector function. The discovery that NK cells are able to "remember" prior certain stimulations indicates they may also contribute to adaptive immunity. After hematopoietic stem cell transplantation (HSCT), NK cells are the first donor-derived lymphogenous cells to reconstitute and alloreactivitiy of donor-derived NK cells have been shown to mediate graft-versus-leukemia (GvL) effect rather than to induce graft-versus-host disease (GvHD). These properties make donor-derived NK cells appealing for applications to benefit the outcome of HSCT. Here, we will review the improved understanding of NK cell biology, discuss characteristics of donor-derived NK cells which are associated with beneficial outcome of HSCT and explore novel methodologies that enhance the therapeutic effect of donor NK cells.

**Keywords:** hematopoietic stem cell transplantation, NK cells, immunotherapy, leukemia, cytomegalovirus, immune memory

## 1. Introduction

Allogeneic hematopoietic stem cell transplantation (allo-HSCT) is one of the most effective therapy for leukemia and other malignant diseases [1]. Its major complications are graft-versus-host disease (GvHD), infections, and leukemia relapse [2, 3]. Natural killer (NK) cells represent a key component of innate lymphoid cells and provide defense against microbial infection and malignant transformation by direct cytotoxicity and cytokine production [4, 5]. The role of NK cells in allo-HSCT was first demonstrated in haploidentical transplants [6]. During T-cell depleted haploidentical HSCT, the rapid recovery of donor-derived NK cells mediated potent graft-versus-leukemia (GvL) effect. Importantly, allore-active NK cells mediated beneficial GvL effect without the occurrence of GvHD, which was consistently caused by donor T cells [7, 8].

Although the rapid reconstitution of donor NK cells plays a critical role in their GvL effect of the graft, they still take about 6 months or more to acquire maturation phenotype and full functionality [9]. This immaturity and insufficient education status may result in impaired function of donor NK cells in the early stage post transplantation. In addition, since the allo-reactivity of donor NK cells was proved to account for the clinical benefit, genotyping the polymorphisms of killer cell immunoglobulin-like receptor (KIR), human leukocyte antigen (HLA) and Fcγ receptor (FcγR) are important for donor selection to maximize the GvL effect [10]. Sufficient numbers of allogeneic NK cells with high purity can also be generated and expanded through several sources including peripheral blood mononuclear cells, umbilical cord blood (UCB), and bone marrow–derived $CD34^+$ cells to be adoptively transferred after allo-HSCT [11, 12]. Many approaches involving the use of different feeder cells, engineered feeder cell, and cytokine stimulation were utilized to achieve sufficient numbers of donor NK cells with the most efficient GvL effect and clinical responses [13, 14]. Moreover, seven NK cell lines have been established to be used effectively during allo-HSCT, among which, NK-92 cell line has been shown to be safe and efficient in clinical trials [15–17]. Recently, genetic modification of NK cells has also been developed to enhance their function. Both gene transfer of chimeric antigen receptors (CARs) and expression of cytokine transgenes in NK cells are performed to improve the efficacy of NK cells therapy [18–20]. Furthermore, although traditionally considered as members of innate branch, increasing studies suggest that NK cells also "remember" prior certain stimulation like antigens, cytomegalovirus (CMV), or cytokines [21–26]. It draws particular interest to evaluate the role of adoptively transferred memory-like donor NK cells in allo-HSCT. Based on these research progresses of donor NK cell-mediated immunotherapy during allo-HSCT, in this chapter, we will describe the present state of donor NK cell therapy during allo-HSCT and its future direction aiming to improve therapeutic benefit of donor NK cells.

## 2. Overview of natural killer cell biology

NK cells represent a key component of innate lymphoid cells (ILC) and provide defense against microbial infection and malignant transformation. They belong to ILC1 group (according to their ability to produce type1 cytokine and transcription factors, they required for differentiation) and are so named for their capacity to mediate cytotoxicity toward cancer cells and virus-infected cells without prior sensitization [27–29]. NK cells constitute 10–15% of human

http://dx.doi.org/10.5772/intechopen.69684

peripheral blood lymphocytes and are defined by expression of CD56 without T cell marker CD3 [30]. Human NK cells can be further divided into two different subsets depending on the expression density of CD56 and CD16 [30]. The $CD56^{dim}$ $CD16^{bright}$ subsets account for majority (90%) of peripheral blood circulating NK cells and display cytotoxic function [31, 32], whereas $CD56^{bright}$ $CD16^{bright}$ subsets are predominantly found in lymph nodes and produce abundant amounts of inflammatory cytokines such as interferon-$\gamma$ (IFN-$\gamma$), tumor necrosis factor alpha (TNF-$\alpha$), tumor necrosis factor beta (TNF-β), IL-10, IL-13, granulocyte-macrophage colony stimulating factor (GM-CSF), etc., thereby promote adaptive immune responses [31, 33].

### 2.1. Natural killer cell receptors

NK cells immune function is mediated through an array of inhibitory and activating cell surface receptors. There are three main types of receptor families: KIR, C-type lectin receptors and natural cytotoxicity receptors (NCR) [34].

KIRs are proteins belonging to immunoglobulin superfamily that are encoded by a gene complex located on chromosome 19q13.4. Individuals may have up to 15 different KIR genes and two pseudogenes encoding for relevant receptors [35]. KIRs express stochastically on mature NK cells and recognize HLA molecules in a manner independent of antigen presentation. When bound to their ligands, these receptors transmit either inhibitory or activating signals. KIR genes are inherited as haplotypes due to the different number of KIR gene, and their high degree of diversity induced by various KIR gene content and allelic polymorphism [36]. Two major groups of KIR haplotypes have been distinguished based on gene content. Group A haplotypes contain a fix number of genes that are mainly inhibitory KIR, including KIR2DL1, KIR2DL3, KIR3DL1, KIR2DS4, and the pseudogene KIR2DP1. On the other hand, group B haplotypes are alterable both in numbers and content of KIR gene and have at least one of the following genes: KIR2DL2, KIR2DL5A, KIR2DL5B, KIR2DS2, KIR2DS5, and KIR3DS1 [37]. Group B haplotypes contain more activating KIR (up to 5) compared with group A haplotypes (only one).

C-type lectin receptors are heterodimers and comprise of two subunits including CD94 protein and a C-type lectin natural killer group 2 (NKG2) molecule [38]. The gene of this receptor family located on chromosome 12 encoding six different NKG2 proteins: NKG2A, NKG2C, NKG2E, NKG2F, NKG2B, NKG2H, as well as CD94 protein. Among these receptors, CD94/NKG2A and CD94/NKG2B are inhibitory receptors and bind HLA-E, whereas other receptors are activating. Activating receptor NKG2D also belongs to NKG2 family and is expressed on the surface of NK cells as a homodimer. NKG2D can recognize two different families of cognate ligands including nonclassical major histocompatibility complex (MHC) molecules (MIC-A and MIC-B) and UL16 binding protein family [39, 40]. The expression of NKG2D ligands is upregulated under the influence of cellular stress such as viral infection, inflammation, and tumor formation.

Natural cytotoxicity receptors including NKp30, NKp44, and NKp46 are activating receptors expressed on the surface of NK cells [41]. NKp30 can recognize ligands expressed on tumor cells such as the nuclear factor HLA-B-associated transcript-3 (BAT-3) and B7-H6 [42]. NKp30 also binds to viral ligands (CMV pp65 protein) [42]. Both NKp46 and NKp44 bind to viral-derived proteins such as influenza hemagglutinin (HA) [43, 44]. Moreover, NKp44 has been shown to recognize the envelope glycorpoteins from West Nile and dengue viruses and NKp46 has been shown to recognize vimentin expressed on *Mycobacterium tuberculosis*–infected human monocytes [45]. However, the ligands of NCR have not been well identified yet.

### 2.2. Natural killer cell function

Upon education, the "licensed" NK cells acquire cytotoxic activity toward target cells lacking self MHC class-I molecules, meanwhile they are tolerant to normal cells expressing self MHC class-I molecules, namely "missing self" hypothesis. However, this hypothesis seems to oversimplify NK function regulation. Activating receptors have also been shown to play an important role to make the decision "to kill or not." For example, during murine allo-HSCT model, alloreactive donor NK cells do not respond to host's epithelial cells although donor NK cells lacking inhibitory receptors specific for host MHC class-I, mainly due to their low expression level of ligands specific for activating receptors of donor NK cells [6]. In some cases, the extremely high strength of activating signals may even overcome weaker inhibitory signals resulting in activation of NK cells [46, 47]. Therefore, triggering of NK cell activation is finally depended on the balance of activating and inhibitory receptors of NK cells.

Once NK cells are activated, they respond to target cells with function similar to $CD8^+$ T cells. Immune synapse forms and perforin and granzyme are released to induce apoptosis of target cells through activation of Caspase 3 [48]. NK cell activation also upregulates the expression of factor associated suicide (FAS) and tumor necrosis factor-related apoptosis-inducing ligand (TRAIL) and kill the target cells through Caspase 8 activation induced apoptosis [49, 50]. Furthermore, NK cells can also crosstalk with adaptive immune system through cytokine release and antibodies. Virus infected cells and tumor cells are recognized by B cells. These cells are then marked with antibodies covering their cell surface. NK cells recognize and bind to these cells through the interaction between activating receptor CD16 and the Fc end of antibodies [51]. This recognition mediates a potent activating signal in NK cells and results in target cells lysis. Moreover, NK cells are able to secret cytokines and chemokines upon activation, such as TNF-$\alpha$, IFN-$\gamma$, regulated upon activation, norma, T-cell expressed and secreted (RANTES), GM-CSF, macrophage inflammatory protein-1-alpha and beta (MIP1-$\alpha$ and-$\beta$). NK cells can promote dendritic cells maturation through TNF-$\alpha$ and IFN-$\gamma$ secretion [52]. IFN-$\gamma$ production also affects helper T cell subset 1 (Th1) migration and effector function. Additionally, Th1 polarization in secondary lymphogenous organs is enhanced by IFN-$\gamma$ secretion [53]. Thus, IFN-$\gamma$ secretion of NK cells is critical for forming a bridge between the innate and adaptive immune responses.

## 3. Natural killer cell development and education

### 3.1. Natural killer cell development

NK cells develop from $CD34^+$ hematopoietic progenitor cells which can also give rise to T cells, B cells, and dendritic cells [54]. Particular transcription factors such as purine rich box-1 (PU.1), E26 transformation-specific (ETS-1), thymocyte selection-associated HMG box factor (TOX), the

http://dx.doi.org/10.5772/intechopen.69684

mammalian transcription factor E4 binding protein 4 (E4BP4), eomesodermin (Eomes), and T-box transcription factor (T-bet) are required for NK cell maturation stages [55–58]. Among these transcription factors, Eomes and T-bet are responsible for cytotoxicity and IFN-γ production in mature NK cells [59]. Furthermore, CD56$^{dim}$ NK cells express higher levels of T-bet and lower levels of Eomes than CD56$^{bright}$ NK cells, and T-bet/Eomes ratio increases with NK cells maturation [60]. A central cytokine required for NK cell development *in vivo* is IL-15, as mice lacking IL-15, CD122 (IL-15β-chain receptor), interleukin 15 receptor alpha (IL-15Rα), or signal transducer and activator of transcription 5 (STAT5) do not generate mature NK cells [61]. Stem cell factor (SCF), IL-7, and fms-like tyrosine kinase 3-ligand (Flt3-L) are also necessary for NK cell maturation since they induce pro-NK cell to express CD122 and CD132 (the common γ-chain receptor) so as to render cell to respond to IL-15 [62, 63]. Intriguingly, IL-15 is primarily accompanied by IL-15Rα and trans-presented by accessory cells to support NK cell differentiation and proliferation *in vivo* rather than affecting NK cell in a soluble form [64].

After maturation in the bone marrow, NK cells migrate to peripheral circulation and take part in the defense against cancers and viral infections. Two major subsets in the peripheral blood are CD56$^{dim}$ and CD56$^{bright}$ NK cells [30]. These subsets differ in receptor expressions, functional capabilities, and tissue distribution. Although CD56$^{dim}$ NK cells have been considered to be cytotoxic population, it is now clearly proved that they also produce large amounts of cytokines upon receptor-induced NK cell triggering [65, 66]. These functional differences can be partly explained by different expression pattern of surface receptors. CD56$^{dim}$ NK cells express CD16, KIR and other activating or inhibitory receptors which are critical for their cytolytic functions, whereas CD56$^{birght}$ NK cells rarely express KIR and CD16 [67]. Interestingly, CD56$^{bright}$ NK cells could express KIR and CD16 after stimulation of IL-2 or IL-12 suggesting CD56$^{bright}$ NK cells are NK cell subsets in the stage of maturation [68, 69]. Thereafter, recent studies confirm that CD56$^{dim}$ NK cells indeed differentiate from CD56$^{bright}$ NK cells which display longer telomerase [70]. Due to different expression of chemokine receptors and adhesion molecules, CD56$^{dim}$ NK cells account for around 90% of peripheral blood NK cells, while CD56$^{bright}$ NK cells primarily exist in secondary lymphoid tissues or decidual tissues during early pregnancy [71].

### 3.2. Generation of memory-like natural killer cells

Immune memory is previously considered as an exclusive property of T cells and B cells and defined as quicker and more robust responses to recurrent antigens [72]. However, accumulating evidence proved NK cell also have memory-like feature after certain modes of challenge including antigen-specific stimulation and antigen-independent activation. The hepatic NK cell memory was first observed by the Von Andrian's group [73]. They found NK cells can mediate delayed-type hypersensitivity (DTH) reactions in *Rag2*$^{-/-}$ mice model. These hapten-specific NK cells are exclusively recruited to the liver and identified as CD49a$^{+}$ DX5$^{-}$ NK cell population, expressing chemokine receptor CXCR6 [21, 73, 74]. The mechanism that generate this antigen-specific NK cells whose receptors cannot be somatically rearranged remain unknown. Moreover, similar hepatic memory response has not been proved to occur in humans.

Another differentiation pathway for antigen-specific NK cell memory response is CMV infection. CMV-triggered NK cell memory was first observed by the Lanier laboratory demonstrating that Ly49H$^+$ NK cells can rapidly expand and response robustly after murine CMV (MCMV) re-infection [75]. NK cell co-activating receptor DNAX adhesion molecule-1 (DNAM-1) is required for the initial expansion of MCMV-induced memory NK cells [76]. Furthermore, transcription factor Zbtb32 and pro-inflammatory cytokine pathway also play important role in MCMV-induced expansion [77, 78]. In human, natural killer Group 2, member C positive (NKG2C$^+$) NK cells also expand during acute human CMV (HCMV) infection and display a CD56$^{dim}$CD57$^+$NKG2A$^-$ phenotype [79, 80]. These HCMV-induced memory NK cells have increased expression of IFN-$\gamma$, which may be induced by epigenetic remodeling of *IFNG* locus [81, 82]. The role of HCMV-induced NK memory during HSCT will be described in section 6 of this chapter.

Antigen-independent NK cell memory response was first observed by the Yokoyama laboratory [24]. They showed mouse NK cells which were pre-activated with the combination of IL-12/15/18 overnight produced increased level of IFN-$\gamma$ upon re-stimulation. Additionally, these cytokine-induced memory-like NK cells displayed enhanced proliferation and upregulation of CD25 expression in response to re-stimulation with cytokines [24, 25]. Intriguingly, human NK cells also can give rise to cytokine-induced memory-like NK cells with similar key properties [26]. Series of studies explored the antitumor responses of cytokine-induced memory-like NK cells, and we will discuss their role during HSCT in section 7 and 9 of this chapter.

### 3.3. Natural killer cell education

#### *3.3.1. Inhibitory receptors are critical for natural killer cell education*

The genes encoding for KIR are located on chromosome 19, while HLA genes are on chromosome 6 [83]. Therefore, KIR genes and HLA genes are inherited independently, and this randomness may result in the expression of KIR on NK cells in the absence of their corresponding HLA ligands, thereby NK cells may have chance to attack normal cells. In fact, NK cells are tolerant to our body most of the time. It is interesting to understand how NK cells are educated to become tolerant? Inhibitory receptors have been shown to play an important role in this education process. During NK cell maturation, when the inhibitory receptors recognize self-MHC class I, the stochastic expression of KIR genes is switched off, and signals are transmitted to promote NK cell maturation and generate effector function. Oppositely, when the inhibitory receptors of NK cells fail to recognize self-MHC class I, they remain in a state of hyporesponsiveness and are not able to attack normal autologous cells [35, 84]. Collectively, only NK cells expressing "at least one" self-recognizing inhibitory receptor are "licensed" and acquire effector function, whereas "unlicensed" NK cells that recognize non-self-MHC are hyporesponsive and tolerant to normal cells. This process of "licensing" was proved in "peptide transporter-associated antigen processing" (TAP)-deficient patients [85]. Cells from these patients hardly express HLA class I molecules on their surface, thereby potentially render self-cells to be targets of NK cells. However, most of these patients do not have autoimmune disorders because of the hyporesponsiveness of NK cells. Additionally, NK cells isolated from TAP-deficient patients are also unresponsive to autologous HLA class I-negative B lymphoblastoid cell lines [86].

### 3.3.2. *The state of "unlicensed" natural killer cells is reversible*

It is important to note that the hyporesponsive state of "unlicensed" NK cells is reversible. During viral infection, "unlicensed" NK cells regain cytotoxic activity and are even more effectively in controlling murine cytomegalovirus (MCMV) infection compared with "licensed" NK cells owing to the lack of inhibitory effect of self MHC class-I expression on target cells [87]. The activity of "unlicensed" NK cells can also be restored after *in vitro* culture in the presence of IL-2 or IL-12+IL-18 or through activating receptors mediated strong signals [88].

The education process is more complex during allo-HSCT as donor-derived progenitors of NK cells posses both possibilities to undergo either donor type or host type education. Besides this, adoptively transferred mature NK cells can undergo "re-education" following MHC mismatched HSCT. It is now believed that donor HSC-derived NK cells generate a KIR repertoire of donor type, thanks to the high number of infused donor cells during haplo-HSCT and both nonhematopoietic as well as hematopoietic cells may present self MHC class-I molecules to precursors of NK cells thereby are involved in NK cell education [34, 89].

## 4. Donor natural killer cell reconstitution after hematopoietic stem cell transplantation

NK cells need to develop *in vivo* to acquire effector function following HSCT. Accordingly, they are the first donor-derived lymphogenous cells to reconstitute and can be detected as early as the first month post-transplant [90]. The reconstitution kinetics and functional properties of NK cells are variable due to the primary activity of NK cells in the graft and different graft source including bone marrow, G-CSF-mobilized peripheral blood stem cell, and UCB. Series studies demonstrated that different grant source did not affect the rate of NK cell reconstitution and during the early stage post-HSCT, the primary NK cell subsets were $CD56^{bright}$ donor NK cells [91, 92]. These results indicated that the early reconstituting NK cells after HSCT were mainly generated from the differentiation and maturation of NK precursors but not the expansion of mature NK cells in the graft. Nevertheless, the expansion of adoptive transferred NK cells also influences the reconstitution of donor NK cells since Eissens et al. find that in HLA-matched allogeneic peripheral blood stem cell transplantation, $CD3^+/CD19^+$-depleted grafts which contain more mature NK cells than $CD34^+$-selected grafts lead to more rapid NK cell reconstitution [93].

Although donor-derived NK cells are observed very early post-HSCT, they have an immature $CD56^{bright}$ $KIR^-$ $NKG2A^+$ phenotype for at least 3-6 months [94]. Interestingly, the ability of these immature $CD56^{bright}$ NK cells to produce IFN-$\gamma$ is significantly impaired in response to tumor cell line or primary leukemia cells [95, 96]. The expression of T-bet and mucin-containing domain-3 (Tim-3) is much lower in the patients post-HSCT compared with the healthy individuals [97]. Both of these two molecules are critical for induction of IFN-$\gamma$ production, thus their reduced expression may partly account for the decreased recovery of cytokine production.

It is difficult to clearly define the effect of T cell content in the graft on NK cell reconstitution as it is also depended on immunosuppressive therapy. By far, graft T cell content is thought to significantly influence functional reconstitution of NK cells rather than numerical reconstitution. One study observed donor-derived NK cells reconstitution following HSCT with three different kinds of donor source including T-cell-replete adult grafts, T-cell-deplete adult grafts, and UCB [95]. Both of the T-cell-replete group and UCB group were treated with immunosuppression. They found KIR expression in T-cell-replete group was the highest among these three groups indicated donor-derived NK cells in this group may have better effector function. Accordingly, in an earlier study by the same group, they found IFN-γ production was more potent following HSCT with T-cell-replete grafts compared to T-cell-deplete transplantation [98]. These results were consistent with the observations by Nguyen et al. which demonstrated that without immunosuppression, recovery NK cells in the partial T-cell-depleted group had lower cytotoxicity than NK cells in the full T-cell-depleted group [92]. In summary, graft T cell content trends to enhance functional reconstitution of NK cells irrespective of immunosuppression. This promotion effect may be due to activation from T-cell-derived IL-2, or stimulation from other inflammatory cytokine such as IL-12 and IL-18, which are increased following donor T cell engraftment. Finally, CMV infection and GvHD may also have potent effect on NK cell reconstitution, and we will discuss this in the following sections.

## 5. Association between natural killer cell alloreactivity and graft-versus-leukemia effect

### 5.1. The complexity of hematopoietic stem cell transplantation may affect the graft-versus-leukemia effects of alloreactive natural killer cells

HSCT is well-established curative treatment for hematologic malignances. The major limitation of HSCT is the absence of HLA-matched donor. Therefore, the HLA-haploidentical relatives are increasingly used as donor sources of HSCs. During the haplo-HSCT, donor and recipient share one identical HLA haplotype, while other haplotype is fully mismatched [99]. The GvL effect of NK cells was first observed in a landmark study which demonstrated that NK cells rapidly reconstituted and displayed potent anti-leukemia activity after extensive T-cell depleted haplo-HSCT [6]. After inhibitory receptor KIR was identified as a mediator of missing-self response, the GvL effect of NK cells was assumed to be mainly due to mismatches between donor KIR and recipient HLA class I which increase NK cell function thereby effectively lyse residual leukemia cells in the recipient. This hypothesis was first verified by Ruggeri L et al. [100]. They isolated donor-derived NK cells from haplotype-mismatched HCT recipients and tested their cytotoxicity toward recipient lymphocytes. Their results demonstrated donor alloreactive NK cells indeed effectively killed recipient myeloid leukemia cells. The follow-up study of this group demonstrated therapeutic utility of NK cell alloreactivity. They found transplants with KIR ligand mismatch were associated with decreased probability of relapse and increases in disease-free survival in the absence of GvHD [6].

Series studies subsequently tested NK cell alloreactivity-mediated GvL effect in the KIR ligand incompatibility model. However, not all studies supported the benefit role of alloreactive NK cells. During haplotype-HCT with less T cell depletion, KIR ligand mismatch patients even developed more acute GvHD (aGvHD), and the overall survival was poor. In a cohort using unrelated donors, no effect of predicted NK cell alloreactivity was observed, whereas in another similar cohort with T-cell depletion, KIR ligand mismatch prolonged overall survival [101, 102]. Frag et al. examined the clinical impact of NK cell alloreactivity in over 1500 unrelated transplants and found KIR ligand mismatch was not associated with relapse prevention [103]. In a retrospective study, data from 2062 unrelated transplant recipients were analyzed for acute myelocytic leukemia (AML), chronic myeloid leukemia (CML), and myelodysplastic syndrome (MDS) [104]. Missing one or more KIR ligands in the recipient were associated with less relapse in patients with early myeloid leukemia and in CML patients during first chronic phase. Nevertheless, KIR ligand mismatch was also associated with an increased risk of chronic GvHD (cGvHD) in CML patients.

The effect of NK alloreactivity in recipients of UCB grafts has also been tested. Willemze et al. evaluated the impact of KIR ligand incompatibility in recipients of UCB grafts with T-cell depletion and found KIR ligand mismatch was associated with relapse prevention and improved overall survival [105]. However, Brunstein et al. reported different results [106]. They investigated the impact of KIR ligand mismatch in patients of UCB grafts after different intensity conditioning regimens. After myeloablative conditioning, KIR ligand mismatch did not exert protective effect on GvHD, relapse, transplantation-related mortality, or survival. Following reduced intensity conditioning, KIR ligand mismatch patients developed more aGvHD and poorer overall survival.

The different results among these studies using either adult grafts or UCB grafts may be explained by the complexity of HCT, such as variable preparative regimens, donor sources, and degree of HLA mismatch with the donor. For instance, the degree of T-cell depletion was different among these studies, the grafts were extensively T-cell depleted in some studies, whereas only were partially depleted in others. T cell content may outcompete NK cells for cytokines and thereby influence the beneficial effect of alloreactive NK cells. Additionally, different intensity of preparative regimens also affects numeral and functional reconstitution of alloreactive NK cells after HSCT thus influences HSCT outcomes. Finally, the origin of leukemic blasts also affects HSCT outcomes. No beneficial effects of alloreactive NK cells in adult acute lymphoblastic leukemia (ALL) patients were observed probably due to the lack of expression of activating ligands [100]. However, allorecative NK cells have been proved to positively affect the outcome of HSCT in children with ALL [107]. Accordingly, the intensity of HLA expression on the leukemic lymphoblasts was shown to be critical for NK-mediated cytotoxicity in an experimental study [108].

### 5.2. Donor killer immunoglobulin-like receptors affect beneficial effects of alloreactive natural killer cells and outcome after hematopoietic stem cell transplantation

As we have mentioned above, KIR genes can be simplified into two main haplotypes: haplotype A and haplotype B. A hapltotype consists of main inhibitory KIR and single-activating KIR, KIR2DS4. B haplotype contains variable KIR gene encoding both inhibitory and activating KIRs which can be further divided into either centromeric (Cen) or telomeric (Tel) regions. The role of these haplotypes in HSCT is also evaluated. Mc Queen et al. first demonstrated grafts from KIR A/A genotype donors into KIR B recipients resulted in poorer survival in HLA-matched T-cell-replete sibling transplants [109]. In contrast, Stringaris et al. reported transplants from KIR B haplotype donors including genes for KIR2DS1, KIR3DS1, and KIR2DL5 improved overall survival and prevented relapse specific for AML patients with T-cell depletion during HLA identical siblings HSCT [110]. A larger cohort was performed to further evaluate the effect of KIR B haplotype in AML patients. The results indicated that grafts from donors with KIR B haplotype significantly reduced the risk of relapse and improved overall survival [111]. A follow-up study expanded numbers of AML patients with T-cell-depleted unrelated donor transplants and found that donor KIR B haplotype-mediated relapse prevention was enhanced in recipients who have HLA-C1 alleles rather than C2 homozygous recipients [36]. Michaelis SU et al. reported transplants from KIR B haplotype donors resulted in better HSCT outcome in ALL patients [112].

Collectively, it is logical to hypothesize that the presence of activating KIR in donor KIR B haplotype is favorably associated with better transplant outcome. However, it is difficult to evaluate the contribution of each activating KIR to relapse protection and better overall survival due to their unknown ligands. KIR2DS1 has been proved to interact with HLA-C group 2 alleles and involved in the killing of leukemic blasts from HLA-C2 patients. The interaction between KIR2DS1 and HLA-C2 was found to overcome NKG2A mediated inhibitory signals in vitro [113, 114]. These results suggested KIR2DS1-mediated activating signal may break the barrier of NKG2A and exert positive effect during HSCT. Venstrom et al. investigated the role of KIR2DS1 from donor in unrelated HSCT in 1277 patients with AML and found that KIR2DS1 expression in donor mediated a significant GvL effect [114]. Notably, no beneficial effect was observed when donors were HLA C2 homozygous as in those donors, NK cells expressing KIR2DS1 cannot be educated and acquire effector function. Therefore, at least one copy of HLA-C1 in donor is needed for KLR2DS1-dependent GvL effect. In addition, KIR3DS1 was also found to associate with lower rate of relapse and infection. Mancusi A et al. reported KIR3DS1 was associated with reduced infection mortality [115]. Further studies are still needed to identify ligands for activating KIR so as to confirm the effect of each activating KIR gene on allo-HSCT outcome.

The intensity of interaction between KIR and HLA may also influence the alloreactivity of NK cells during allo-HSCT. HLA alleles have been shown to bind NK cells with different affinities. The HLA class I molecules are highly polymorphic, and HLA-B alleles can be divided into HLA-B alleles with an isoleucine at position 80 (80I) and with a theonine (80T). The affinity between certain HLA-B alleles with an 80I and KIR3DL1 was found to be much stronger than those with an 80T [116, 117]. The impact of this different affinity was tested in HIV patients [118]. Presence of 80I but not 80T in HIV patients associated with slower AIDS progression. These results indicated strong interaction with KIR3DL1 may promote NK cell education and enhance their effector function. HLA-C1 alleles can also bind to NK cells with different affinity [119]. Donors who were homozygous for HLA-C*07 produce higher level of IFN-$\gamma$ compared to donors expressing either HLA-C*01, 03*,*08, *1402, or 1403*. Since the strength of the interaction between KIR and HLA is critical for NK cell education and function, it is tempting to speculate that during allo-HSCT certain HLA combination may enhance NK cell activity and contribute to better outcome of HSCT. The differing KIR/HLA affinity also can be generated by KIR allelic differences. KIR3DL1 is one of the most polymorphic KIR genes with more than 60 alleles [120]. KIR3DL1*01052 binds to Bw4 more firmly than KIR3DL*007 due to their high-expression level [119]. Although the surface expression of KIR3DL1*002 is similar to KIR3DL*007, the former generates stronger interaction with Bw4 than the latter [121]. KIR-recognizing HLA-C alleles also have varying interactions. KIR2DL1 has been shown to be the strongest KIR for HLA-C2 followed by KIR2DL2 then KIR2DL3 [122]. These differing affinities may explain the beneficial effect of haplotype B from donors as these donors are homozygous for KIR2DL2 which may account for the generation of NK cells with enhanced function.

Besides using "missing self" model to predict alloreactivites of NK cells as described above, "missing ligand" model has also been used to speculate alloreactivites. According to this model, NK cell alloreactivity may also be observed when the KIR on the surface of donor NK cells cannot recognize the ligands either from donor or recipient [123, 124]. As we have mentioned, these "unlicensed" NK cells are hyporesponsive in situ but can have potential to acquire effector function in recipients. Thus, NK cell alloreactivity can occur even after autologous HSCT. This model is supported by the observation that most individuals have 3 inhibitory KIR, but only 1 or 2 corresponding HLA KIR ligands are expressed on the surface of their own cells [125, 126]. Several comparative analyses have been performed to test the prediction rate of this model. Some groups found the selection of donors based on this model indeed was associated with better outcome, while others reported opposite results [127–129]. These variable results may be due to the complexity and variables of HSCT.

## 6. The impact of cytomegalovirus infection on natural killer cell-mediated graft-versus-leukemia effect: reconstitution promotion and memory induction

### 6.1. The impact of cytomegalovirus infection on natural killer cell reconstitution

Although in healthy individuals, CMV infection is potentially controlled by T cells and NK cells, it can cause life-threatening complication in immunodeficient transplant recipients. Lethal CMV-caused illness is now uncommon thanks to the use of drugs such as ganciclovir and foscarnet. In view of the strong immune response caused by CMV, it is attractive to investigate whether CMV reactivation can reduce the risk of relapse in patients after HSCT. As early as 30 years ago, Lonnqvist et al. reported that CMV infection was associated with lower relapse in BMT recipients with various hematological malignancies [130]. Subsequently, a number of reports confirmed that CMV reactivation following HSCT resulted in reduced relapse in AML patients. Among these reports, Elmaagacli et al. found CMV reactivation occurred within the first 100 days after HSCT significantly reduce the rate of AML relapse from 42 to 9% [131]. Remarkably, this CMV reactivation-mediated relapse prevention effect was independent of aGvHD. Furthermore, in another study of large cohort of 2566 patients with variable hematological malignancies, Green et al. comprehensively analyzed the results among all kinds of disease with adjustment for potential variables and reported that CMV reactivation was significantly associated with a decreased risk of relapse [132].

Upon the association between CMV reactivation and decreased rate of relapse after HSCT was confirmed, several studies next tried to test whether CMV-specific donor T cells accounted for this beneficial effect. However, CMV-specific donor T cells appeared not to impact relapse rates after HSCT [133]. On the other hand, NK cells have been shown to play an important role in CMV reactivation-mediated relapse prevention. Foley et al. demonstrated that the beneficial effect of CMV reactivation was specifically associated with the clonal-like expansion of NK cells characterized by the NKG2C$^{+}$ NKG2A$^{-}$ self-KIR$^{+}$ CD57$^{+}$ CD56$^{dim}$ signature [80]. These NK cells have been shown to exhibit enhanced cytolytic activity and cytokine production. During CMV reactivation, both NKG2C$^{+}$ NK cell percentages and numbers are significantly increased with enhanced capability of producing IFN-γ upon the stimulation of myeloid leukemia cell line K562. Nevertheless, the mechanisms underlie the increased expansion and functions of NKG2C$^{+}$ NK cells are not entirely clear. Guma et al. reported that after *ex vivo* stimulation with CMV-infected fibroblasts, NKG2C$^{+}$ NK cells from seropositive healthy donors rapidly proliferated [134]. These results indicated that NKG2C may play a unique role in NKG2C$^{+}$ NK cell expansion. However, the exact ligands of NKG2C on CMV infected cells are not completely confirmed. Although HLA-E has been shown to be a ligand for NKG2C [135], other undefined ligands may also take part in NKG2C-mediated effect. Leukemic cells can retain HLE expression while downregulate the level of classical class I HLA molecule [136]. Therefore, it is now believed that the change in receptor repertoire from inhibitory receptor NKG2A to activating receptor NKG2C may play a crucial role in this NK cell subset-mediated GvL effect [137].

It has been shown that NK cells from UCB transplants will undergo slower reconstitution compared with NK cells from adult grafts. In contrast, in CMV-infected UCB transplantation patients, NK cells are found to reconstitute rapidly with decreased NKG2A expression and increased KIR expression [138]. Their functional reconstitution is also promoted as they can produce high level of IFN-γ in response to K562 cells. Intriguingly, during CMV-infected UCB transplantation, Della Chiesa et al. detected a unique subset of hyporesponsive NK cells which shared similar surface markers with the expanded NKG2C$^{+}$ NK cells except for CD56 expression [139]. Briefly, this NK cell subset does not express CD56. IL-2 stimulation can reverse the hyporesponsive state of CD56$^{-}$ NK cells thereby this NK cells subset may represent a stage of NK cell differentiation in the case of cytokine deficiencies.

The effect of CMV reactivation was also investigated in recipients received grafts either from peripheral blood or bone marrow [140]. Strikingly, the expansion of NKG2C$^{+}$ NK cells seemed to be dependent on the serostatus of recipient. The percentage of NKG2C$^{+}$ NK cells was significantly increased when CMV seropositive recipients received grafts from CMV seronegative donors. Oppositely, when grafts from CMV seropositive donors were infused into CMV seronegative recipients, NKG2C$^{+}$ NK cells failed to expand, and their percentage was declined to the levels similar to CMV seronegative donor/recipient pairs.

Besides NKG2C, activating KIR may also contribute to CMV-induced NK cell expansion. Della Chiesa et al. proved that when donor grafts were lack of NKG2C, NKG2C$^{-}$ NK cells can rapidly expanded expressing activating KIR in the recipients following CMV infection [141]. These data indicated that activating KIR can recognize CMV and promote NK cell reconstitution

http://dx.doi.org/10.5772/intechopen.69684

independent of NKG2C. Correspondingly, the increased presence of donor activating KIR has been shown to result in reduced risk of CMV infection [142, 143]. However, the ligands expressed on the CMV infected cells specific for activating KIR are still elusive, which become an obstacle to explore the actual role of activating KIR in CMV-infected HSCT.

Additionally, CMV seropositivity has been shown to be associated with presence of a population of NK cells which does not express FcγRIγ [144]. FcγRIγ is an adapter molecule that is used by CD16, NKP30, and NKp46 for signal transmitting. CD3ζ is also required for CD16 associated signal transduction. Lack of both FcγRIγ and CD3ζ in HIV-infected patients was proved to diminish CD16 signaling [145], while single down-regulation of FcγRIγ in CMV seropositive healthy donors resulted in enhanced CD16 signaling [146]. The deficiency of FcγRIγ induced NK cells hyporesponsive to CMV infected fibroblasts, whereas CMV specific antibody can reverse NK cells to degranulate and produce IFN-γ and TNF-α against CMV infected fibroblasts.

### 6.2. Cytomegalovirus infection induces natural killer cell memory

Although traditionally viewed as a member of innate immune cells, NK cells have been demonstrated to mount memory response to hapten and mediate hapten-induced contact hypersensitivity responses [21]. In MCMV model, NK cells were also observed to develop memory-like properties including viral ligand m157 specific expansion, persisting over time and enhanced effector function after rechallenge with MCMV [22, 23]. This MCMV-induced memory-like population of NK cells is characterized by the expression Ly49H. Intriguingly, during acute human CMV, the expanded $NKG2C^+$ $NKG2A^-$ self-$KIR^+$ $CD57^+$ $CD56^{dim}$ NK cells which we have described above was proved to be human analog of $Ly49H^+$ memory-like NK cells [139, 147]. After HSCT, these CMV-specific memory-like NK cells can be detected in peripheral blood of CMV-infected HSCT recipients. As we have mentioned, when CMV-seropositive recipients received grafts from CMV-seropositive donors, these $NKG2C^+$ NK cells underwent expansion even in the absence of detectable viremia, which meant a nonclassical recall response was developed [140]. However, the mechanisms underlined the generation of memory NK cells have not been exactly defined. Recently, two studies demonstrated that CMV infection resulted in modified effector function through driving epigenetic alterations in these "adaptive" NK cells [148]. These memory-like NK cells were proved to lack expression of signaling proteins such as Fc epsilon receptor I (FcεRIγ), spleen tyrosine kinase (Syk), ewing's sarcoma-associated transcript 2 (EAT2) and exhibit increased capacity to mediate ADCC as well as produce IFN-γ in response to tumor targets. In contrast, memory-like NK cells produced extremely less level of IFN-γ in response to cytokines such as IL-12 and IL-18 mainly due to the downregulation of cytokine receptors.

In summary, $NKG2C^+$ NK cells expanded after CMV-infected HSCT display memory-like properties and associated with reduced risk of relapse. Nevertheless, it is still unclear whether the GvL effect observed in CMV-infected HSCT is mainly due to $NKG2^+C$ NK cells cytotoxicity toward leukemic blasts or primarily due to the cytolytic effect of CMV. This potent effect of CMV reactivation in shaping immune response after HSCT may provide new choice for therapeutic strategies, such as utilizing CMV vaccine to mimic this beneficial effect, isolating $NKG2C^+$ NK cells for adoptive transfer setting and optimizing the criterion for donor selection.

## 7. The effects of natural killer cells on graft-versus-host disease

Allo-HSCT has curative potential through donor immune effectors-mediated GvL effects. However, the donor versus host direction effect of alloreactive T cells also causes GvHD which is a major complication of allo-HSCT [2]. Depletion of donor T cells in grafts and application of immunosuppressive pretreatment are often used to eliminate GvHD; however, these treatments also hampers GvL effects at the same time. NK cells have also been shown to play an important role in GvHD. In murine models, alloreactive NK cells are shown to kill antigen presenting cells (APCs) thereby prevent the initiation of aGvHD [100]. Correspondingly, another study demonstrated that alloreactive NK cells can be recruited into the lymph nodes and suppress T cells activation through cytotoxicity toward allogeneic dentritic cells (DCs) [149]. Donor NK cells may also mediate suppression of aGvHD through the direct killing of activated donor alloreactive T cells [150]. The possible mechanism involves the interactions between activating receptor NKG2D and its ligand highly expressed on the surface of activated T cells, which help NK cells to discriminate activated T cells from normal T cells and initiate killing [151, 152]. NK cells were also found to inhibit aGvHD through cytokine production such as TGF-β [153]. Furthermore, NK cells were able to inhibit the proliferation of donor $CD4^{+}$T cells and reduce the risk of cGvHD [154]. Remarkably, donor NK cells are believed not to attack normal host tissues mainly due to the absence of activating receptor ligands on normal nonhematopoietic cells [155].

Although these previous experimental studies suggested that donor NK cells may have potential role in modulating GvHD, the clinical results are variable. Ruggeri L et al. reported NK cell alloreactivity was favorably associated with the lower risk of aGvHD [6]. However, this benefit effect cannot be observed in most groups, some groups even found KIR mismatch may worsen GvHD [156, 157]. Notably, in a recent clinical trial, IL-15/4-1BBL-activated donor NK cell infusion was found to contribute to aGvHD in T-cell depleted HSCT [158]. Collectively, these contradictory results indicated the role of alloreactive NK cells in GvHD may be variable. They could either aggravate or attenuate GvHD probably depended on different immune microenvironment in HSCT. Correspondingly, in our study of murine acute GvHD model, IL-12/15/18-preactivated donor NK cells significantly inhibited severe aGvHD, whereas they accelerated the development of aGvHD in a mild aGvHD model (unpublished data).

## 8. Donor selection based on killer cell immunoglobulin-like receptor typing

Since alloreactive NK cells play a critical role in the successful treatment of leukemia patients receiving alloreactive grafts, it is crucial to ensure sufficient number of NK cells in the best possible donor. As we have discussed above, the polymorphisms of KIR and its ligand HLA obviously affect NK cell alloreactivity. Therefore, genotyping of these two families of genes provides the probability to identify the size of alloreactive NK cell populations in donor. Up to now, there are three levels of KIR typing. The first level is genotyping to test the gene content of KIR families [159]. Based on these results, the KIR haplotype of donor is confirmed and scored.

The preferable donors defined in this level are those possess inhibitory KIR specific for HLA-I alleles absent in the recipients with highest haplotype B score [128, 160]. The second level of KIR typing is using flow cytometry and quantitative PCR to assess the number of KIR mismatched NK cells and the expression of KIR gene [125]. Based on the results of this level, the donors possess the largest number of KIR mismatched NK cells with high frequency of KIR gene expression are preferable. The third level is KIR typing of alleles [161]. As we have discussed above, different alleles of KIR gene may result in different intensity of NK cell alloreactivity. Therefore, donors with stronger KIR alleles should be selected. Finally, FcγR polymorphisms are also needed to analyze when the treatment is associated with ADCC effect of NK cells [162]. Additionally, the assess of NK cell cytotoxicity toward leukemic blasts from patients could also help to predict the outcome of HSCT.

## 9. Adoptive transfer of donor natural killer cells and natural killer cell expansion

Despite their potential beneficial role in allo-HSCT, donor NK cells derived from the hematopoietic stem cells may be functionally impaired due to their immaturity and insufficient education. Thus, adoptively transfer of mature donor NK cells has been employed to provide the immunotherapeutic benefits for allo-HSCT. The first trial of utilizing allogeneic NK cells as immunotherapy in humans was published in 2005 focused on the impact of different chemotherapy preparative regimens on infused donor NK cells [163]. Three different chemotherapy preparative regimens were used in their study: high cyclophosphamide and fludarabine (Hi-Cy/Flu), low cylcophosphamide and methylprednisone, or fludarabine alone. Their results demonstrated that the infusion of NK cells was well tolerated by patients, donor-derived NK cells expansion can only be detected in patients receiving Hi-Cy/Flu. Furthermore, long-term remission was observed in 5 of 19 patients. An obvious increase in endogenous IL-15 concentration was detected in patients receiving high intensity of the conditioning regimen and was associated with the expansion of adoptive transferred donor NK cells. These results indicated the Hi-Cy/Flu treatment may eliminate recipient's lymphocytes thereby provide "space" and adequate cytokines for expansion of transferred donor NK cells. These results also suggested besides IL-2, IL-15 might be a good choice to promote NK cell expansion *in vivo*. In the follow-up study, the criteria for successful donor NK cell expansion were defined as a measurement of more than 100 donor NK cells/μl of peripheral blood 12–16 days after infusion [113].

Although remission of patients was observed in the above studies, this benefit effect was not permanent as patients ultimately relapsed. To test whether host-mediated rejection affected the expansion of donor NK cells thereby resulted in remission, total body irradiation was added to Hi-Cy/Flu to deplete recipient cells [138]. The results demonstrated that measurable NK cell expansion was obviously increased in patients received total body irradiation, which was associated with better leukemia clearance effect. These data again indicated the importance of enough "space" for successful expansion of donor NK cells during HSCT. In a pediatric study, Rubnitz et al. reported after high intensity of lymphodepeleting chemotherapy, infused donor NK cells could successfully expand in the patients of AML [164]. Remarkably, among 10 patients, three patients were observed to have detectable NK cells up to 1 month after infusion and have a disease-free survival rate of 100% at a median of 2 years. This promising outcome may due to the higher cell dose of transferred donor NK cells used in this study; thus, higher doses of infused NK cells may be important for better HSCT outcome.

To produce sufficient number of donor NK cells and achieve the optimal expansion of NK cells *ex vivo*, numbers of studies were performed with variable approaches, such as cytokine stimulation and utilizing engineered feeder cells. Up to now, clinical NK cell doses can be reached even up to $10^8$ NK cells/kg [165]. However, there are numerous factors that may affect the effector function of expanded NK cells. A crucial factor among these complicated production protocol is how to activate NK cells *ex vivo*. Addition of cytokines such as IL-2 or IL-15 was used to promote survival and expansion of NK cells. Although IL-2 stimulation may result in activation-induced cell death (AICD) of NK cells *in vivo*, IL-15 stimulation does not have this side effect [166, 167]. Subsequently, human-derived feeder cells were used to develop approaches in expanding NK cells. Fujisaki et al. first reported the use of genetically modified APCs that could expand NK cells from peripheral blood 500- to 1000-fold [13]. These artificial APCs can be further modified with costimulatory molecules and membrane-bound cytokines [168, 169]. The expanded NK cells express high level of activating receptors and CD16 molecule and are proved to be potent mediators of cytotoxicity. However, these activated NK cells often become "exhausted" and cannot maintain their effector function and expansion *in vivo* [170]. Denman CJ et al. used APCs modified with membrane-bound form of IL-21 to break this barrier [168]. However, after cytokine withdrawal, these *ex vivo* expanded NK cells have been shown to have shorter survival *in vivo* compared with freshly activated NK cells [171].

Another alternative approach is to generate "memory-like" NK cells *ex vivo*. Cooper et al. reported that IL-12/15/18-preactivated NK cells obtained the ability to produce increased IFN-γ upon restimulation for up to 4 months after adoptive transfer [24]. Therefore, cytokine preactivation before infusion may amplify and sustain the beneficial effects of NK cells during allo-HSCT. The enhanced antitumor activity of murine IL-12/15/18-preactivated NK cells was first demonstrated in a murine tumor model [172]. Similar to murine NK cells, human IL-12/15/18-preactivated NK cells have been recently shown to have memory-like properties, including increased IFN-γ production, enhanced proliferation, and high expression of IL-2 receptor [26]. Recently, a phase I study of adoptively transferred cytokine-induced memory-like NK cells has demonstrated sustained anti-leukemia responses in patients with relapsed or refractory AML [173]. Therefore, cytokine-induced memory-like NK cells may possess long-lasting effector function *in vivo*, which can be harnessed in the treatment of leukemia patients. However, the safety of such therapy could be complicated by the induction of aGvHD after allo-HSCT. Adoptively transfer of donor-derived IL-15/4-1BBL-activated donor NK cells contributed to aGvHD [158], likely through upregulation of activating receptor expression and inflammatory cytokine production. Therefore, the effect of IL-12/15/18-preactivated NK cell infusion on GvL and GvHD after allo-HSCT needs further investigation.

## 10. Methods to enhance natural killer cell function and future perspectives

Monoclonal antibodies are now increasingly being studied for their effect on enhancement of NK cell activity. The isotype IgG1 subclass is often used to induce ADCC through stimulating activating Fc receptors on NK cells. The most effective monoclonal antibody used in hematological malignancy is Rituximab, which targets antigen CD20 on B cells [174]. Notably, it was proved that such antibodies should be administered at appropriate time point as NK cells reconstituted early after HSCT are immature with lower expression of CD16 [95]. Interactions between inhibitory KIRs and HLA molecules transmit a potent inhibitory signal to the NK cell, thus monoclonal antibodies blocking inhibitory KIR receptors are used to enhance NK cell activity. The preclinical results demonstrated these antibodies appear safe and do not induce autoimmunity [175]. Additionally, a disintegrin and metalloprotease-17 (ADAM17) was demonstrated to induce activated NK cells to lose expression of CD16 and CD62L [176]. Therefore, pharmacologic inhibition of ADAM17 is used to enhance the cytotoxicity of NK cells toward Rituximab bound lymphoma cells. Following the improvement of antibody production, bispecific killer engagers (BiKE) and trispecific killer engagers (TriKE) are used to crosslink specific tumor antigens such as CD19, CD20 with a potent stimulator on NK cell such as CD16 [177–179]. CD16 × 19 BiKEs and CD16 × 19 × 22 TriKEs have been constructed and shown to significantly activate CD16 signaling of NK cells [180, 181]. Furthermore, a CD16 × 33 BiKEs was constructed recently and proved to result in potent cytotoxicity of NK cells in patients of refractory AML [182]. However, the very short half-life of bi- and trispecific antibodies might limit their therapeutic effect [179].

Another important focus is to enhance the immune response of NK cells through sensitizing target cells. Bortezomib is a drug classically used to treat multiple myeloma and mantle cell lymphoma. As a proteosome inhibitor, Bortezomib can sensitize tumor cells to TRAIL-mediated apoptosis [14]. Moreover, drugs such as doxorubicin and depsipeptide have been proved to upregulate the expression of death receptors including Fas, TRAIL-R1, TNFR1, thereby sensitize tumor cells to the cytotoxicity of NK cells [183, 184].

Recently, NK cells are also genetic engineered to express CARs which represent an effective therapy. The preclinical studies demonstrated that primary NK cells expressed CAR constructs can result in potent killing of B cell tumors [185, 186]. However, it is difficult to express exogenous genes in primary NK cells and to reach enough number for immunotherapy. Therefore, human NK-like cell line, NK-92 becomes another candidate for genetic engineering. Based on the results of phase I clinical trials of NK-92 cells [187], CAR-expressing NK-92 cells may be easily expanded *ex vivo* and well tolerated in patients.

## 11. Conclusions

A number of recent studies demonstrated that NK cells played a critical role in disease-relapse prevention. Based on the progress made in the field of NK cell therapy, the criteria for choosing HSCT donor have been significantly changed and shown to be associated with better outcomes. However, the role of NK cells in HSCT is not fully understood. The GvL effect of NK alloreactivity may be affected by the complexity of HSCT including the degree of T-cell depletion, donor sources, degree of HLA mismatch, different intensity of preparative regimens, and the origin of leukemic blasts. Furthermore, the haplotype of donor KIR genes and the intensity of interaction between KIR and HLA may also influence the GvL effect of NK cells. Donor KIR B haplotype may be favorably associated with better overall survival. The education of NK cells is also critical for their beneficial effect. The stronger KIR/HLA affinity may contribute to the generation of NK cells with enhanced GvL effect. Intriguingly, "unlicensed" NK cells may also have chance to undergo "re-education" and acquire potent effector function after HSCT. Several studies reported the favorable association between CMV reactivation and better HSCT outcome. This beneficial effect of CMV reactivation was mainly due to the expansion of NKG2C$^+$ NK cells. Moreover, these NKG2C$^+$ NK cells display memory-like properties and enhanced cytotoxicity toward leukemic blasts. NK alloreactivity has been demonstrated to play potential role in suppression of aGvHD. However, some groups found KIR mismatch or alloreactive donor NK cell infusion also worsen aGvHD. Therefore, the role of NK alloreactivity in GVHD still needs to be carefully studied.

Since the GvL effect of NK alloreactiviy is affected in various aspects. Some critical questions are still remained to answer so as to ensure NK cells play the most desirable role during HSCT. The fate of NK cells is still unpredictable after transfusion. The optimal approach to expand most powerful NK cells which can maintain their proliferative potential and effector function *in vivo* is still not confirmed. The risk of the clinical usage of these activated NK cells is still needed for evaluation. The ligands of several activating receptors are undefined and the interactions between NK cells and other immune cells need further investigation. Further studies are also required to explore the mechanism underlying the process of NK cell "education" and "memory". Recently, monoclonal antibodies and immunomodulatory drugs are utilized to modulate NK cell function and proved to have benefit effect on the outcome of HSCT, whereas it is still needed to confirm the suitable hematopoietic malignancies for these treatments. The answers to these questions and continuous progress in understanding NK cells biology will optimize donor NK cells-based therapy and benefit the outcomes of HSCT.

## Author details

Bo Hu[1,2,3] and Haiyan Liu[4*]

*Address all correspondence to: micliuh@nus.edu.sg

1 Institute of Blood and Marrow Transplantation, Soochow University, Suzhou, China

2 Collaborative Innovation Center of Hematology, Soochow University, China

3 The First Affiliated Hospital of Soochow University, Suzhou, China

4 Immunology Programme, Life Sciences Institute and Department of Microbiology and Immunology, National University of Singapore, Singapore

http://dx.doi.org/10.5772/intechopen.69684

## References

[1] Hamilton BK, Copelan EA. Concise review: The role of hematopoietic stem cell transplantation in the treatment of acute myeloid leukemia. Stem cells. 2012;**30**(8):1581-1586

[2] Parkman R. Getting a handle on graft-versus-host disease. The New England Journal of Medicine. 2004;**350**(6):614-615

[3] Beilhack A, Schulz S, Baker J et al. *In vivo* analyses of early events in acute graft-versus-host disease reveal sequential infiltration of T-cell subsets. Blood. 2005;**106**(3):1113-1122

[4] Ljunggren HG, Malmberg KJ. Prospects for the use of NK cells in immunotherapy of human cancer. Nature Reviews Immunology. 2007;**7**(5):329-339

[5] Terme M, Ullrich E, Delahaye NF et al. Natural killer cell-directed therapies: Moving from unexpected results to successful strategies. Nature Immunology 2008;**9**(5):486-494

[6] Ruggeri L, Capanni M, Urbani E et al. Effectiveness of donor natural killer cell alloreactivity in mismatched hematopoietic transplants. Science. 2002;**295**(5562):2097-2100

[7] Olson JA, Zeiser R, Beilhack A et al. Tissue-specific homing and expansion of donor NK cells in allogeneic bone marrow transplantation. Journal of Immunology. 2009;**183**(5): 3219-3228

[8] Symons HJ, Fuchs EJ. Hematopoietic SCT from partially HLA-mismatched (HLA-haploidentical) related donors. Bone Marrow Transplantation. 2008;**42**(6):365-377

[9] Yu J, Freud AG, Caligiuri MA. Location and cellular stages of natural killer cell development. Trends Immunology. 2013;**34**(12):573-582

[10] Koehl U, Kalberer C, Spanholtz J et al. Advances in clinical NK cell studies: Donor selection, manufacturing and quality control. Oncoimmunology. 2016;**5**(4):e1115178

[11] Klingemann H. Challenges of cancer therapy with natural killer cells. Cytotherapy. 2015; **17**(3):245-249

[12] Schonberg K, Fischer JC, Kogler G, Uhrberg M. Neonatal NK-cell repertoires are functionally, but not structurally, biased toward recognition of self HLA class I. Blood. 2011; **117**(19):5152-5156

[13] Fujisaki H, Kakuda H, Shimasaki N et al. Expansion of highly cytotoxic human natural killer cells for cancer cell therapy. Cancer Research. 2009;**69**(9):4010-4017

[14] Berg M, Lundqvist A, McCoy P, Jr. et al. Clinical-grade *ex vivo*-expanded human natural killer cells up-regulate activating receptors and death receptor ligands and have enhanced cytolytic activity against tumor cells. Cytotherapy. 2009;**11**(3):341-355

[15] Spanholtz J, Preijers F, Tordoir M et al. Clinical-grade generation of active NK cells from cord blood hematopoietic progenitor cells for immunotherapy using a closed-system culture process. PloS One. 2011;**6**(6):e20740

[16] Tonn T, Schwabe D, Klingemann HG et al. Treatment of patients with advanced cancer with the natural killer cell line NK-92. Cytotherapy. 2013;**15**(12):1563-1570

[17] Tam YK, Martinson JA, Doligosa K, Klingemann HG. *Ex vivo* expansion of the highly cytotoxic human natural killer-92 cell-line under current good manufacturing practice conditions for clinical adoptive cellular immunotherapy. Cytotherapy. 2003;**5**(3):259-272

[18] Binyamin L, Alpaugh RK, Hughes TL et al. Blocking NK cell inhibitory self-recognition promotes antibody-dependent cellular cytotoxicity in a model of anti-lymphoma therapy. Journal of Immunology. 2008;**180**(9):6392-6401

[19] Clemenceau B, Vivien R, Pellat C et al. The human natural killer cytotoxic cell line NK-92, once armed with a murine CD16 receptor, represents a convenient cellular tool for the screening of mouse mAbs according to their ADCC potential. mAbs. 2013;**5**(4):587-594

[20] Romanski A, Uherek C, Bug G et al. CD19-CAR engineered NK-92 cells are sufficient to overcome NK cell resistance in B-cell malignancies. Journal of Cellular and Molecular Medicine. 2016;**20**(7):1287-1294

[21] Paust S, Gill HS, Wang BZ et al. Critical role for the chemokine receptor CXCR6 in NK cell-mediated antigen-specific memory of haptens and viruses. Nature Immunology. 2010;**11**(12):1127-1135

[22] Kuijpers TW, Baars PA, Dantin C et al. Human NK cells can control CMV infection in the absence of T cells. Blood. 2008;**112**(3):914-915

[23] Cheng TP, French AR, Plougastel BF et al. Ly49h is necessary for genetic resistance to murine cytomegalovirus. Immunogenetics. 2008;**60**(10):565-573

[24] Cooper MA, Elliott JM, Keyel PA et al. Cytokine-induced memory-like natural killer cells. Proceedings of the National Academy of Sciences of the United States of America. 2009;**106**(6):1915-1919

[25] Keppel MP, Yang L, Cooper MA. Murine NK cell intrinsic cytokine-induced memory-like responses are maintained following homeostatic proliferation. Journal of Immunology. 2013;**190**(9):4754-4762

[26] Romee R, Schneider SE, Leong JW et al. Cytokine activation induces human memory-like NK cells. Blood. 2012;**120**(24):4751-4760

[27] Herberman RB, Nunn ME, Lavrin DH. Natural cytotoxic reactivity of mouse lymphoid cells against syngeneic acid allogeneic tumors. I. Distribution of reactivity and specificity. International Journal of Cancer Journal International du Cancer. 1975;**16**(2):216-229

[28] Kiessling R, Klein E, Wigzell H. "Natural" killer cells in the mouse. I. Cytotoxic cells with specificity for mouse Moloney leukemia cells. Specificity and distribution according to genotype. European Journal of Immunology. 1975;**5**(2):112-117

[29] Montaldo E, Vacca P, Moretta L, Mingari MC. Development of human natural killer cells and other innate lymphoid cells. Seminars in Immunology. 2014;**26**(2):107-113

[30] Caligiuri MA. Human natural killer cells. Blood. 2008;**112**(3):461-469

[31] Jacobs R, Hintzen G, Kemper A et al. CD56bright cells differ in their KIR repertoire and cytotoxic features from CD56dim NK cells. European Journal of Immunology. 2001;**31**(10):3121-3127

[32] Robertson MJ, Manley TJ, Donahue C et al. Costimulatory signals are required for optimal proliferation of human natural killer cells. Journal of Immunology. 1993;**150**(5):1705-1714

[33] Baume DM, Robertson MJ, Levine H et al. Differential responses to interleukin 2 define functionally distinct subsets of human natural killer cells. European Journal of Immunology. 1992;**22**(1):1-6

[34] Moretta L, Locatelli F, Pende D et al. Killer Ig-like receptor-mediated control of natural killer cell alloreactivity in haploidentical hematopoietic stem cell transplantation. Blood. 2011;**117**(3):764-771

[35] Valiante NM, Uhrberg M, Shilling HG et al. Functionally and structurally distinct NK cell receptor repertoires in the peripheral blood of two human donors. Immunity. 1997;**7**(6):739-751

[36] Cooley S, Trachtenberg E, Bergemann TL et al. Donors with group B KIR haplotypes improve relapse-free survival after unrelated hematopoietic cell transplantation for acute myelogenous leukemia. Blood. 2009;**113**(3):726-732

[37] Pyo CW, Guethlein LA, Vu Q et al. Different patterns of evolution in the centromeric and telomeric regions of group A and B haplotypes of the human killer cell Ig-like receptor locus. PloS One. 2010;**5**(12):e15115

[38] Bryceson YT, March ME, Ljunggren HG, Long EO. Activation, coactivation, and costimulation of resting human natural killer cells. Immunol Reviews. 2006;**214**(73-91)

[39] Pende D, Cantoni C, Rivera P et al. Role of NKG2D in tumor cell lysis mediated by human NK cells: Cooperation with natural cytotoxicity receptors and capability of recognizing tumors of nonepithelial origin. European Journal of Immunology. 2001;**31**(4):1076-1086

[40] Cosman D, Mullberg J, Sutherland CL et al. ULBPs, novel MHC class I-related molecules, bind to CMV glycoprotein UL16 and stimulate NK cytotoxicity through the NKG2D receptor. Immunity. 2001;**14**(2):123-133

[41] Hershkovitz O, Rosental B, Rosenberg LA et al. NKp44 receptor mediates interaction of the envelope glycoproteins from the West Nile and dengue viruses with NK cells. Journal of Immunology. 2009;**183**(4):2610-2621

[42] Pende D, Parolini S, Pessino A et al. Identification and molecular characterization of NKp30, a novel triggering receptor involved in natural cytotoxicity mediated by human natural killer cells. The Journal of Experimental Medicine. 1999;**190**(10):1505-1516

[43] Vitale M, Bottino C, Sivori S et al. NKp44, a novel triggering surface molecule specifically expressed by activated natural killer cells, is involved in non-major histocompatibility complex-restricted tumor cell lysis. The Journal of Experimental Medicine. 1998;**187**(12):2065-2072

[44] Mandelboim O, Lieberman N, Lev M et al. Recognition of haemagglutinins on virus-infected cells by NKp46 activates lysis by human NK cells. Nature. 2001;**409**(6823): 1055-1060

[45] Baychelier F, Sennepin A, Ermonval M et al. Identification of a cellular ligand for the natural cytotoxicity receptor NKp44. Blood. 2013;**122**(17):2935-2942

[46] Yokoyama WM. Specific and non-specific natural killer cell responses to viral infection. Advances in Experimental Medicine and Biology. 2005;**560**(57-61)

[47] Torelli GF, Guarini A, Palmieri G et al. Expansion of cytotoxic effectors with lytic activity against autologous blasts from acute myeloid leukaemia patients in complete haematological remission. British Journal of Haematology. 2002;**116**(2):299-307

[48] Trapani JA, Smyth MJ. Killing by cytotoxic T cells and natural killer cells: Multiple granule serine proteases as initiators of DNA fragmentation. Immunology and cell biology 1993;**71**(Pt 3):201-208

[49] Screpanti V, Wallin RP, Ljunggren HG, Grandien A. A central role for death receptor-mediated apoptosis in the rejection of tumors by NK cells. Journal of Immunology. 2001;**167**(4):2068-2073

[50] Smyth MJ, Takeda K, Hayakawa Y et al. Nature's TRAIL—on a path to cancer immunotherapy. Immunity. 2003;**18**(1):1-6

[51] Lanier LL, Ruitenberg JJ, Phillips JH. Functional and biochemical analysis of CD16 antigen on natural killer cells and granulocytes. Journal of Immunology. 1988;**141**(10):3478-3485

[52] Gerosa F, Baldani-Guerra B, Nisii C et al. Reciprocal activating interaction between natural killer cells and dendritic cells. The Journal of Experimental Medicine. 2002;**195**(3): 327-333

[53] Martin-Fontecha A, Thomsen LL, Brett S et al. Induced recruitment of NK cells to lymph nodes provides IFN-gamma for T(H)1 priming. Nature Immunology. 2004;**5**(12): 1260-1265

[54] Montaldo E, Del Zotto G, Della Chiesa M et al. Human NK cell receptors/markers: A tool to analyze NK cell development, subsets and function. Cytometry Part A: The Journal of the International Society for Analytical Cytology 2013;**83**(8):702-713

[55] Boos MD, Yokota Y, Eberl G, Kee BL. Mature natural killer cell and lymphoid tissue-inducing cell development requires Id2-mediated suppression of E protein activity. The Journal of Experimental Medicine. 2007;**204**(5):1119-1130

[56] Aliahmad P, de la Torre B, Kaye J. Shared dependence on the DNA-binding factor TOX for the development of lymphoid tissue-inducer cell and NK cell lineages. Nature Immunology. 2010;**11**(10):945-952

[57] Gascoyne DM, Long E, Veiga-Fernandes H et al. The basic leucine zipper transcription factor E4BP4 is essential for natural killer cell development. Nature Immunology. 2009;**10**(10):1118-1124

[58] Kamizono S, Duncan GS, Seidel MG et al. Nfil3/E4bp4 is required for the development and maturation of NK cells *in vivo*. The Journal of Experimental Medicine. 2009;**206**(13): 2977-2986

[59] Gordon SM, Chaix J, Rupp LJ et al. The transcription factors T-bet and Eomes control key checkpoints of natural killer cell maturation. Immunity. 2012;**36**(1):55-67

[60] Pradier A, Simonetta F, Waldvogel S et al. Modulation of T-bet and eomes during maturation of peripheral blood NK cells does not depend on licensing/educating KIR. Frontiers Immunology. 2016;**7**:299

[61] Minagawa M, Watanabe H, Miyaji C et al. Enforced expression of Bcl-2 restores the number of NK cells, but does not rescue the impaired development of NKT cells or intraepithelial lymphocytes, in IL-2/IL-15 receptor beta-chain-deficient mice. Journal of Immunology. 2002;**169**(8):4153-4160

[62] Yu H, Fehniger TA, Fuchshuber P et al. Flt3 ligand promotes the generation of a distinct CD34(+) human natural killer cell progenitor that responds to interleukin-15. Blood. 1998;**92**(10):3647-3657

[63] Carson WE, Haldar S, Baiocchi RA et al. The c-kit ligand suppresses apoptosis of human natural killer cells through the upregulation of bcl-2. Proceedings of the National Academy of Sciences of the United States of America. 1994;**91**(16):7553-7557

[64] Bulfone-Paus S, Bulanova E, Budagian V, Paus R. The interleukin-15/interleukin-15 receptor system as a model for juxtacrine and reverse signaling. BioEssays: News and Reviews in Molecular, Cellular and Developmental Biology. 2006;**28**(4):362-377

[65] Fauriat C, Long EO, Ljunggren HG, Bryceson YT. Regulation of human NK-cell cytokine and chemokine production by target cell recognition. Blood. 2010;**115**(11):2167-2176

[66] De Maria A, Bozzano F, Cantoni C, Moretta L. Revisiting human natural killer cell subset function revealed cytolytic CD56(dim)CD16+ NK cells as rapid producers of abundant IFN-gamma on activation. Proceedings of the National Academy of Sciences of the United States of America. 2011;**108**(2):728-732

[67] Hallett WH, Murphy WJ. Positive and negative regulation of Natural Killer cells: Therapeutic implications. Seminars in Cancer Biology. 2006;**16**(5):367-382

[68] Ferlazzo G, Thomas D, Lin SL et al. The abundant NK cells in human secondary lymphoid tissues require activation to express killer cell Ig-like receptors and become cytolytic. Journal of Immunology. 2004;**172**(3):1455-1462

[69] Fehniger TA, Cooper MA, Nuovo GJ et al. CD56bright natural killer cells are present in human lymph nodes and are activated by T cell-derived IL-2: A potential new link between adaptive and innate immunity. Blood. 2003;**101**(8):3052-3057

[70] Romagnani C, Juelke K, Falco M et al. CD56brightCD16- killer Ig-like receptor- NK cells display longer telomeres and acquire features of CD56dim NK cells upon activation. Journal of Immunology. 2007;**178**(8):4947-4955

[71] Zhang J, Chen Z, Smith GN, Croy BA. Natural killer cell-triggered vascular transformation: Maternal care before birth? Cellular & Molecular Immunology. 2011;**8**(1):1-11

[72] Macallan DC, Borghans JA, Asquith B. Human T cell memory: A dynamic view. Vaccines. 2017;**5**(1)

[73] O'Leary JG, Goodarzi M, Drayton DL, von Andrian UH. T cell- and B cell-independent adaptive immunity mediated by natural killer cells. Nature Immunology. 2006;**7**(5): 507-516

[74] Peng H, Jiang X, Chen Y et al. Liver-resident NK cells confer adaptive immunity in skin-contact inflammation. The Journal of Clinical Investigation. 2013;**123**(4):1444-1456

[75] Sun JC, Beilke JN, Lanier LL. Adaptive immune features of natural killer cells. Nature. 2009;**457**(7229):557-561

[76] Nabekura T, Kanaya M, Shibuya A et al. Costimulatory molecule DNAM-1 is essential for optimal differentiation of memory natural killer cells during mouse cytomegalovirus infection. Immunity. 2014;**40**(2):225-234

[77] Madera S, Rapp M, Firth MA et al. Type I IFN promotes NK cell expansion during viral infection by protecting NK cells against fratricide. The Journal of Experimental Medicine. 2016;**213**(2):225-233

[78] Beaulieu AM, Zawislak CL, Nakayama T, Sun JC. The transcription factor Zbtb32 controls the proliferative burst of virus-specific natural killer cells responding to infection. Nature Immunology. 2014;**15**(6):546-553

[79] Lopez-Verges S, Milush JM, Schwartz BS et al. Expansion of a unique CD57(+) NKG2Chi natural killer cell subset during acute human cytomegalovirus infection. Proceedings of the National Academy of Sciences of the United States of America. 2011;**108**(36):14725-14732

[80] Foley B, Cooley S, Verneris MR et al. Cytomegalovirus reactivation after allogeneic transplantation promotes a lasting increase in educated NKG2C+ natural killer cells with potent function. Blood. 2012;**119**(11):2665-2674

[81] Rolle A, Brodin P. Immune adaptation to environmental influence: The case of NK cells and HCMV. Trends Immunology. 2016;**37**(3):233-243

[82] Luetke-Eversloh M, Hammer Q, Durek P et al. Human cytomegalovirus drives epigenetic imprinting of the IFNG locus in NKG2Chi natural killer cells. PLoS Pathogens. 2014;**10**(10):e1004441

[83] Raulet DH, Vance RE, McMahon CW. Regulation of the natural killer cell receptor repertoire. Annual Review of Immunology. 2001;**19**:291-330

[84] Raulet DH, Held W, Correa I et al. Specificity, tolerance and developmental regulation of natural killer cells defined by expression of class I-specific Ly49 receptors. Immunology Reviews. 1997;**155**:41-52

[85] Zimmer J, Donato L, Hanau D et al. Activity and phenotype of natural killer cells in peptide transporter (TAP)-deficient patients (type I bare lymphocyte syndrome). The Journal of Experimental Medicine. 1998;**187**(1):117-122

[86] Zimmer J, Donato L, Hanau D et al. Inefficient protection of human TAP-deficient fibroblasts from autologous NK cell-mediated lysis by cytokines inducing HLA class I expression. European Journal of Immunology. 1999;**29**(4):1286-1291

[87] Orr MT, Murphy WJ, Lanier LL. 'Unlicensed' natural killer cells dominate the response to cytomegalovirus infection. Nature Immunology. 2010;**11**(4):321-327

[88] Kim S, Poursine-Laurent J, Truscott SM et al. Licensing of natural killer cells by host major histocompatibility complex class I molecules. Nature. 2005;**436**(7051):709-713

[89] Pende D, Marcenaro S, Falco M et al. Anti-leukemia activity of alloreactive NK cells in KIR ligand-mismatched haploidentical HSCT for pediatric patients: Evaluation of the functional role of activating KIR and redefinition of inhibitory KIR specificity. Blood 2009;**113**(13):3119-3129

[90] Small TN, Papadopoulos EB, Boulad F et al. Comparison of immune reconstitution after unrelated and related T-cell-depleted bone marrow transplantation: Effect of patient age and donor leukocyte infusions. Blood. 1999;**93**(2):467-480

[91] Bjorklund AT, Schaffer M, Fauriat C et al. NK cells expressing inhibitory KIR for non-self-ligands remain tolerant in HLA-matched sibling stem cell transplantation. Blood. 2010;**115**(13):2686-2694

[92] Nguyen S, Kuentz M, Vernant JP et al. Involvement of mature donor T cells in the NK cell reconstitution after haploidentical hematopoietic stem-cell transplantation. Leukemia. 2008;**22**(2):344-352

[93] Eissens DN, Schaap NP, Preijers FW et al. CD3+/CD19+-depleted grafts in HLA-matched allogeneic peripheral blood stem cell transplantation lead to early NK cell cytolytic responses and reduced inhibitory activity of NKG2A. Leukemia. 2010;**24**(3):583-591

[94] Shilling HG, McQueen KL, Cheng NW et al. Reconstitution of NK cell receptor repertoire following HLA-matched hematopoietic cell transplantation. Blood. 2003;**101**(9): 3730-3740

[95] Foley B, Cooley S, Verneris MR et al. NK cell education after allogeneic transplantation: Dissociation between recovery of cytokine-producing and cytotoxic functions. Blood. 2011;**118**(10):2784-2792

[96] Vago L, Forno B, Sormani MP et al. Temporal, quantitative, and functional characteristics of single-KIR-positive alloreactive natural killer cell recovery account for impaired graft-versus-leukemia activity after haploidentical hematopoietic stem cell transplantation. Blood. 2008;**112**(8):3488-3499

[97] Gleason MK, Lenvik TR, McCullar V et al. Tim-3 is an inducible human natural killer cell receptor that enhances interferon gamma production in response to galectin-9. Blood. 2012;**119**(13):3064-3072

[98] Fehniger TA, Shah MH, Turner MJ et al. Differential cytokine and chemokine gene expression by human NK cells following activation with IL-18 or IL-15 in combination with IL-12: Implications for the innate immune response. Journal of Immunology. 1999;**162**(8):4511-4520

[99] Locatelli F, Pende D, Maccario R et al. Haploidentical hemopoietic stem cell transplantation for the treatment of high-risk leukemias: How NK cells make the difference. Clinical Immunology. 2009;**133**(2):171-178

[100] Ruggeri L, Capanni M, Casucci M et al. Role of natural killer cell alloreactivity in HLA-mismatched hematopoietic stem cell transplantation. Blood. 1999;**94**(1):333-339

[101] Davies SM, Ruggieri L, DeFor T et al. Evaluation of KIR ligand incompatibility in mismatched unrelated donor hematopoietic transplants. Killer immunoglobulin-like receptor. Blood. 2002;**100**(10):3825-3827

[102] Giebel S, Locatelli F, Lamparelli T et al. Survival advantage with KIR ligand incompatibility in hematopoietic stem cell transplantation from unrelated donors. Blood. 2003;**102**(3):814-819

[103] Farag SS, Bacigalupo A, Eapen M et al. The effect of KIR ligand incompatibility on the outcome of unrelated donor transplantation: A report from the center for international blood and marrow transplant research, the European blood and marrow transplant registry, and the Dutch registry. Biology of Blood and Marrow Transplantation: Journal of the American Society for Blood and Marrow Transplantation. 2006;**12**(8):876-884

[104] Miller JS, Cooley S, Parham P et al. Missing KIR ligands are associated with less relapse and increased graft-versus-host disease (GVHD) following unrelated donor allogeneic HCT. Blood. 2007;**109**(11):5058-5061

[105] Willemze R, Rodrigues CA, Labopin M et al. KIR-ligand incompatibility in the graft-versus-host direction improves outcomes after umbilical cord blood transplantation for acute leukemia. Leukemia. 2009;**23**(3):492-500

[106] Brunstein CG, Wagner JE, Weisdorf DJ et al. Negative effect of KIR alloreactivity in recipients of umbilical cord blood transplant depends on transplantation conditioning intensity. Blood. 2009;**113**(22):5628-5634

[107] Almalte Z, Samarani S, Iannello A et al. Novel associations between activating killer-cell immunoglobulin-like receptor genes and childhood leukemia. Blood. 2011;**118**(5): 1323-1328

[108] Pfeiffer M, Schumm M, Feuchtinger T et al. Intensity of HLA class I expression and KIR-mismatch determine NK-cell mediated lysis of leukaemic blasts from children with acute lymphatic leukaemia. British Journal of Haematology. 2007;**138**(1):97-100

[109] McQueen KL, Dorighi KM, Guethlein LA et al. Donor-recipient combinations of group A and B KIR haplotypes and HLA class I ligand affect the outcome of HLA-matched, sibling donor hematopoietic cell transplantation. Human Immunology. 2007;**68**(5):309-323

[110] Stringaris K, Adams S, Uribe M et al. Donor KIR Genes 2DL5A, 2DS1 and 3DS1 are associated with a reduced rate of leukemia relapse after HLA-identical sibling stem cell transplantation for acute myeloid leukemia but not other hematologic malignancies. Biology of Blood and Marrow Transplantation : Journal of the American Society for Blood and Marrow Transplantation. 2010;**16**(9):1257-1264

[111] Venstrom JM, Gooley TA, Spellman S et al. Donor activating KIR3DS1 is associated with decreased acute GVHD in unrelated allogeneic hematopoietic stem cell transplantation. Blood. 2010;**115**(15):3162-3165

[112] Michaelis SU, Mezger M, Bornhauser M et al. KIR haplotype B donors but not KIR-ligand mismatch result in a reduced incidence of relapse after haploidentical transplantation using reduced intensity conditioning and CD3/CD19-depleted grafts. Annals of Hematology. 2014;**93**(9):1579-1586

[113] Foley B, De Santis D, Lathbury L et al. KIR2DS1-mediated activation overrides NKG2A-mediated inhibition in HLA-C C2-negative individuals. International Immunology. 2008;**20**(4):555-563

[114] Venstrom JM, Pittari G, Gooley TA et al. HLA-C-dependent prevention of leukemia relapse by donor activating KIR2DS1. The New England Journal of Medicine. 2012;**367**(9):805-816

[115] Mancusi A, Ruggeri L, Urbani E et al. Haploidentical hematopoietic transplantation from KIR ligand-mismatched donors with activating KIRs reduces nonrelapse mortality. Blood. 2015;**125**(20):3173-3182

[116] Cella M, Longo A, Ferrara GB et al. NK3-specific natural killer cells are selectively inhibited by Bw4-positive HLA alleles with isoleucine 80. The Journal of Experimental Medicine. 1994;**180**(4):1235-1242

[117] Draghi M, Yawata N, Gleimer M et al. Single-cell analysis of the human NK cell response to missing self and its inhibition by HLA class I. Blood. 2005;**105**(5):2028-2035

[118] Martin MP, Gao X, Lee JH et al. Epistatic interaction between KIR3DS1 and HLA-B delays the progression to AIDS. Nature Genetics. 2002;**31**(4):429-434

[119] Yawata M, Yawata N, Draghi M et al. MHC class I-specific inhibitory receptors and their ligands structure diverse human NK-cell repertoires toward a balance of missing self-response. Blood. 2008;**112**(6):2369-2380

[120] Pando MJ, Gardiner CM, Gleimer M et al. The protein made from a common allele of KIR3DL1 (3DL1*004) is poorly expressed at cell surfaces due to substitution at positions 86 in Ig domain 0 and 182 in Ig domain 1. Journal of Immunology. 2003;**171**(12):6640-6649

[121] Carr WH, Pando MJ, Parham P. KIR3DL1 polymorphisms that affect NK cell inhibition by HLA-Bw4 ligand. Journal of Immunology. 2005;**175**(8):5222-5229

[122] Moesta AK, Norman PJ, Yawata M et al. Synergistic polymorphism at two positions distal to the ligand-binding site makes KIR2DL2 a stronger receptor for HLA-C than KIR2DL3. Journal of Immunology. 2008;**180**(6):3969-3979

[123] Ljunggren HG, Karre K. In search of the 'missing self': MHC molecules and NK cell recognition. Immunology Today. 1990;**11**(7):237-244

[124] Karre K. Immunology. A perfect mismatch. Science. 2002;**295**(5562):2029-2031

[125] Leung W, Iyengar R, Triplett B et al. Comparison of killer Ig-like receptor genotyping and phenotyping for selection of allogeneic blood stem cell donors. Journal of Immunology. 2005;**174**(10):6540-6545

[126] Hsu KC, Gooley T, Malkki M et al. KIR ligands and prediction of relapse after unrelated donor hematopoietic cell transplantation for hematologic malignancy. Biology of Blood and Marrow Transplantation: Journal of the American Society for Blood and Marrow Transplantation. 2006;**12**(8):828-836

[127] Hsu KC, Keever-Taylor CA, Wilton A et al. Improved outcome in HLA-identical sibling hematopoietic stem-cell transplantation for acute myelogenous leukemia predicted by KIR and HLA genotypes. Blood. 2005;**105**(12):4878-4884

[128] Leung W, Iyengar R, Turner V et al. Determinants of antileukemia effects of allogeneic NK cells. Journal of Immunology. 2004;**172**(1):644-650

[129] Ruggeri L, Mancusi A, Capanni M et al. Donor natural killer cell allorecognition of missing self in haploidentical hematopoietic transplantation for acute myeloid leukemia: Challenging its predictive value. Blood. 2007;**110**(1):433-440

[130] Lonnqvist B, Ringden O, Ljungman P et al. Reduced risk of recurrent leukaemia in bone marrow transplant recipients after cytomegalovirus infection. British Journal of Haematology. 1986;**63**(4):671-679

[131] Elmaagacli AH, Steckel NK, Koldehoff M et al. Early human cytomegalovirus replication after transplantation is associated with a decreased relapse risk: Evidence for a putative virus-versus-leukemia effect in acute myeloid leukemia patients. Blood. 2011;**118**(5):1402-1412

[132] Green ML, Leisenring WM, Xie H et al. CMV reactivation after allogeneic HCT and relapse risk: Evidence for early protection in acute myeloid leukemia. Blood. 2013;**122**(7):1316-1324

[133] Thomson KJ, Mackinnon S, Peggs KS. CMV-specific cellular therapy for acute myeloid leukemia? Blood. 2012;**119**(4):1088-1090; author reply 1090-1081

[134] Guma M, Budt M, Saez A et al. Expansion of CD94/NKG2C+ NK cells in response to human cytomegalovirus-infected fibroblasts. Blood. 2006;**107**(9):3624-3631

[135] Braud VM, Allan DS, O'Callaghan CA et al. HLA-E binds to natural killer cell receptors CD94/NKG2A, B and C. Nature. 1998;**391**(6669):795-799

[136] Hosseini E, Schwarer AP, Ghasemzadeh M. Do human leukocyte antigen E polymorphisms influence graft-versus-leukemia after allogeneic hematopoietic stem cell transplantation? Experimental Hematology 2015;**43**(3):149-157

[137] Della Chiesa M, Moretta L, Muccio L et al. Haploidentical haematopoietic stem cell transplantation: Role of NK cells and effect of cytomegalovirus infections. Current Topics in Microbiology and Immunology. 2016;**395**:209-224

[138] Foley B, Felices M, Cichocki F et al. The biology of NK cells and their receptors affects clinical outcomes after hematopoietic cell transplantation (HCT). Immunol Reviews. 2014;**258**(1):45-63

[139] Della Chiesa M, Falco M, Podesta M et al. Phenotypic and functional heterogeneity of human NK cells developing after umbilical cord blood transplantation: A role for human cytomegalovirus? Blood. 2012;**119**(2):399-410

[140] Foley B, Cooley S, Verneris MR et al. Human cytomegalovirus (CMV)-induced memory-like NKG2C(+) NK cells are transplantable and expand *in vivo* in response to recipient CMV antigen. Journal of Immunology 2012;**189**(10):5082-5088

[141] Della Chiesa M, Falco M, Bertaina A et al. Human cytomegalovirus infection promotes rapid maturation of NK cells expressing activating killer Ig-like receptor in patients transplanted with NKG2C-/- umbilical cord blood. Journal of Immunology. 2014;**192**(4):1471-1479

[142] Di Bona D, Scafidi V, Plaia A et al. HLA and killer cell immunoglobulin-like receptors influence the natural course of CMV infection. The Journal of Infectious Diseases 2014;**210**(7):1083-1089

[143] Stern M, Ruggeri L, Mancusi A et al. Survival after T cell-depleted haploidentical stem cell transplantation is improved using the mother as donor. Blood. 2008;**112**(7):2990-2995

[144] Hwang I, Zhang T, Scott JM et al. Identification of human NK cells that are deficient for signaling adaptor FcRgamma and specialized for antibody-dependent immune functions. International Immunology 2012;**24**(12):793-802

[145] Lichtfuss GF, Cheng WJ, Farsakoglu Y et al. Virologically suppressed HIV patients show activation of NK cells and persistent innate immune activation. Journal of Immunology. 2012;**189**(3):1491-1499

[146] Zhang T, Scott JM, Hwang I, Kim S. Cutting edge: Antibody-dependent memory-like NK cells distinguished by FcRgamma deficiency. Journal of Immunology. 2013;**190**(4): 1402-1406

[147] Guma M, Angulo A, Vilches C et al. Imprint of human cytomegalovirus infection on the NK cell receptor repertoire. Blood. 2004;**104**(12):3664-3671

[148] Cichocki F, Verneris MR, Cooley S et al. The past, present, and future of NK cells in hematopoietic cell transplantation and adoptive transfer. Current topics in Microbiology and Immunology. 2016;**395**:225-243

[149] Laffont S, Seillet C, Ortaldo J et al. Natural killer cells recruited into lymph nodes inhibit alloreactive T-cell activation through perforin-mediated killing of donor allogeneic dendritic cells. Blood. 2008;**112**(3):661-671

[150] Olson JA, Leveson-Gower DB, Gill S et al. NK cells mediate reduction of GVHD by inhibiting activated, alloreactive T cells while retaining GVT effects. Blood. 2010;**115**(21): 4293-4301

[151] Lang PA, Lang KS, Xu HC et al. Natural killer cell activation enhances immune pathology and promotes chronic infection by limiting CD8+ T-cell immunity. Proceedings of the National Academy of Sciences of the United States of America. 2012;**109**(4):1210-1215

[152] Waggoner SN, Cornberg M, Selin LK, Welsh RM. Natural killer cells act as rheostats modulating antiviral T cells. Nature. 2011;**481**(7381):394-398

[153] Asai O, Longo DL, Tian ZG et al. Suppression of graft-versus-host disease and amplification of graft-versus-tumor effects by activated natural killer cells after allogeneic bone marrow transplantation. The Journal of Clinical Investigation. 1998;**101**(9):1835-1842

[154] Noval Rivas M, Hazzan M, Weatherly K et al. NK cell regulation of CD4 T cell-mediated graft-versus-host disease. Journal of Immunology. 2010;**184**(12):6790-6798

[155] Tsirigotis PD, Resnick IB, Shapira MY. The role of natural killer cells in hematopoietic stem cell transplantation. Annals of Medicine 2012;**44**(2):130-145

[156] De Santis D, Bishara A, Witt CS et al. Natural killer cell HLA-C epitopes and killer cell immunoglobulin-like receptors both influence outcome of mismatched unrelated donor bone marrow transplants. Tissue Antigens. 2005;**65**(6):519-528

[157] Yabe T, Matsuo K, Hirayasu K et al. Donor killer immunoglobulin-like receptor (KIR) genotype-patient cognate KIR ligand combination and antithymocyte globulin preadministration are critical factors in outcome of HLA-C-KIR ligand-mismatched T cell-replete unrelated bone marrow transplantation. Biology of Blood and Marrow Transplantation: Journal of the American Society for Blood and Marrow Transplantation. 2008;**14**(1):75-87

[158] Shah NN, Baird K, Delbrook CP et al. Acute GVHD in patients receiving IL-15/4-1BBL activated NK cells following T-cell-depleted stem cell transplantation. Blood. 2015;**125**(5):784-792

[159] Leung W. Use of NK cell activity in cure by transplant. British Journal of Haematology. 2011;**155**(1):14-29

[160] Cooley S, Weisdorf DJ, Guethlein LA et al. Donor selection for natural killer cell receptor genes leads to superior survival after unrelated transplantation for acute myelogenous leukemia. Blood. 2010;**116**(14):2411-2419

[161] Bari R, Bell T, Leung WH et al. Significant functional heterogeneity among KIR2DL1 alleles and a pivotal role of arginine 245. Blood. 2009;**114**(25):5182-5190

[162] Cartron G, Dacheux L, Salles G et al. Therapeutic activity of humanized anti-CD20 monoclonal antibody and polymorphism in IgG Fc receptor FcgammaRIIIa gene. Blood. 2002;**99**(3):754-758

[163] Miller JS, Soignier Y, Panoskaltsis-Mortari A et al. Successful adoptive transfer and *in vivo* expansion of human haploidentical NK cells in patients with cancer. Blood. 2005;**105**(8):3051-3057

[164] Rubnitz JE, Inaba H, Ribeiro RC et al. NKAML: A pilot study to determine the safety and feasibility of haploidentical natural killer cell transplantation in childhood acute myeloid leukemia. Journal of Clinical Oncology: Official Journal of the American Society of Clinical Oncology. 2010;**28**(6):955-959

[165] Szmania S, Lapteva N, Garg T et al. *Ex vivo*-expanded natural killer cells demonstrate robust proliferation *in vivo* in high-risk relapsed multiple myeloma patients. Journal of Immunotherapy. 2015;**38**(1):24-36

[166] Waldmann TA, Dubois S, Tagaya Y. Contrasting roles of IL-2 and IL-15 in the life and death of lymphocytes: Implications for immunotherapy. Immunity. 2001;**14**(2):105-110

[167] Rodella L, Zamai L, Rezzani R et al. Interleukin 2 and interleukin 15 differentially predispose natural killer cells to apoptosis mediated by endothelial and tumour cells. British Journal of Haematology. 2001;**115**(2):442-450

[168] Denman CJ, Senyukov VV, Somanchi SS et al. Membrane-bound IL-21 promotes sustained *ex vivo* proliferation of human natural killer cells. PloS One. 2012;**7**(1):e30264

[169] Somanchi SS, Somanchi A, Cooper LJ, Lee DA. Engineering lymph node homing of *ex vivo*-expanded human natural killer cells via trogocytosis of the chemokine receptor CCR7. Blood. 2012;**119**(22):5164-5172

[170] Fujisaki H, Kakuda H, Imai C et al. Replicative potential of human natural killer cells. British Journal of Haematology. 2009;**145**(5):606-613

[171] Knorr DA, Bachanova V, Verneris MR, Miller JS. Clinical utility of natural killer cells in cancer therapy and transplantation. Seminars in Immunology. 2014;**26**(2):161-172

[172] Ni J, Miller M, Stojanovic A et al. Sustained effector function of IL-12/15/18-preactivated NK cells against established tumors. The Journal of Experimental Medicine. 2012;**209**(13):2351-2365

[173] Romee R, Rosario M, Berrien-Elliott MM et al. Cytokine-induced memory-like natural killer cells exhibit enhanced responses against myeloid leukemia. Science Translational Medicine. 2016;**8**(357):357ra123

[174] Skarbnik AP, Faderl S. The role of combined fludarabine, cyclophosphamide and rituximab chemoimmunotherapy in chronic lymphocytic leukemia: Current evidence and controversies. Therapeutic Advances in Hematology. 2017;**8**(3):99-105

[175] Benson DM, Jr., Bakan CE, Zhang S et al. IPH2101, a novel anti-inhibitory KIR antibody, and lenalidomide combine to enhance the natural killer cell versus multiple myeloma effect. Blood. 2011;**118**(24):6387-6391

[176] Romee R, Foley B, Lenvik T et al. NK cell CD16 surface expression and function is regulated by a disintegrin and metalloprotease-17 (ADAM17). Blood. 2013;**121**(18):3599-3608

[177] Scott AM, Wolchok JD, Old LJ. Antibody therapy of cancer. Nature Reviews Cancer. 2012;**12**(4):278-287

[178] Baeuerle PA, Reinhardt C. Bispecific T-cell engaging antibodies for cancer therapy. Cancer Research. 2009;**69**(12):4941-4944

[179] Bargou R, Leo E, Zugmaier G et al. Tumor regression in cancer patients by very low doses of a T cell-engaging antibody. Science. 2008;**321**(5891):974-977

[180] Gleason MK, Verneris MR, Todhunter DA et al. Bispecific and trispecific killer cell engagers directly activate human NK cells through CD16 signaling and induce cytotoxicity and cytokine production. Molecular Cancer Therapeutics. 2012;**11**(12):2674-2684

[181] Vallera DA, Zhang B, Gleason MK et al. Heterodimeric bispecific single-chain variable-fragment antibodies against EpCAM and CD16 induce effective antibody-dependent cellular cytotoxicity against human carcinoma cells. Cancer Biotherapy & Radiopharmaceuticals. 2013;**28**(4):274-282

[182] Wiernik A, Foley B, Zhang B et al. Targeting natural killer cells to acute myeloid leukemia in vitro with a CD16 x 33 bispecific killer cell engager and ADAM17 inhibition. Clinical Cancer Research: An Official Journal of the American Association for Cancer Research. 2013;**19**(14):3844-3855

[183] Lundqvist A, Abrams SI, Schrump DS et al. Bortezomib and depsipeptide sensitize tumors to tumor necrosis factor-related apoptosis-inducing ligand: A novel method to potentiate natural killer cell tumor cytotoxicity. Cancer Research. 2006;**66**(14):7317-7325

[184] Wennerberg E, Sarhan D, Carlsten M et al. Doxorubicin sensitizes human tumor cells to NK cell- and T-cell-mediated killing by augmented TRAIL receptor signaling. International Journal of Cancer Journal International du Cancer. 2013;**133**(7):1643-1652

[185] Altvater B, Landmeier S, Pscherer S et al. 2B4 (CD244) signaling by recombinant antigen-specific chimeric receptors costimulates natural killer cell activation to leukemia and neuroblastoma cells. Clinical Cancer Research: An Official Journal of the American Association for Cancer Research. 2009;**15**(15):4857-4866

[186] Imai C, Iwamoto S, Campana D. Genetic modification of primary natural killer cells overcomes inhibitory signals and induces specific killing of leukemic cells. Blood. 2005;**106**(1):376-383

[187] Arai S, Meagher R, Swearingen M et al. Infusion of the allogeneic cell line NK-92 in patients with advanced renal cell cancer or melanoma: A phase I trial. Cytotherapy. 2008;**10**(6):625-632

Chapter 8

# Natural Killer Cells Interaction with Carbon Nanoparticles

Anwar Alam and Rajiv K Saxena

Additional information is available at the end of the chapter

http://dx.doi.org/10.5772/intechopen.69731

**Abstract**

The increased use of nanomaterials for biomedical purposes has warranted the need to introspect their toxicological properties and assess their utility to human health, particularly the immune system. Natural killer (NK) cells hold a pivotal position in innate immunity and serve as first line of defense against foreign bodies. Acid functionalized Carbon nanotubes (CNTs) that easily polydisperse in aqueous solution and could be coupled with fluorescent molecules were used to study the effect of carbon nanoparticles on NK cells *in vitro* and *in vivo*. Flow cytometry-based assays were used to study the effect of CNTs on various physiological parameters of NK cells, such as cell recovery, apoptosis, cell cycle, and generation of reactive oxygen species. A downregulation of the cytotoxicity of IL-2-activated murine NK cells was observed in the presence of acid-functionalized CNTs. The mechanistic basis of this downregulation was studied by assessing markers of NK cell activation (CD69), generation (NLK1.1), degranulation (CD107a) and apoptosis (annexin V assay). This chapter provides a blueprint for assessing the effect of carbon nanoparticles on NK cells. The assays mentioned in this chapter can be extrapolated to study the effect of other nanoparticles on different cell types as well.

**Keywords:** NK cell cytotoxicity, carbon nanotube, flow cytometry, apoptosis, NK cell degranulation, YT-INDY

## 1. Introduction

Carbon nanoparticles (CNPs) have size less than 100 nm in at least one dimension and can be engineered in allotropic forms, such as nanodiamonds, fullerenes, nanobuds, and nanotubes. Each of these CNPs exhibits unique physicochemical properties and by virtue of their extremely low size can effectively interact with cells and tissues. Carbon nanoparticles, specifically carbon nanotubes (CNTs), are being tested for their potential use in the field of nanomedicine including medicinal chemistry, imaging, vaccine delivery, etc. [1]. How these CNPs affect the living systems and the risks or benefits associated with their environmental, occupational, or therapeutic exposure is a matter of active research [2]. This chapter focuses on the interaction of an important component of innate immunity, the natural killer cells, with carbon nanotube.

### 1.1. Natural killer cells

Natural killer (NK) cells are important effector cells of the innate immune system and constitute about 5–15% of peripheral blood lymphocytes [3]. NK cells originate from lymphoid progenitors in the bone marrow and require IL-15-mediated signaling for development and survival [4]. NK cells can be identified through a set of markers, such as NK1.1 in mice or CD56 and CD16 in humans [5, 6]. The absence of CD3 on NK cells is a useful marker to differentiate between NK and natural killer T cells (NKT) [7].

NK cells kill syngeneic or allogeneic cells through mechanisms that require neither a prior sensitization with target cells nor the presentation of antigen in association with MHC-I. NK cell functions through an array of germline-encoded inhibitory or activating receptors that recognize MHC-I expressed in steady state on normal cells or altered ligands on dysregulated cells, respectively. Killer inhibitory receptor (KIR) in humans, the lectin-like Ly49 molecules in mice, and CD94/NKG2A heterodimers in both species detect MHC-I molecules on normal cells [8]. Perturbations in expression of MHC-I molecules on viral-infected cells or malignant transformed cells lead to loss of inhibitory signals causing activation of NK cells. Additionally, NK cells also require signaling through activating receptors, such as NKp30, NKp44, NKp46, NKp65, and NKp80 to trigger effector functions, such as cytokine production and cytolytic activity. Stimulation with inflammatory cytokines, such as IL-2, IL-15, IL-12, or IL-18 evokes differentiation into effector NK cells. CD16 or constant Fc$\gamma$-receptor IIIa (Fc$\gamma$RIIIa) exerts antibody-dependent cell-mediated cytotoxicity (ADCC) against various antibody coated cellular targets, leading to the exocytosis of perforin and granzyme-loaded vesicles. By integrating activating and inhibitory signals, NK cells contribute to the elimination of stressed cells expressing modified motifs while sparing healthy cells [9].

Upon recognition, target cells can get killed by NK cells through one of two pathways: either via the perforin and granzyme secretion pathway or via membrane-bound death receptors. NK cells store preformed perforin and granzyme in secretory vesicles that when triggered by activating signals causes formation of microtubule-organizing center (MTOC) which guides the vesicles, containing perforin and granzyme, in a directed way toward the target cell to prevent damage to bystander cells. Perforin forms pores in the target cell membrane, disrupts membrane integrity, and allows the entry of the apoptosis-inducing granzymes. The importance of the lytic perforin/granzyme pathway is evident in perforin knockout animals that exhibit lesser efficiency in ADCC or tumor control after transplantation of tumor cells. Perforin-/granzyme-containing cytoplasmic vesicles express CD107a or lysosomal-associated membrane protein (LAMP-1). Upon degranulation, CD107a is transferred transiently on the surface of NK cells and protects NK cells from damage from their own perforin or granzyme release [10].

NK cytotoxicity via its membrane-bound death receptors occurs upon binding with ligands, expressed on target cells. Receptor-ligand pairs, such as Fas-FasL, TNFR-TNF, and TRAILR-TRAIL, induce recruitment of various adaptor proteins leading to the formation of the death-inducing signaling complex (DISC). Subsequently, the caspases 8 and 10 get activated via proteolysis and initiate apoptosis. In addition to the cytotoxic response, NK cells are important sources of various cytokines, such as IFN-γ, TNF-α, or IL-10 and of chemokines, such as CCL3/CCL4/CCL5 or CXCL8. Natural killer (NK) cells basally express high levels of the signal transducer and activator of transcription 4 (STAT4) and produce the cytokine gamma interferon (IFN-γ). Type 1 interferons could potentially activate STAT4 and promote IFN-γ expression; however, concurrent elevated expression of STAT1 negatively regulates access to this pathway. IFN-γ due to its pleiotropic functions is considered to be the signature cytokine of NK cells [11]. IFN-γ has been shown to have antiproliferative effects on tumor cells and exert anti-angiogenic activity. A combination of TNF-α and IFN-γ has been shown to trigger tumor senescence and activates macrophages and dendritic cells [12]. Cytokine secretion is mediated via recycling endosomes using a distinct pathway from cytolytic vesicles, which allows for differential regulation.

## 2. Carbon nanotube

Carbon nanotubes resemble rolled-up tubes of graphite sheet of $sp^2$ hybridized carbon atoms. A single cylindrical form of CNTs is designated as single-walled nanotubes (SWCNTs) that are 0.4–3.0 nm in diameter and up to 1000 nm in length. CNTs display a unique combination of extraordinary mechanical, thermal, and electronic properties. CNTs, by virtue of their exceptional high aspect ratio (surface area to volume ratio), can carry high amounts of ligands on the outer as well as in inner surface of their tubular backbone for tissue-/cell-specific drug delivery. These are therefore conceptualized as nano-bullets capable of carrying different drugs for targeting multiple microorganisms or diseases simultaneously. However, the use of CNTs in biological system poses practical problems due to their inherent tendency to form aggregate as a result of high intermolecular hydrophobic force arising out of unit graphene rings. Within the aqueous phase of the biological system, the hydrophobic behavior of CNTs could result not only in poor biodistribution but also pose a serious challenge due to agglomeration and cause tissue lesions or granulomas. In order to circumvent hydrophobicity of CNTs so that it is rendered biocompatible, their backbone can be chemically modified with functional groups or linkers that impart solvable properties to CNTs. This process is known as functionalization of CNTs.

### 2.1. Acid functionalization of SWCNT

SWCNTs may be acid functionalized by suspension in sulfuric acid and nitric acid and subjecting to high-pressure microwave as described before [13–15]. As a result the side walls of SWCNTs are decorated with high density of various oxygen-containing groups (mainly carboxyl groups). The carboxyl groups impart negative charge to SWCNTs, which facilitate the separation of nanotube bundles into individual tubes and enhance their dispersibility in aqueous solutions. The carboxyl groups represent useful sites for covalent coupling of molecules, through the creation of amide or ester bonds, thereby facilitating further addition of wide range of bifunctional linker molecules, nucleic acids, peptides, or other nanoparticles, such as polyethylene glycol (PEG) [16].

The process of acid functionalization of CNTs is outlined in **Figure 1A**. Briefly, SWCNTs were suspended in equimolar ratio of nitric acid ($HNO_3$) and sulfuric acid ($H_2SO_4$) in high-pressure microwave digester that provide 450 W power for 3 min, resulting in an internal pressure of 20 ± 2 psi and temperature of 138–150°C. The suspension was cooled and dialyzed in excess milli-Q water till it attained neutral pH. Dialyzed suspensions of acid-functionalized SWCNTs (AF-SWCNTs) were lyophilized, weighed, and resuspended at the desired concentration in phosphate buffer saline (PBS) or water.

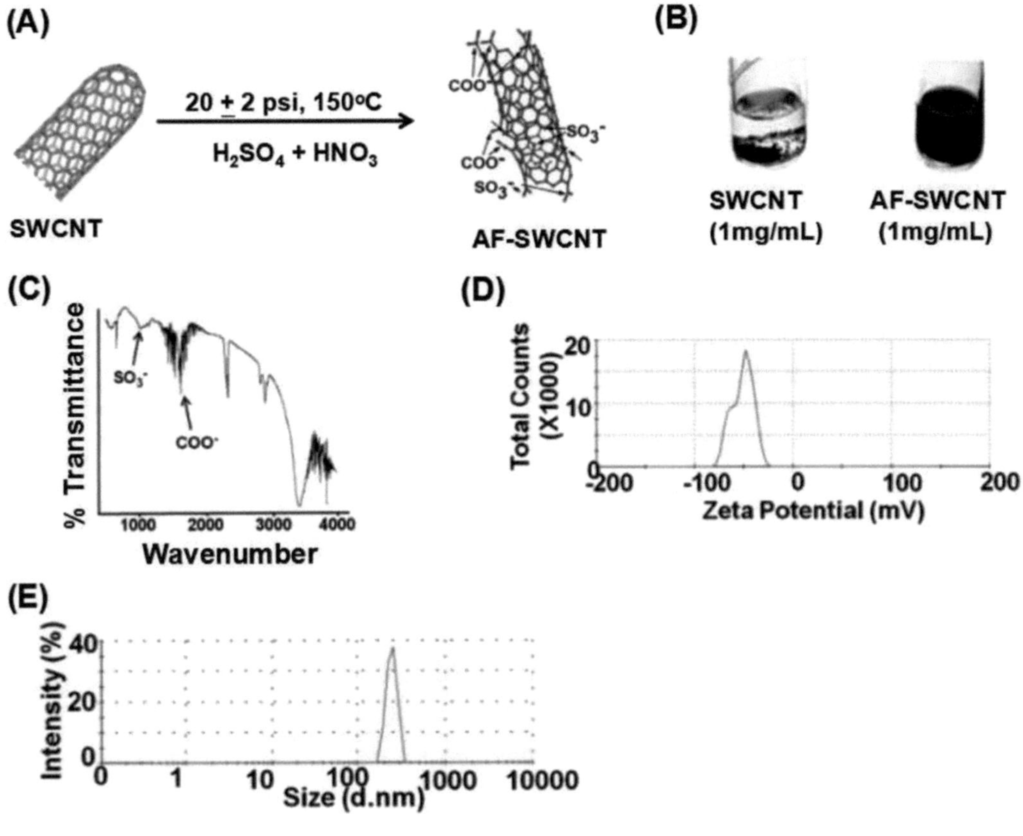


**Figure 1.** Functionalization of SWCNT and characterization of acid-functionalized SWCNT (AF-SWCNT): schematic overview of the process of acid functionalization of SWCNT is depicted in Panel A. Functionalization of SWCNT in the presence of equimolar $H_2SO_4$ and $HNO_3$ generates carboxyl and sulfonate groups on the backbone of SWCNT. Panel B shows that AF-SWCNT (1 mg/mL) homogenously dissolves in aqueous solution as compared to SWCNT. The physiochemical properties of AF-SWCNT were tested using fourier transmission infrared (FTIR) spectroscopy and Zetasizer. FTIR spectra of AF-SWCNT showed distinct bands in the range 1740 and 1350 $cm^{-1}$, characteristic of carboxyl and sulfonate groups, respectively (Panel C). These groups are negatively charged and affect the electrical properties of AF-SWCNT. Data obtained from Zetasizer showed that the mean charge and size of AF-SWCNT were −55 mV (Panel D) and 350 nm (Panel E), respectively.

In comparison to SWCNTs that agglomerate in aqueous solution, AF-SWCNTs (1 mg/mL) remain stably suspended. The physiochemical properties of AF-SWCNTs are influenced mainly by the duration of acid functionalization. Increasing the duration of functionalization reaction resulted in smaller sized particles and decreased recovery of functionalized nanotubes due to oxidative degradation. The recovery of AF-SWCNTs was relatively better with lower acid concentrations; the size and charge distribution of the resultant particles were comparable. Particles generated under constant temperature for different time durations did not differ significantly in their size or zeta potential. The zeta potential provides an estimate whether the particles within a liquid will tend to flocculate or not. A high positive or negative zeta potential of particle corresponds to greater dispersibility within the liquid, while values close to zero correspond to greater aggregation potential. Zeta potential of the AF-SWCNTs depends on the suspension media. AF-SWCNTs suspended in water had the higher zeta potential than PBS followed by culture media. Greater dispersion of AF-SWCNTs in water is due to formation of electrical double layer in which ionic accumulation of few-angstrom thick prevents particle aggregation. For details of physiochemical properties of AF-SWCNTs, see **Figure 1C–E**.

### 2.2. Attachment of fluorescent probes to AF-SWCNTs

CNTs, due to their nanosized structure, cannot be visualized using normal light microscope. The carboxylic groups generated on the AF-SWCNTs were exploited to attach fluorescent probes to the particles for the purpose of studying their uptake by cells [17]. **Figure 2A** shows the schematic overview of attachment of fluorescent probes to AF-SWCNTs. In our experiment, polydispersed AF-SWCNTs were treated with 1-ethyl 3-(3-dimethyl aminopropyl) carbodiimide (EDAC) and N-hydroxysuccinimide (NHS) in order to get succinimidyl intermediate. The mixture was continually shaken for 2 h and dialyzed in water using 3 kDa cutoff Centricon to remove excess NHS, EDAC, and urea by-product. AF-SWCNTs thus activated were incubated with Alexa Fluor 488/633 hydrazide in 1:1 ratio in the dark with continuous mixing for 12 h, followed by dialysis to remove free dye. Attachment of fluorescent probe to AF-SWCNTs can be confirmed using spectrophotometer or flow cytometer.

The interaction of fluorescently tagged AF-SWCNTs (FAF-SWCNTs) with cells could be easily quantified using flow cytometer (**Figure 2B**), and their localization within the cell can be visualized using confocal microscopy (**Figure 2C**). Although earlier studies on the uptake and localization of CNTs could be performed on fixed cells using transmission electron microscope (TEM), preparation of fluorescently tagged AF-SWCNTs was a significant step in this direction because it enabled us to directly observe the interaction of CNTs with live cells. Thus, FAF-SWCNTs in conjugation with organelle markers provided an important tool to observe the effect of CNTs on the cellular process like exocytosis, actin-myosin assembly, cell division, etc. For example, FAF-SWCNTs used in combination with LysoTracker and MitoTracker can be used to observe the actual interaction of CNTs with these organelles and the attendant effects on exocytosis and mitochondrial potential, respectively. Our studies showed that activated NK cells internalize higher amounts of AF-SWCNTs than resting NK cells. Our studies further indicated that internalized AF-SWCNTs are essentially localized in the cytoplasm of NK cells. Previous studies by our group on the uptake of diesel exhaust particles (another category of carbon nanoparticles) by macrophages and alveolar epithelial cells showed that

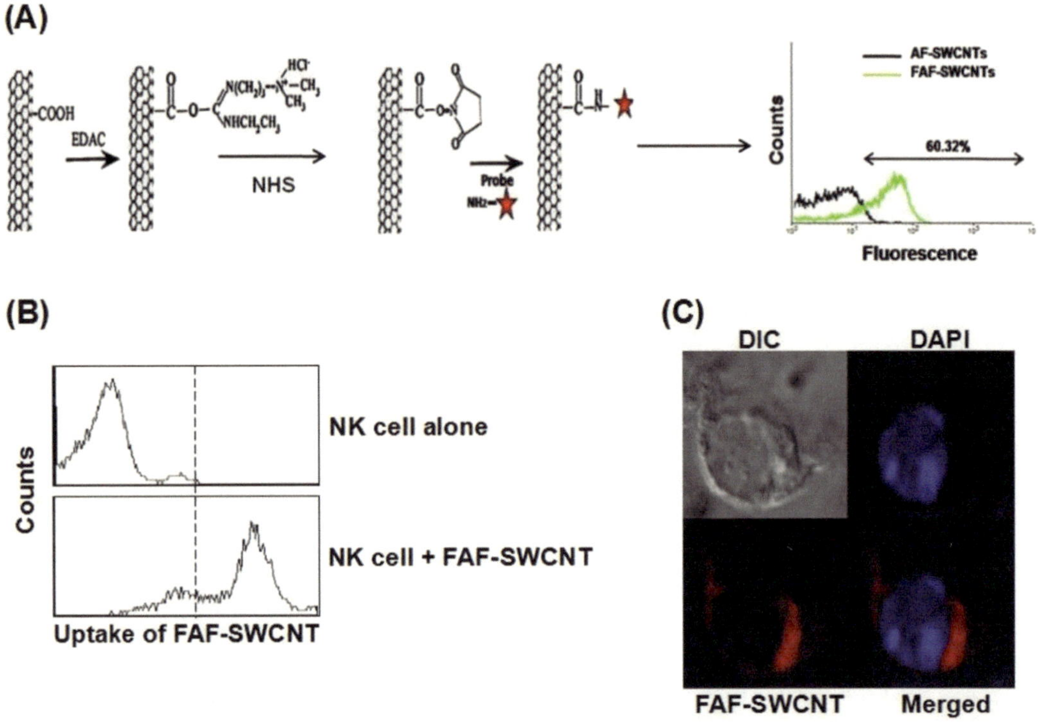


**Figure 2.** Attachment of fluorescent probe to AF-SWCNT. Panel A shows the schematic diagram of preparation of fluorescent-coupled AF-SWCNT (FAF-SWCNT). The carboxyl group provided a pivotal point to which amide containing fluorescent molecules could be attached. Flow cytometric data shows that 60% of AF-SWCNT particles got tagged with the fluorescence probe (denoted by green line). The interaction of NK1.1$^+$ cells with AF-SWCNT was studied by incubating the IL-2-activated splenocytes with FAF-SWCNT. Panel B shows that NK1.1$^+$ sorted cells sequestered FAF-SWCNT and generated positive signal for fluorescence. The localization of FAF-SWCNT in NK cells was visualized using confocal microscopy. NK1.1$^+$FAF-SWCNT$^+$ cells were isolated using fluorescence-activated cell sorter and cultured on poly-L-lysine coated cover slips. Cells were fixed using 4% paraformaldehyde, incubated with DAPI (0.2 mg/mL) and examined microscopically. Panel C shows the DIC, DAPI, and merged image of FAF-SWCNT in NK1.1$^+$ cells.

active uptake was blocked in the presence of Cytochalasin D, an inhibitor of actin-myosin assembly system [17]. Internalization of AF-SWCNTs has also been demonstrated in erythrocytes that lack membrane phagocytic functions [18]. Internalization of AF-SWCNTs in NK cells may therefore involve active transport, or by the virtue of their long needle-like structure, these nanoparticles may pierce cell membranes and enter into the cytoplasm.

## 3. Interaction of CNTs with NK cell

CNTs act as adjuvant or haptens and allow formation of protein bio-corona on their surface. When proteins unfold, they reveal hidden epitopes that may act as nanomaterial-associated molecular patterns (NAMPs) [19]. These molecular signatures are recognized by pattern recognition receptors (PRPs) present on the surface of innate immune cells. The activation of

PRPs may induce adaptive immune system causing inflammation, allergic reactions, complement activation, susceptibility to diseases, or autoimmune diseases [20, 21]. The prospects of CNTs as a magic bullet in cancer therapy are due to their ability to act passively or actively at site of tumor or for improving bioavailability of insoluble drugs. Besides, CNTs have unique anisotropic and spectroscopic properties that make them suitable for detection and radiation-guided ablation of tumors.

The ability of the immune system to successfully eliminate cancer cells or viral-infected cells is mediated mainly by cytotoxic T cells and NK cells. Therefore the inadvertent interaction of CNTs with NK cells in the body, particularly at site of tumor, cannot be ignored. This situation warrants extensive studies to assert that CNTs have minimal effect on the effector functions of NK cells so that the benefits achieved by the use of CNTs in cancer therapy are not outweighed by the toxic effect of CNTs on NK cells itself. The effects of nanoparticle on NK cell cytotoxicity should be examined to determine whether there is an association between NK cell activity and nanoparticle treatment. A decreased NK cell activity is often associated with chronic fatigue immune dysfunction syndrome (CFIDS), characterized by acute and chronic conditions that predispose individuals toward an immunocompromised state leading to AIDS [22].

Although the mechanistic details of NK-mediated killing of target cells is well established, little is known in literature about the interaction of NK cells with CNTs, and hence there is no consensus to evaluate immunomodulatory effects of CNTs on NK cells. We have established three models to assess the interaction of CNTs with NK cells and evaluate the effect of CNTs on effector function of NK cells *in vitro* and *in vivo*. *In vitro* assessment of the effect of CNTs on NK cells was performed using YT-INDY human NK cell line and IL-2-activated mouse spleen cells. *In vivo* effects of CNTs were studied in C57BL/6 inbred mice treated with poly I:C, a synthetic analogue of viral RNA. We have extensively used flow cytometry to assess these parameters because it provides accurate, reproducible, and quick quantitative estimation of cell subpopulations in the mixed culture of cells.

### 3.1. *In vitro* assessment of effect of CNTs on a NK cell line

YT-INDY, a NK cell line of human origin, proliferates continuously *in vitro* without being supplemented with cytokines or conditioned medium. *In vitro* assessment of the effect of CNTs on YT-INDY cells provides us preliminary estimation of dosage that may be deemed fit to explore on actual NK cells derived from primary cell cultures.

### 3.2. Cell viability assay

Cell viability assays are used for screening nanoparticles in order to determine if these affect cell proliferation or show direct cytotoxic effects causing cell death. Trypan Blue assay was used for staining dead cells, and viability was determined by counting the unstained cells microscopically. As is evident from **Figure 3A**, exposure of AF-SWCNTs resulted in decrease of cell recovery although the effect was marginally less in SWCNT treatment. YT-INDY, which has a doubling time of nearly 42 h, shows decreased proliferation rate in the presence of SWCNTs, the effect being more enhanced with AF-SWCNTs.

Trypan Blue staining does not distinguish between the healthy cells and the cells that are alive but losing cell functions. MTT is a water-soluble yellow dye that is readily cleaved and converted into insoluble purple formazan by the activity of mitochondrial dehydrogenase of living cells [23]. Results in **Figure 3B** clearly indicate that AF-SWCNTs above 25 μg/mL reduce cell viability, whereas SWCNTs show the same effect above 50 μg/mL.

Reduced cell viability in the presence of CNTs could be attributed not only to reduction in proliferation of cells but also due to accumulation of dead cells in the culture. The activity of cytoplasmic enzyme, such as lactate dehydrogenase (LDH), released upon plasma membrane damage, can be detected in culture supernatant and correlates with the proportion of lysed or dead cells [23]. Results in **Figure 3C** show that AF-SWCNTs caused increase in LDH release from YT-INDY cells. These results of LDH assay complement the data obtained from MTT assay.

### 3.3. Effect of CNTs on cell cycle

Increase in doubling time of YT-INDY cells in the presence of AF-SWCNTs pointed to a possible alteration in cell cycle. The effect of SWCNTs or AF-SWCNTs on cell cycle of YT-INDY

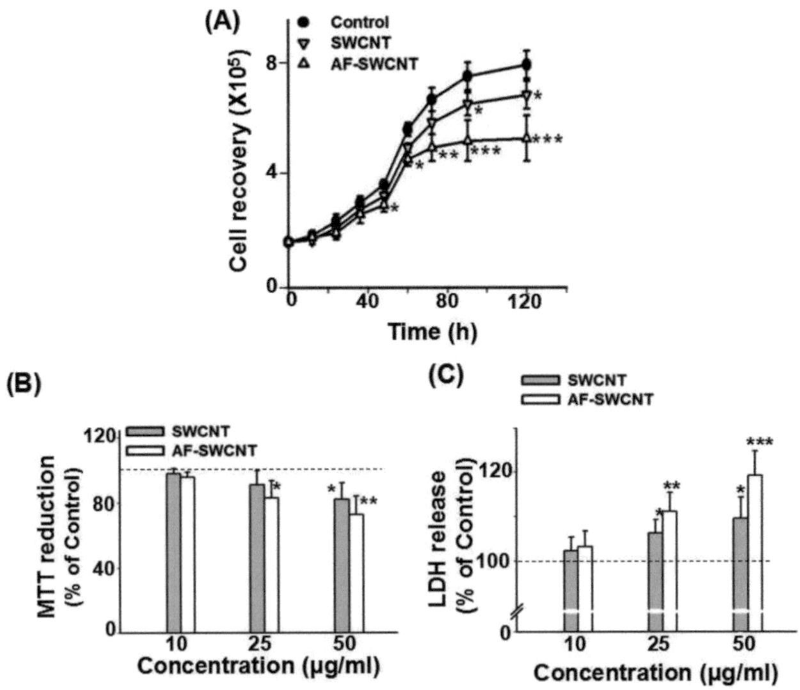


**Figure 3.** Effect of SWCNT and AF-SWCNT on viability of NK cells *in vitro*. YT-INDY cells were cultured in the presence of 10, 25, and 50 μg/mL of SWCNT or AF-SWCNT. Panel A shows the cell recovery of viable cells using Trypan Blue exclusion assay. Panel B shows the results of MTT assay in terms of percent cell recovery. Panel C depicts the percent LDH released from nonviable cells in cultures treated with 10, 25, and 50 μg/mL of SWCNT or AF-SWCNT. *$p < 0.05$, **$p < 0.01$, ***$p < 0.005$ by Student's *t* test.

http://dx.doi.org/10.5772/intechopen.69731

cells was examined. A fourfold decrease in proportion of cells in S-phase indicated that AF-SWCNT treatment caused cell cycle arrest in YT-INDY cells (**Figure 4**).

### 3.4. Flow cytometric assessment of apoptosis using annexin V/7-AAD assay

Cellular toxicity evokes sequential steps leading to apoptosis and ultimately causing cell death. Apoptotic and necrotic response of YT-INDY to AF-SWCNTs was examined by using annexin V/7-AAD stainings described before [24]. Results in **Figure 5A** show that the treatment of YT-INDY cells with SWCNTs or AF-SWCNTs led to an increase in apoptotic cell by twofold and threefold, respectively.

Apoptosis can be brought about by a loss of calcium ($Ca^{2+}$) homeostatic control but can also be finely tuned, positively or negatively, by more subtle changes in $Ca^{2+}$ distribution within intracellular compartments. An aberrant increase in intracellular calcium can trigger initiation of apoptosis. The levels of calcium in the cell have to be kept at an optimum level to maintain cellular homeostasis. Intracellular levels of calcium can be monitored using Fluo-3AM dye. The levels of calcium can be examined by flow cytometrically. Mean fluorescence intensity (MFI) values for Fluo-3AM signals gave an estimate of average levels of calcium per cell in the population of cells. AF-SWCNT treatment caused increased intracellular calcium indicating that they caused off of the signaling process that regulates apoptosis (**Figure 5B**).

### 3.5. Generation of reactive oxygen species

Reactive oxygen species (ROS) are continuously generated in living cells and play a key role in cellular homeostasis. ROS is principally produced and regulated in mitochondria and may affect the mitochondrial health and activity in a cell. The production of ROS in the cell is regulated as excessive ROS production leads to cascade of signaling processes that may trigger cell

| Control | SWCNT | AF-SWCNT | |
|---|---|---|---|
| 44 | 54 | 88 | G1 |
| 38 | 33 | 9 | S |
| 18 | 13 | 3 | G2/M |

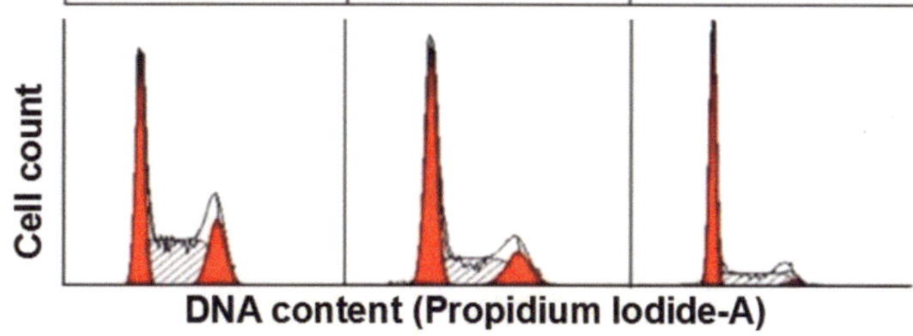


**Figure 4.** Effect of SWCNT and AF-SWCNT on cell cycle of YT-INDY cells. YT-INDY cells were cultured in the presence of SWCNT or AF-SWCNT. Cells were harvested, fixed with 70% ethanol, and treated with RNase. The fixed cells were stained with propidium iodide (2 μg/mL), and cell cycle was assessed flow cytometrically. Data shows percentage of cells in G1, S, and G2/M stages of cell cycle.

(A)

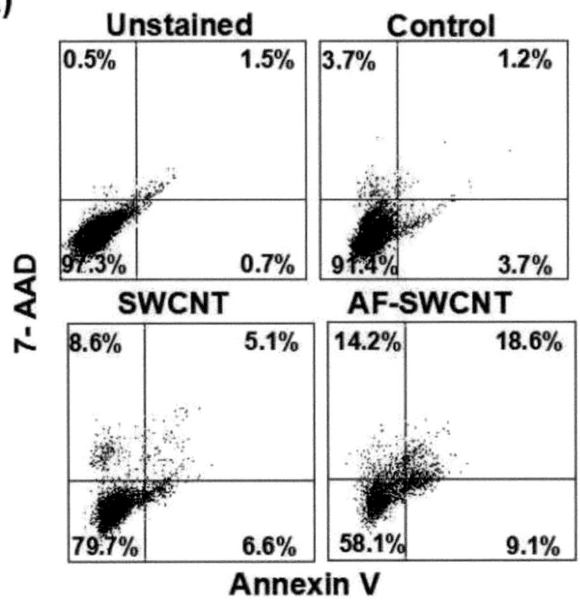


(B)

| | Control | SWCNT | AF-SWCNT |
|---|---|---|---|
| Fluo-3AM (MFI) | 100.6 | 114.7 | 120.1 |

**Figure 5.** Effect of SWCNT and AF-SWCNT on apoptotic response in YT-INDY cells. YT-INDY cells were cultured in the presence of 50 μg/mL of SWCNT or AF-SWCNT for 48 h. Cellular apoptosis was assessed flow cytometrically by staining cells with annexin V and 7-AAD dye. Percent dead, necrotic and apoptotic cells obtained from cultures treated with SWCNT or AF-SWCNT are shown in Panel A. Increased levels of calcium in cells as an initiator for apoptotic response are assessed using Fluo-3AM dye. Intracellular levels of calcium in YT-INDY cells treated with SWCNT or AF-SWCNT (50 μg/mL) are assessed flow cytometrically (Panel B).

to undergo apoptosis, cell cycle arrest, and modulation in cytokine production [25]. Results shown in **Figure 6** indicate that control cells produce basal levels of ROS (MFI 198). A 63% increase in ROS generation is observed in the presence of AF-SWCNTs as compared to a 21% increase in the presence of SWCNTs. Generation of ROS is an indication of cellular stress that corresponds to greater toxic potential of AF-SWCNTs as compared to SWCNTs.

### 3.6. Mitochondrial membrane potential

Generation of ROS causes disturbance in mitochondrial membrane potential ($\Delta\psi$). Mitochondrial potential is important for the proper functioning of mitochondria [26]. AF-SWCNTs being negatively charged could modulate the potential of mitochondria once it is taken up by cells. Effect of SWCNTs and AF-SWCNTs on mitochondrial potential in

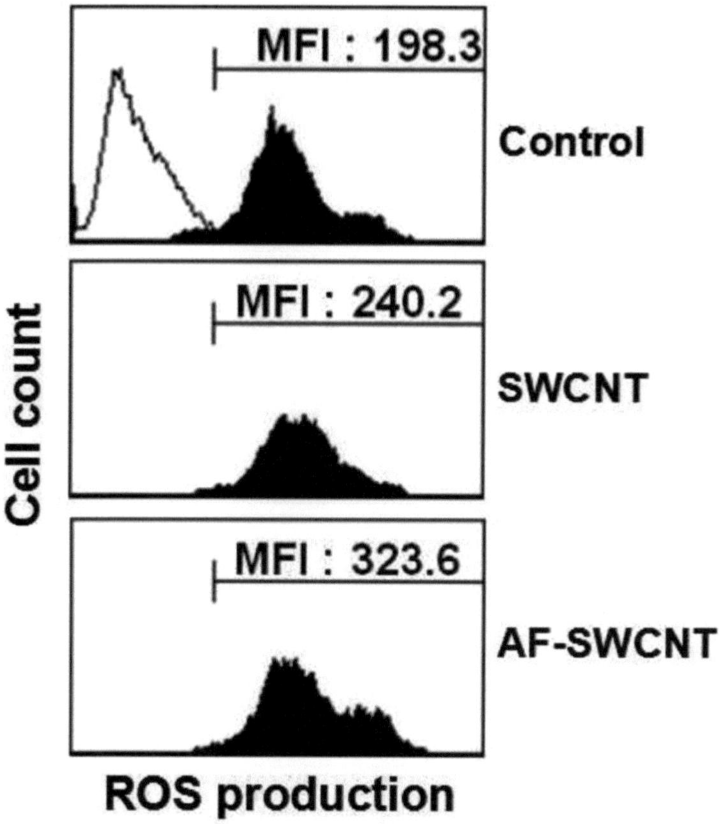


**Figure 6.** Generation of reactive oxygen species in YT-INDY cells treated with SWCNT and AF-SWCNT. YT-INDY cells were cultured with or without SWCNT or AF-SWCNT (50 μg/mL) for 24 h and ROS levels assessed by using $H_2$DCFDA dye. Fluorescent signals due to basal level of ROS in control cells are depicted as open histogram.

YT-INDY cells was examined using dyes: JC-1 and MitoTracker. JC-1 is a dimeric molecule which is converted to a monomeric form upon change in mitochondrial membrane potential. Change of JC-1 from dimeric form to monomeric form can be estimated by a shift from red fluorescence to green fluorescence. Increase in green fluorescence is an indicator for decrease in mitochondrial potential. MitoTracker red stain mitochondria in live cell and its accumulation are dependent upon membrane potential. The MFI of MitoTracker red emission therefore gives an estimate of the overall accumulation of MitoTracker red in live cells.

Results in **Figure 7** show that the treatment with SWCNTs or AF-SWCNTs resulted in an increase in JC-1 green fluorescence to 22 and 47%, respectively, indicating a significant decrease in mitochondrial potential. The corresponding reduction in MFI values of MitoTracker red fluorescence of SWCNTs and AF-SWCNTs culture were 20 and 54%, respectively.

Taken together, toxicity of SWCNTs and AF-SWCNTs was adjudged by a significant ($p < 0.05$) decrease in cell recovery, increased apoptosis, S-phase arrest in cell cycle, increased generation of ROS, poor mitochondrial health, and loss of cellular integrity.

(A)

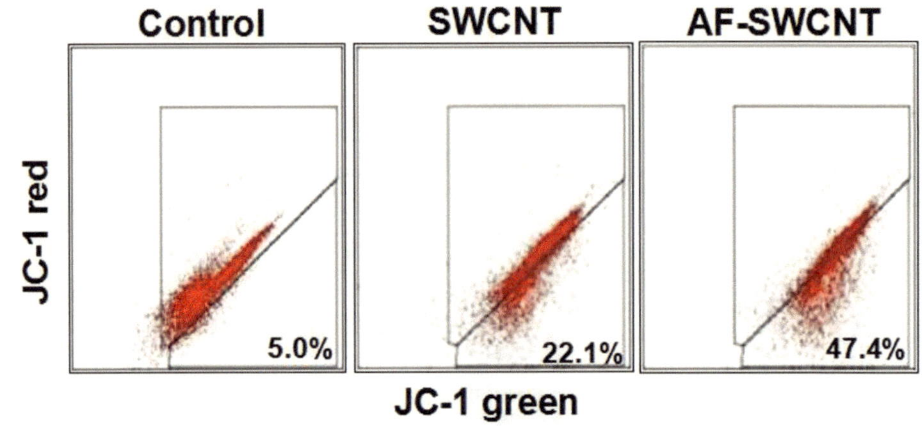


(B)

| | Control | SWCNT | AF-SWCNT |
|---|---|---|---|
| Mitotracker (MFI) | 320.3 | 256.1 | 147.1 |

**Figure 7.** Estimation of mitochondrial potential in YT-INDY cells treated with SWCNT or AF-SWCNT. YT-INDY cells cultured with SWCNT or AF-SWCNT were harvested, centrifuged, and rinsed twice with PBS, resuspended in 5 mM JC-1 or 10 mM MitoTracker red in serum-free media. Fluorescence emission was analyzed flow cytometrically (JC-1 monomers, excitation wavelength 488 nm, emission filter 530/30 nm; JC-1 aggregates, excitation wavelength 488 nm, emission filter 585/42 nm). Decrease in red fluorescence or increase in green fluorescence is indicative of depolarization of mitochondria. Panel A shows the percent increase in green fluorescence of JC-1 in YT-INDY cells treated with SWCNT or AF-SWCNT. The uptake of mitochondrial dye, MitoTracker, depends on membrane potential. Data in Panel B shows the mean fluorescent intensity (MFI) of MitoTracker red in control and SWCNT- and AF-SWCNT-treated cells.

## 4. *In vitro* assessment of the effect of CNTs on splenic NK cells

Studies described above used NK cell lines for assessing the toxicity of various nanoparticles *in vitro*. This was followed by a detailed investigation into the effect of AF-SWCNTs on mouse spleen-derived NK cells.

### 4.1. NK cell cytotoxicity assay

While a basal level of NK cells exists in the mouse spleen, proliferation and activation of these cells can be induced *in vitro* by culturing with IL-2, IL-12, IL-15, or IL-18 [27]. NK cells achieve maximal activation after 3 days of activation with IL-2, and the activity gradually subsidizes within 5 days [28, 29]. Effect of CNTs on basal as well as IL-2-induced NK response was examined *in vitro*.

Spleen cells (5 × $10^6$/mL) obtained from C57BL/6 mice were treated with tris ammonium chloride buffer (ACK lysis buffer) to remove red blood cells (RBCs). Splenocytes, devoid of RBCs, were cultured with 500 U/mL IL-2 in complete medium (RPMI1640 + 10% FCS), with or without SWCNTs or AF-SWCNTs for 3 days. Control and activated spleen cells were washed, counted, and used as effector cells (E). YAC-1, a NK-sensitive murine lymphoma cell line, was used to examine the cytolytic potential of NK cells by using a 4 h $^{51}Cr$ release assay as described before [30, 31].

Lytic units (LU) per $10^7$ effector cells were calculated from the E/T ratio versus percent lysis plots [32]. Briefly, E/T ratios corresponding to a 20% target lysis were determined from the E/T ratio versus percent lysis plots, and the number of lymphocytes corresponding to this E/T ratio in the assay well was taken as one lytic unit.

Results in **Figure 8B** show that addition of SWCNTs or AF-SWCNTs during the chromium release assay had no significant effect on the killing of target cells by NK cells indicating that SWCNTs and AF-SWCNTs did not directly interfere with the E/T interaction in chromium release assay. A significant decrease in the NK activity by treatment with AF-SWCNTs is shown in **Figure 8A**.

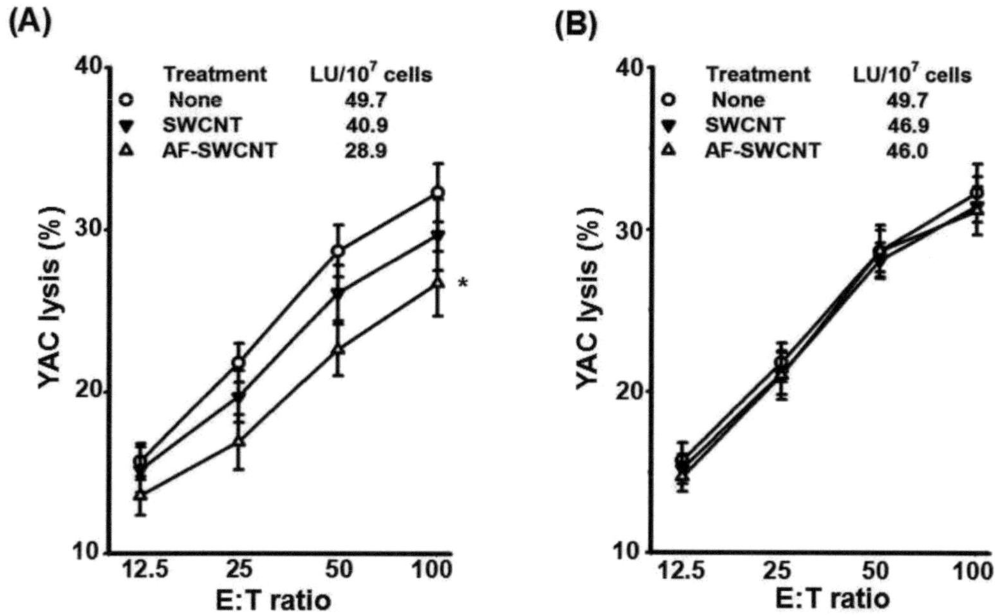


**Figure 8.** Effect of SWCNT and AF-SWCNT on the generation of NK cell response *in vitro*. NK cells were activated *in vitro* by culturing spleen cells with IL-2 in the presence or absence of SWCNT or AF-SWCNT (50 μg/mL). Anti-YAC-1 cytotoxic activity was assessed in a 4 h chromium release assay (CRA) at E/T ratios of 100, 50, 25, and 12.5 and lytic units/$10^7$ cells calculated (Panel A). Data in Panel B denoted the effect of addition of SWCNT and AF-SWCNT, during chromium release assay, on the cytotoxicity of NK cell response *in vitro*. *$p < 0.05$ by ANOVA.

### 4.2. Effect of CNTs on the recovery of IL-2-activated NK1.1⁺ cells *in vitro*

Suppression of IL-2-induced NK cell cytotoxicity by AF-SWCNTs could be due to a possible interference with the NK cell proliferation and/or activation process or a loss of NK cells due to toxic effect of AF-SWCNTs or both. In order to assess the possible toxic effect of SWCNTs and AF-SWCNTs on NK cells, recoveries of NK1.1⁺ cells from control and IL-2-activated spleen cultures were examined. Results in **Figure 9** indicate that the recovery of NK cells (percentage of NK 1.1⁺ cells by flow cytometry) in IL-2-activated spleen cell cultures declined by 17% if AF-SWCNTs were added to cultures.

### 4.3. Effect of SWCNTs and AF-SWCNTs on activated NK cells

Spleen cells express early activation marker CD69 on the surface as early as 12 h after *in vitro* stimulation with IL-2 [33]. Results in **Figure 10** show that in IL-2-treated spleen cell cultures, 53% of NK1.1⁺ cells expressed CD69 marker. Treatment with AF-SWCNTs significantly reduced the expression of CD69 on NK1.1⁺ cells by 23%.

Induction of apoptosis in NK cells activated by IL-2 in the presence of SWCNTs or AF-SWCNTs was also examined by using annexin V staining. Our results indicated that as compared to 11% apoptotic NK cells in control IL-2-activated spleen cells, the presence of SWCNTs and AF-SWCNTs increased the percentage of apoptotic cell to 17 and 22%, respectively (data not shown). Taken together, our results point to the possibility of decreased NK cell proliferation as well induction of apoptotic cell death resulting from exposure to AF-SWCNTs. In addition, expression of CD69, an early cell activation marker, was significantly lower in NK cells treated with AF-SWCNTs, indicating that the AF-SWCNTs interfered with NK cell activation process. Increased apoptosis of IL-2-activated NK cells indicates that activated NK cells are more prone to lysis than resting NK cells.

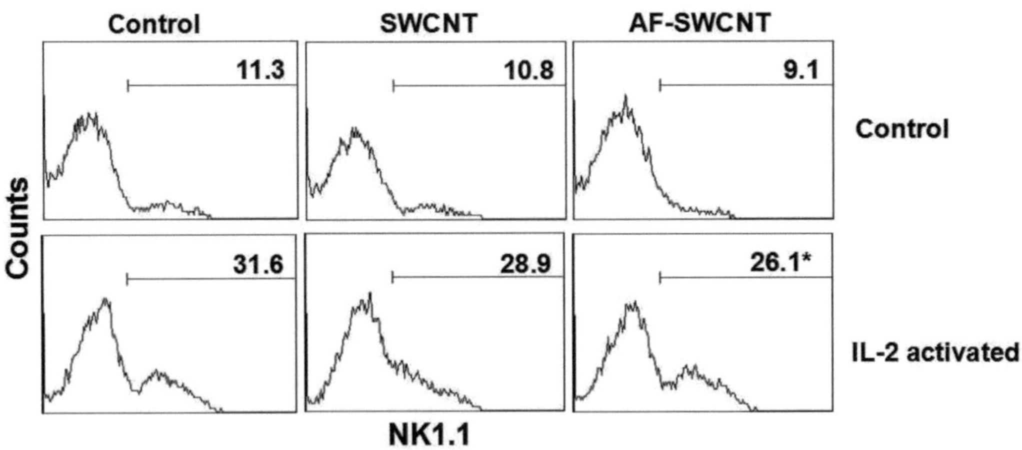


**Figure 9.** Effect of SWCNT and AF-SWCNT on recovery of NK1.1⁺ cells *in vitro*. Spleen cells activated by IL-2 in the presence and absence of 50 μg/mL of SWCNT or AF-SWCNT were stained with NK1.1 mAb and analyzed on flow cytometer. Illustrative flow cytometry histograms for percent NK cell recovery in control and activated NK cells have been shown. *$p<0.05$, by Student's *t* test.

http://dx.doi.org/10.5772/intechopen.69731

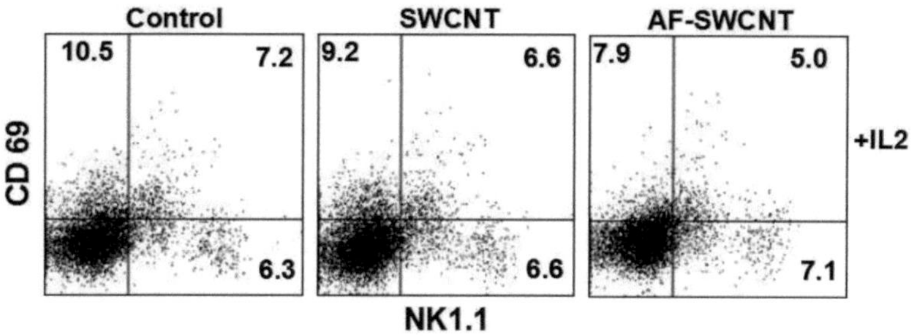


**Figure 10.** Effect of SWCNT and AF-SWCNT on the expression of CD69 activation marker on NK cells. Splenocytes cultured in the absence or presence of 500 U/mL of IL-2 were simultaneously treated with 50 μg/mL of SWCNT or AF-SWCNT. After 12 h, the splenocytes were harvested, double stained with antimouse NK1.1 and CD69 mAbs, and analyzed on a flow cytometer.

### 4.4. Effect of CNTs on effector functions of NK cells

NK cell cytotoxicity is mediated by release of cytotoxic granules like perforin or through Fas-FasL mechanism. Perforins are stored in preformed granules within the cytoplasm of NK cell and are released when NK cells are triggered by interaction with target cells. Granule release is correlated with the lysosomal marker CD107a (lysosomal-associated membrane protein or LAMP-1) [34].

Results in **Figure 11** show that addition of AF-SWCNTs to IL-2-activated culture resulted in downregulation in expression of CD107a on YAC cocultured NK1.1$^{+}$ cells from 57 to 44% (22% decline) indicating that AF-SWCNT treatment impaired the process of degranulation of activated NK cells, which may be a contributing factor in suppressing cell-mediated cytotoxicity seen in AF-SWCNT-treated NK cells.

FasL expression on IL-2-activated NK cells was also examined. Our results showed that 74% of IL-2-activated NK1.1$^{+}$ cells expressed FasL, and this significantly declined by 31% upon treatment with AF-SWCNTs (data not shown) (see **Figure 11**).

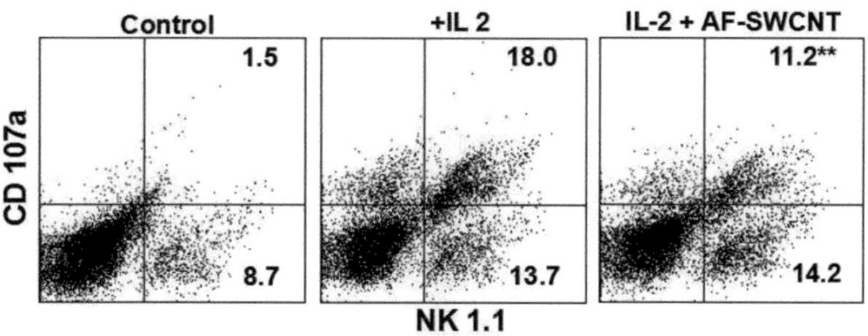


**Figure 11.** Effect of AF-SWCNT on NK cell degranulation. Splenocytes (2 × 10$^{6}$) cultured in the absence or presence of 500 U/mL of IL-2 were simultaneously treated with 50 μg/ml of AF-SWCNT. After 72 h, the activated splenocytes used as effector cells were harvested and cocultured with YAC-1 target cells to induce NK cell degranulation. The cells were stained with antimouse CD107a mAb and counterstained with antimouse NK1.1 mAb. **p < 0.01 by Student's *t* test.

## 5. *In vivo* assessment of the effect of CNTs on the NK cell in murine model

Effect of AF-SWCNTs was also examined on NK cell activation *in vivo*. For *in vivo* studies, mice were treated with poly I:C, a RNA analogue, which activates splenic NK cells. Poly I:C induces NK cell activation through the release of interferons [35–39]. The maximum activity of splenic NK cells upon stimulation with poly I:C occurs after 3 days of exposure [40, 41]. Intravenous treatment of AF-SWCNTs resulted in suppression of NK1.1⁺ cells by 15% and reduction in NK cytotoxicity by 46% (data not shown). NK cell mediates cytolytic activity through release of cytokines-IFN-$\gamma$ and TNF-$\alpha$ [42]. The effect of AF-SWCNTs was examined on expression of IFN-$\gamma$ and TNF-$\alpha$ by coculturing splenocytes with YAC cells. Intracellular expression of IFN-$\gamma$ and TNF-$\alpha$ in splenocytes obtained from mice treated with AF-SWCNTs was assessed flow cytometrically by coculturing with YAC cells *ex vivo*. Our results showed that treatment with AF-SWCNTs resulted in decline of IFN-$\gamma$ and TNF-$\alpha$ in NK1.1⁺ cells by 31 and 41%, respectively (**Figure 12**).

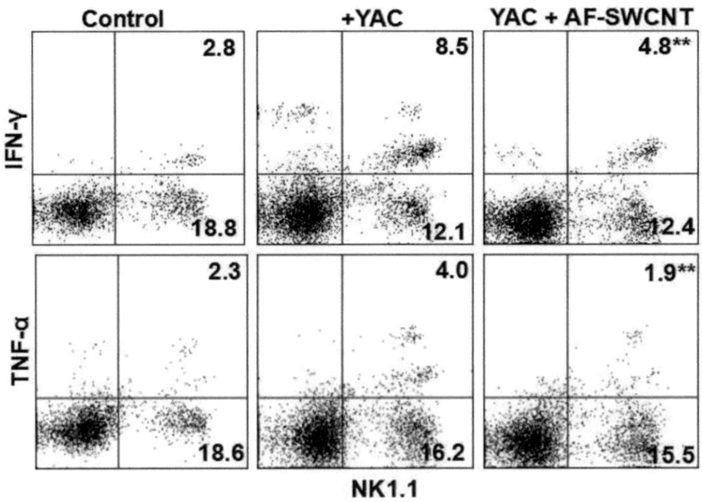


**Figure 12.** Intracellular expression levels of IFN-$\gamma$ and TNF-$\alpha$ in NK cells. Splenocytes were obtained from mice administered with poly I:C and treated with AF-SWCNT. Splenocytes ($1 \times 10^6$) were cocultured *ex vivo* with YAC cells ($2 \times 10^5$) for 5 h and treated with brefeldin and monensin. Cells were stained with antimouse IFN-$\gamma$ or antimouse TNF-$\alpha$ mAbs and counterstained with antimouse NK1.1 mAb. Percentages of NK1.1⁺ cells expressing IFN-$\gamma$ or TNF-$\alpha$ (upper right quadrant) in the presence and absence of YAC-1 target cells are shown. **$p < 0.01$ by Student's *t* test.

## 6. Conclusions

NK cells possess inherent ability to kill tumor cells without requiring a prior sensitization. NK cells and cytotoxic T lymphocytes (CTLs) both exhibit cytolytic activity involving secretory (perforin and granzymes) and nonsecretory mechanisms (Fas-FasL interaction). SWCNTs as such are insoluble and do not interact efficiently with cells. We have prepared an acid-derivatized form of SWCNTs by subjecting them to high pressure and temperature in the presence of concentrated sulfuric acid and nitric acid. Acid-functionalized SWCNTs (AF-SWCNTs) are not only polydispersed in aqueous solution but are also amenable to be attached with fluorescent ligands to their carboxyl groups created on the backbone of SWCNTs. As a result we could visualize the interaction of AF-SWCNTs with live NK cells. This was a significant step as it opened a vast arena to explore the activity of NK cells *in vitro* and *in vivo* without fixing them, as required for transmission electron microscopy. The various physiological parameters of NK cells, such as apoptosis, cell cycle, activation, generation, and degranulation have been studied using flow cytometry. This technique is superior to other conventional spectrometric techniques as the results obtained have higher reproducibility and even minor changes in subpopulation can be monitored.

AF-SWCNT treatment showed greater toxicity which was dose and time dependent. At higher dose of 50 μg/mL, AF-SWCNTs exerted toxic effects that led to decrease in cell proliferation and cell cycle arrest. Mechanistic details showed that AF-SWCNT treatment caused greater generation of ROS that led to fluctuations in mitochondrial potential and calcium concentration. These changes offset the homeostatic mechanisms of the cells, which led to their killing. Previous studies by our group had showed that AF-SWCNTs show significant inflammatory effects in mouse lungs induced anemia in mice and caused suppression of cytotoxic response *in vitro* and *in vivo* [43–46]. This chapter demonstrated the inhibitory effects of AF-SWCNTs on activated NK cells. AF-SWCNTs induced inhibition of NK activation by suppressing cellular proliferation, activation processes, and increased apoptosis. AF-SWCNT treatment led to decreased degranulation of NK cells, lower Fas-FasL interaction, and lower production of inflammatory cytokines, including IFN-$\gamma$ and TNF-$\alpha$. Taken together AF-SWCNT treatment led to downregulation of NK cell system and stipulates further research for their prospective use in autoimmune disorder or hypersensitive conditions.

## Acknowledgements

The work was funded by the Department of Science and Technology (DST), Government of India, to RKS. AA received Senior Research Fellowship from Indian Council of Medical Research (ICMR), New Delhi.

## Abbreviations

| | |
|---|---|
| 7-AAD | 7-Aminoactinomycin D |
| $^{51}Cr$ | Radioactive chromium |
| ADCC | Antibody-dependent cell-mediated cytotoxicity |
| AF-SWCNT | Acid-functionalized single-walled carbon nanotube |

| | |
|---|---|
| AIDS | Acquired immune deficiency syndrome |
| ANOVA | Analysis of variance |
| CD | Cluster of differentiation |
| CTL | Cytotoxic T lymphocyte |
| DAPI | 4′,6-Diamidino-2-phenylindole dye |
| DIC | Differential interference contrast microscopy |
| H2DCFDA | 2′,7′-Dichlorodihydrofluorescein diacetate dye |
| IFN-$\gamma$ | Interferon gamma |
| IL | Interleukin |
| mAb | Monoclonal antibody |
| MHC-I | Major histocompatibility complex class I |
| MTT | 3-(4,5-Dimethylthiazol-2-yl)-2,5-diphenyltetrazolium bromide dye |
| RNA | Ribonucleic acid |
| SWCNT | Single-walled carbon nanotube |
| TNF-$\alpha$ | Tissue necrosis factor alpha |
| TNFR | Tissue necrosis factor alpha receptor |
| TRAIL | TNF-related apoptosis-inducing ligand |
| TRAILR | TNF-related apoptosis-inducing ligand receptor |

## Author details

Anwar Alam and Rajiv K Saxena*

*Address all correspondence to: rksaxena@sau.int

Faculty of Life Sciences and Biotechnology, South Asian University, New Delhi, India

## References

[1] Kumar S, Rani R, Dilbaghi N, Tankeshwar K, Kim KH. Carbon nanotubes: A novel material for multifaceted applications in human healthcare. Chemical Society Reviews. 2017;**46**(1):158-196

[2] Lam CW, James JT, McCluskey R, Arepalli S, Hunter RL. A review of carbon nanotube toxicity and assessment of potential occupational and environmental health risks. Critical Reviews in Toxicology. 2006;**36**(3):189-217

[3] Merkt W, Sturm P, Lasitschka F, Tretter T, Watzl C, Saure D, Hundemer M, Schwenger V, Blank N, Lorenz HM, Cerwenka A. Peripheral blood natural killer cell percentages in granulomatosis with polyangiitis correlate with disease inactivity and stage. Arthritis Research and Therapy. 2015;**17**:337

[4] Ranson T, Vosshenrich CA, Corcuff E, Richard O, Müller W, Di Santo JP. IL-15 is an essential mediator of peripheral NK-cell homeostasis. Blood. 2003;**101**(12):4887-4893

[5] Lai L, Alaverdi N, Maltais L, Morse HC 3rd. Mouse cell surface antigens: Nomenclature and immunophenotyping. The Journal of Immunology. 1998;**160**(8):3861-3868

[6] Bryceson YT, Fauriat C, Nunes JM, Wood SM, Björkström NK, Long EO, Ljunggren HG. Functional analysis of human NK cells by flow cytometry. Methods in Molecular Biology. 2010;**612**:335-352

[7] Lanier LL. NK cell receptors. Annual Review of Immunology. 1998;**16**:359-393

[8] Kim S, Iizuka K, Kang HS, Doken A, French AR, Greco S, Yokoyama WM. *In vivo* development of murine natural killer cell maturation. Nature Immunology. 2002;**3**:523-528

[9] Vivier E, Nunès JA & Vély F. Natural killer cell signaling pathways. Science. 2004;**306**: 1517-1519

[10] Cohnen A, Chiang SC, Stojanovic A, Schmidt H, Claus M, Saftig P, JanBen O, Cerwenka A, Bryceson YT, Watzl C. Surface CD107a/LAMP-1 protects natural killer cells from degranulation-associated damage. Blood. 2013;**122**(8):1411-1418

[11] Ascierto ML, Idowu MO, Zhao Y, Khalak H, Payne KK, Wang XY, Dumur CI, Bedognetti D, Tomei S, Ascierto PA, Shanker A, Bear HD, Wang E, Marincola FM, De Maria A, Manjili MH. Molecular signatures mostly associated with NK cells are predictive of relapse free survival in breast cancer patients. Journal of Translational Medicine. 2013;**11**:145

[12] Dunn GP, Koebel CM, Schreiber RD. Interferons, immunity and cancer immunoediting. Nature Reviews Immunology. 2006;**6**(11):836-848

[13] Wang Y, Iqbal Z, Mitra S. Rapidly functionalized, water-dispersed carbon nanotubes at high concentration. Journal of the American Chemical Society. 2006;**128**(1):95-99

[14] Saxena RK, Williams W, McGee JK, Daniels MJ, Boykin E, Gilmour MI. Enhanced *in vitro* and *in vivo* toxicity of poly-dispersed acid-functionalized single-wall carbon nanotubes. Nanotoxicology. 2007;**1**:291-300

[15] Tong H, McGee JK, Saxena RK, Kodavanti UP, Devlin RB, Gilmour MI. Influence of acid functionalization on the cardiopulmonary toxicity of carbon nanotubes and carbon black particles in mice. Toxicology and Applied Pharmacology. 2009;**239**(3):224-232

[16] Kaur S, Mehra NK, Jain K, Jain NK. Development and evaluation of targeting ligand-anchored CNTs as prospective targeted drug delivery system. Artificial Cells, Nanomedicine, and Biotechnology. 2017;**45**(2):242-250

[17] Kumari M, Sachar S, Saxena RK. Loss of proliferative and antigen presentation activity following internalization of poly-dispersed single-walled carbon nanotubes by primary lung epithelial cells. PLoS One. 2012;**7**(2):e31890

[18] Sachar S, Saxena RK. Cytotoxic effect of poly-dispersed single walled carbon nano-tubes on mouse erythrocytes. PLoS One. 2011;**6**(7):e22032

[19] Fahmy T. Pathogen associated molecular patterns (PAMPS) on nanomaterials. Paradigms for new vaccines. Trends in Biotechnology. 2011;**29**(6):294-306

[20] Bhattacharya K, Mukherjee SP, Gallud A, Burkert SC, Bistarelli S, Bellucci S, Bottini M, Star A, Fadeel B. Biological interactions of carbon-based nanomaterials: From coronation to degradation. Nanomedicine. 2016;**12**(2):333-351

[21] Orecchioni M, Bedognetti D, Sgarrella F, Marincola FM, Bianco A, Delogu LG. Impact of carbon nanotubes and graphene on immune cells. Journal of Translational Medicine. 2014;**12**:138

[22] Levine PH, Whiteside TL, Friberg D, Bryant J, Colclough G, Herberman RB. Dysfunction of natural killer activity in a family with chronic fatigue syndrome. Clinical Immunology and Immunopathology. 1998;**88**(1):96-104

[23] Kepp O, Galluzzi L, Lipinski M, Yuan J, Kroemer G. Cell death assays for drug discovery. Nature Reviews Drug Discovery. 2011;**10**(3):221-237

[24] Zembruski NC, Stache V, Haefeli WE, Weiss J. 7-Aminoactinomycin D for apoptosis staining in flow cytometry. Analytical Biochemistry. 2012;**429**(1):79-81

[25] Circu ML, Aw TY. Reactive oxygen species, cellular redox systems, and apoptosis. Free Radical Biology and Medicine. 2010;**48**(6):749-762

[26] Zorov DB, Juhaszova M, Sollott SJ. Mitochondrial reactive oxygen species (ROS) and ROS-induced ROS release. Physiological Reviews. 2014;**94**(3):909-950

[27] Saxena RK, Saxena QB, Collins GD, Adler WH. Augmentation of spleen natural killer activity in mice treated with interleukin-2 preparation. Indian Journal of Experimental Biology. 1983;**21**:54-58

[28] Saxena RK, Saxena QB, Adler WH. Interleukin-2 induced activation of natural killer activity in spleen cells from old and young mice. Immunology. 1984;**51**:719-726

[29] Saxena RK, Adler WH. Modulation of natural cytotoxicity by alloantibodies. I. Alloantiserum enhancement of cytotoxicity of mouse spleen cells towards a human myeloid cell line. The Journal of Immunology. 1979;**123**:846-851

[30] Motzer SA, Tsuji J, Hertig V, Johnston SK, Scanlan J. Natural killer cell cytotoxicity: A methods analysis of 51 chromium release versus flow cytometry. Biological Research for Nursing. 2003;**5**(2):142-152

[31] Sarin A, Saxena RK. Interleukin-2 induced changes in the buoyant density of cytotoxic cells and its relationship with proliferative activity. Natural Immunity and Cell Growth Regulation. 1989;**8**:279-289

[32] Saxena RK, Saxena QB, Adler WH. Defective T-cell response in beige mutant mice. Nature. 1982;**295**:240-241

[33] Simms PE, Ellis TM. Utility of flow cytometric detection of CD69 expression as a rapid method for determining poly- and oligoclonal lymphocyte activation. Clinical and Diagnostic Laboratory Immunology. 1996;**3**(3):301-304

[34] Alter G, Malenfant JM, Altfeld M. CD107a as a functional marker for the identification of natural killer cell activity. Journal of Immunological Methods. 2004;**294**(1-2):15-22

[35] Saxena RK, Saxena QB, Adler WH. Regulation of natural killer activity *in vivo*. I. Loss of natural killer activity during starvation. Indian Journal of Experimental Biology. 1980;**18**:1383-1386

[36] Saxena QB, Saxena RK, Adler WH. Regulation of natural killer activity *in vivo*. IV. High natural killer activity in alcohol drinking mice. Indian Journal of Experimental Biology. 1981;**19**:1001-1006

[37] Saxena QB, Saxena RK, Adler WH. Regulation of natural killer activity *in vivo*. III. Effect of hypophysectomy and growth hormone treatment on the natural killer activity of the mouse spleen cell population. International Archives of Allergy and Applied Immunology. 1982;**67**:169-174

[38] Saxena QB, Saxena RK, Adler WH. Effect of protein caloric malnutrition on the level of natural and inducible cytotoxic activities in mouse spleen cells. Immunology. 1984;**51**:727-733

[39] Saxena QB, Saxena RK, Adler WH. Effect of feeding a diet with half of the recommended levels of all vitamins on the natural and inducible levels of cytotoxic activity in mouse spleen cells. Immunology. 1984;**52**:41-47

[40] Saxena RK, Saxena QB, Adler WH. Mechanism of loss of natural killer activity in P815 tumor bearing DBA/2 mice. Natural Immunity and Cell Growth Regulation. 1984;**3**:34-42

[41] Saxena RK, Adler WH, Nordin AA. Modulation of natural cytotoxicity by alloantibodies. IV. A comparative study of the activation of mouse spleen cell cytotoxicity by anti H-2 antisera, interferon and mitogens. Cellular Immunology. 1981;**63**:28-41

[42] Wang R, Jaw JJ, Stutzman NC, Zou Z, Sun PD. Natural killer cell-produced IFN-$\gamma$ and TNF-$\alpha$ induce target cell cytolysis through up-regulation of ICAM-1. Journal of Leukocyte Biology. 2012;**91**(2):299-309

[43] Alam A, Sachar S, Puri N, Saxena RK. Interactions of poly-dispersed single walled Carbon Nanotubes with T cells resulting in down regulation of allogeneic CTL responses *in vitro* and *in vivo*. Nanotoxicology. 2013;**7**:1351-1360

[44] Abbas Z, Puri N, Saxena RK. Lipid antigen presentation through CD1d pathway in mouse lung epithelial cells, macrophages and dendritic cells and its suppression by poly-dispersed single-walled carbon nanotubes. Toxicology *in Vitro*. 2014;**29**:1275-1285

[45] Bhardwaj N, Saxena RK. Selective loss of younger erythrocytes from blood circulation and changes in erythropoietic patterns in bone marrow and spleen in mouse anemia induced by poly-dispersed single wall carbon nanotubes. Nanotoxicology. 2015;**9**(8):1032-1040

[46] Alam A, Puri N, Saxena RK. Uptake of poly-dispersed single-walled carbon nanotubes and decline of functions in mouse NK cells undergoing activation. Journal of Immunotoxicology. 2016;**13**(5):758-765

Chapter 9

# A New Method to Determine Natural Killer Cell Activity Without Target Cells

Yasumitsu Nishimura, Naoko Kumagai-Takei, Suni Lee, Hidenori Matsuzaki, Kei Yoshiotme and Takemi Otsuki

Additional information is available at the end of the chapter

http://dx.doi.org/10.5772/intechopen.71912

**Abstract**

Natural killer (NK) cell activity is a conventional parameter used to determine the performance lytic activity against tumor as well as virus-infected cells in innate immunity. However, use of this parameter has several problems related to bioassay measurements. To measure NK cell activity, target cells and cell culture equipment are required and adequate pre-culture of target cells is needed to maintain constant sensitivity for NK cells. NK cell-activating receptors play an important role in the recognition of targets, which transduce the signals necessary for cellular machinery to induce target injury and cytokine production. We statistically examined the parameters related to the NK cell activity of human peripheral blood mononuclear cells (PBMCs) by multiple regression analysis, and obtained a formula with NK cell % and RNA levels of two genes in isolated NK cells. The score calculated using this formula with the three measured values showed significant correlation with NK cell activity. This prediction score, named the non-incubating natural killer (NINK) score, which is independent of target cells, is not affected by inappropriate preparation of those targets, and allows us to accurately compare the performance of NK cell activity among specimens.

**Keywords:** NK cell activity, activating receptor, NKp46, IFN-$\gamma$

## 1. Introduction

The characteristics of antitumor immunity in the body are of interest not only with respect to healthy individuals but also in relation to patients diagnosed with certain kinds of tumor diseases. With the former, information can be utilized by individuals to assess their lifestyle so as to prevent the occurrence of tumor diseases. If smokers were aware of decreased levels of their antitumor immune functions, they might be more motivated to quit smoking or to have medical checks more often. As these considerations are invaluable in the area of preventive medicine, and have the potential to decrease the national cost of medical expenses, the development of appropriate and easy-to-use devices for measuring the status of tumor immunity would be desirable. In clinical medicine, doctors also hope to determine alterations in immunological status as well as tumor size in the body of patients following cancer therapy. The immunological information obtained following the treatment might contribute to an adequate determination of the therapeutic efficacy by doctors. Natural killer (NK) cell activity testing is one effective approach to determine the status of antitumor immunity in the body, which is reflected from the crosstalk between cancer cells and immune cells and the nature of those immune cells. NK cell activity is a conventional index which represents the ability of cell samples to injure NK cell-sensitive target cells, and we utilized the method of NK cell activity to evaluate the natural cytotoxic activity of peripheral blood mononuclear cells (PBMCs) obtained from patients and an NK cell line [1–5]. A recent 11-year follow-up study from 1986 to 1990 involving 3652 Japanese residents of the general population clearly demonstrated the importance of determining and evaluating NK cell activity. In that report, individuals with low NK cell activity actually showed higher cumulative incidence rates of cancer compared to people with high or medium NK cell activity, regardless of gender [6]. In particular, women showed more differences in the incidence rate of cancer, which represented about a twofold difference between groups with low and high or medium levels of NK cell activity. Thus, NK cell activity is a good index in evaluating the status of antitumor immunity. In fact, our previous studies measuring NK cell activity demonstrated that indoor air conditions have a potential to interfere with NK cell function [7–10]. However, NK cell activity testing possesses several difficulties, which concerns researchers and doctors when considering the potential use of NK cell activity as an index in basic and clinical studies in medical science. In the next section, these issues will be examined.

## 2. The conventional method to examine NK cell activity

Simplicity is the reason why the conventional method of determining NK cell activity has been a standard till date. With this method, NK cell-sensitive targets such as K562 cells are prepared and cell specimens are incubated with the target cells for 4 h at 37°C in a $CO_2$ incubator. The original "$^{51}$Chromium release assay (CRA)" method was developed during the 1960s [11, 12]. With that original method, researchers have to label target cells with the $^{51}$Cr radioisotope in an effort to determine the amount of radioisotope released from targets lysed by NK cells in specimens, which reflects the amount of killed targets or, in other words, the NK cell activity. Although to date, commercial services have been examining NK cell activity by employing the $^{51}$Cr release assay, researchers have the option of using flow cytometry with fluorescence dyes *in lieu* of radioisotopes to measure NK cell activity. This approach can distinguish targets from effectors by labeling targets with a fluorescence dye such as carboxyfluorescein diacetate succinimidyl ester (CFSE) and DiO, which has similar excitation

http://dx.doi.org/10.5772/intechopen.71912

and emission properties as fluorescein isothiocyanate (FITC). Then, since dead targets can be distinguished from viable cells by staining with propidium iodide (PI), the percentage of $PI^+$ targets in the total can be measured using flow cytometry in a radioisotope-free manner. Actually, we have measured NK cell activity in this manner and understand the usability of this conventional method [1, 2], although we became familiar with several kinds of difficulties. In order to assay for NK cell activity, a researcher needs to decide the date for the assay and consequently adjust target cells to an adequate condition by pre-culturing for a fixed number of days at a fixed cell density, to ensure that the target cells operate with consistent sensitivity on the assay day. Therefore, although a researcher can assay for NK cell activity of a scheduled specimen on one day under the same conditions performed on the previous day, it may be difficult to maintain adequate or appropriate conditions in the assay for use of an unscheduled specimen since the pre-culture of target cells has not been accomplished on the day. We demonstrated that differences in pre-culture conditions of target cells leads to alterations in the results obtained from the assay for NK cell activity (**Figure 1**). The specimen comprising PBMCs was prepared from human peripheral blood and used as effectors equally for the assays, while K562 cells were prepared as targets by pre-culturing at two different cell

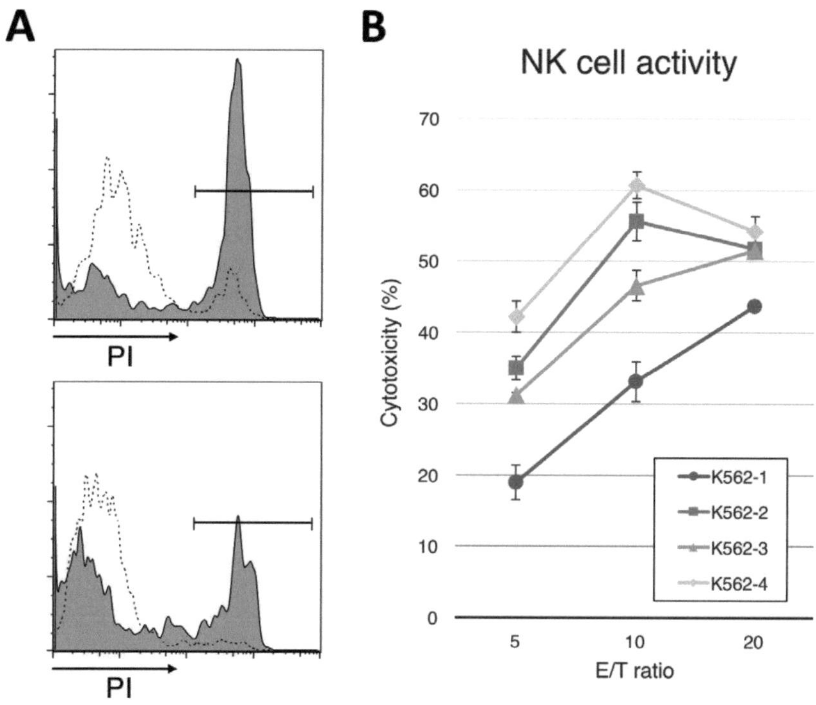


**Figure 1.** Variation in the results of assaying for NK activity due to differences in the pre-culture conditions of target cells. K562 cells were pre-cultured under four different conditions using two different cell densities prepared separately by two individuals. A shows representative histograms of K562 cells obtained by flow cytometry with a high percentage of $PI^+$ dead cells (upper) and low percentage of cells (lower) at an E/T ratio of 10 following incubation with human PBMCs for 4 h. K562 cells were distinguished from PBMCs by positive DiO staining and gated to show the histograms. The bar represents the region defined and measured as the population of $DiO^+PI^+$ cells. Dashed lines represent targets alone. A summarized graph with mean and SD from the three wells is shown in B. It is clear that the cytotoxicity obtained from the assay with K562-1 shows only half the degree of cytotoxicity obtained from the assay with K562-4.

densities prepared separately by two individuals. Following pre-culturing, all targets were stained with DiO and incubated with PBMCs in a 96-well U-bottom culture plate for 4 h. Following incubation, cells were stained with PI before being analyzed by flow cytometry, where the percentage of $DiO^{+}PI^{+}$ cells in the total number of $DiO^{+}$ cells was measured as lysed target cells. Finally, the percentage of natural cytotoxicity was calculated as follows:

$$\text{NK cell activity (\%)} = \big([\text{percentage of lysed cells}] - [\text{percentage of spontaneously dead cells}]\big)/ \big(100 - [\text{percentage of spontaneously dead cells}]\big) \times 100 \quad (1)$$

In this formula, the percentage of spontaneously dead cells represented the percentage of dead cells in target cells harvested from wells without effector cells. In that experiment, the values of NK cell activity clearly differed among the four kinds of pre-cultured K562 cells and showed a maximum twofold difference at an E/T ratio of 10. These results indicate that the values of NK cell activity vary between assays, a phenomenon which is unavoidable when using target cells, that is, bioassay. If researchers were not bound to use target cells for the determination of NK cell activity without targets, the results obtained from the assays might be more stable, and requirements such as a $CO_2$ incubator and a clean bench for cell culture would be unnecessary. Therefore, we attempted to develop a new method to determine NK cell activity without the use of cell culture.

## 3. The importance of NK cell-activating receptors in NK cell cytotoxicity

Although both NK and $CD8^{+}$ T cells have the ability to injure target cells, these cells also possess many different characteristics, one of which is the machinery required for the recognition of targets followed by signal transduction linked to cell injury. The diversity of antigen specificity in T cells is dependent on the T cell receptor (TCR) complex on the cell surface, and accounts for the ability of $CD8^{+}$ T cells to recognize and kill any kind of target cell by the strong interaction between the TCR and MHC antigen peptide complex. However, as naïve T cells are not ready to exert target injury and antigen specificity differs among cells, with only a small amount being present within each clone, $CD8^{+}$ T cells need to be activated before injuring targets. In contrast, NK cells are capable of killing targets with no activation required and are equipped with various kinds of receptors to recognize targets, referred to as NK cell-activating receptors (KARs) [13–16]. NKG2D is the most-studied of these receptors and belongs to the NKG2 family of proteins which are characterized by the presence of a lectin-like domain. NKG2D binds to MHC class I polypeptide-related sequence A and B (MICA/B) and UL16-binding protein (ULBP) [17–22], which are often expressed in tumor cells [23, 24]. Natural cytotoxicity receptors (NCRs) also play a role in killing various kinds of tumors, and NKp30, NKp44, NKp46 and NKp80 are members of the NCR family of proteins [14]. Moreover, the signaling lymphocyte activating molecule (SLAM) family are another group of players involved in the recognition of targets by NK cells, and 2B4 (CD244), a representative member of the SLAM family, recognizes CD48 and leads to cytotoxicity [25–29]. It is thought that the

http://dx.doi.org/10.5772/intechopen.71912

variety of activating receptors on a single cell impart NK cells with the ability to exert cytotoxicity against various target cells without clonal selection and expansion as with T lymphocytes. Those activating receptors share the same mechanism of signal transduction, by which a microtubule organizing center (MTOC) is induced to polarize cytotoxic granules, including perforin and granzymes, near the plasma membrane, and those intragranular molecules are subsequently released against targets *via* degranulation (**Figure 2**). The ligation of those activating receptors allow Src family kinases (SFK) to trigger the pathways from phosphoinositide -3 kinase (PI3K) to extracellular signal-regulated kinase (ERK) and from phospholipase C (PLC) $\gamma$ to c-jun N-terminal kinase (JNK) to facilitate polarization [30–32]. Those findings led us to surmise that some alteration in cell surface expression levels of activating receptors on NK cells might influence lytic activity against targets. We previously investigated the toxicological effects of asbestos on NK cell function, and demonstrated that asbestos exposure caused impaired cytotoxicity of NK cells with altered expression of several activating receptors [1, 2, 4, 5]. Continuous exposure of the human NK cell line YT-A1 to asbestos resulted in decreased levels of cell surface NKG2D and 2B4, as well as impaired cytotoxicity against K562 cells. Furthermore, it was confirmed that the degranulation induced by stimulation with antibodies to NKG2D or

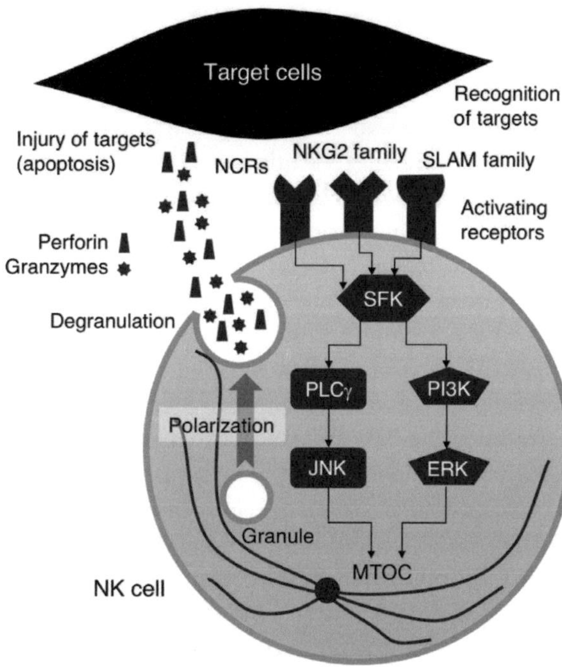


**Figure 2.** The summarized machinery of target cell injury caused by target recognition with activating receptors. Recognition of target cells with various activating receptors induces Src family kinases (SFK) to trigger the two pathways from phosphoinositide-3 kinase (PI3K) to extracellular signal-regulated kinase (ERK) and from phospholipase C (PLC) $\gamma$ to c-jun N-terminal kinase (JNK). Both of these pathways induce polarization of cytotoxic granules *via* a microtubule organizing center (MTOC), whereby granules move to a region near the plasma membrane. Finally, the fusion between plasma membrane and granular membrane occurs to induce degranulation, and perforin and granzymes are released from those granules to induce death of the target cells by apoptosis.

2B4 was low in those asbestos-exposed cells. Moreover, we examined the characteristics of human primary NK cells in PBMCs cultured with asbestos and found a decrease in cell surface NKp46 in patients with malignant mesothelioma, a tumor disease caused by inhalation of asbestos, and also showed impaired natural cytotoxicity. Less information is known about the natural ligands of NKp46. However, a previous investigation demonstrated that cell surface expression levels of NKp46 were correlated with the natural cytotoxicity of K562 and that reverse antibody-dependent cell-mediated cytotoxicity (ADCC) of P815 was correlated with antibodies to NKp46 [33]. Additionally, our previous study demonstrated that NK cells in healthy individuals with high natural cytotoxicity showed high expression of NKG2D, NKp46 and phosphorylation of ERK following stimulation *via* those receptors, whereas NK cells in individuals with low natural cytotoxicity showed the converse [2]. These results led us to surmise that determination of the gene expression level of activating receptors might be one important parameter in estimating the natural cytotoxicity of effector cells such as PBMCs *in lieu* of employing methods involving incubation with NK-sensitive target cells.

## 4. The roles executed by NK cells with molecules in cytotoxic granules, the cell surface ligand and secreted proteins

As mentioned above, the cell surface expression of activating receptors on NK cells is a key event which defines the performance of those cells. What precisely occurs in NK cells following stimulation with KARs? NK cells execute two different events following recognition of target cells with activating receptors (**Figure 3**). The first event exerts natural cytotoxicity against the targets by releasing perforin and granzymes in cytotoxic granules into the space of the immune synapse between NK and target cells. Perforin is thought to function in generating a pore in the plasma membrane as complement proteins, and then granzymes enter through the pore and mediate apoptosis by deploying their serine protease activity [34]. Alternatively, NK cells also express cell surface FasL, which can also induce apoptosis through Fas receptors on the target cells [35]. Moreover, TNF-related apoptosis-inducing ligand (TRAIL) is also produced by NK cells and induces apoptosis of target cells like FasL [36–38]. This natural cytotoxicity itself highlights the importance of early removal of abnormal cells, which transiently appear in the body, and directly contributes to preventing the development of tumor diseases. However, it also has another role linked to antigen-specific cytotoxicity by cytotoxic T lymphocytes (CTLs) in acquired immunity. CTLs have to be primed by dendritic cells (DCs) with a complex comprising antigen peptide and MHC class I molecule before they can become effective cytotoxic cells from naïve cells. In this priming, extracellular antigen is exceptionally presented on MHC class I for CTLs by a particular subset of DCs, in a process referred to as "cross-presentation" [39–41]. These type of DCs endocytose dead target cells, digest their antigens and express a complex of MHC class I and antigen peptide on the cell surface [42], and the dead cells can be provided from early injury of target cells by NK cells to DCs [43]. That is why NK cells are linked to acquired

http://dx.doi.org/10.5772/intechopen.71912

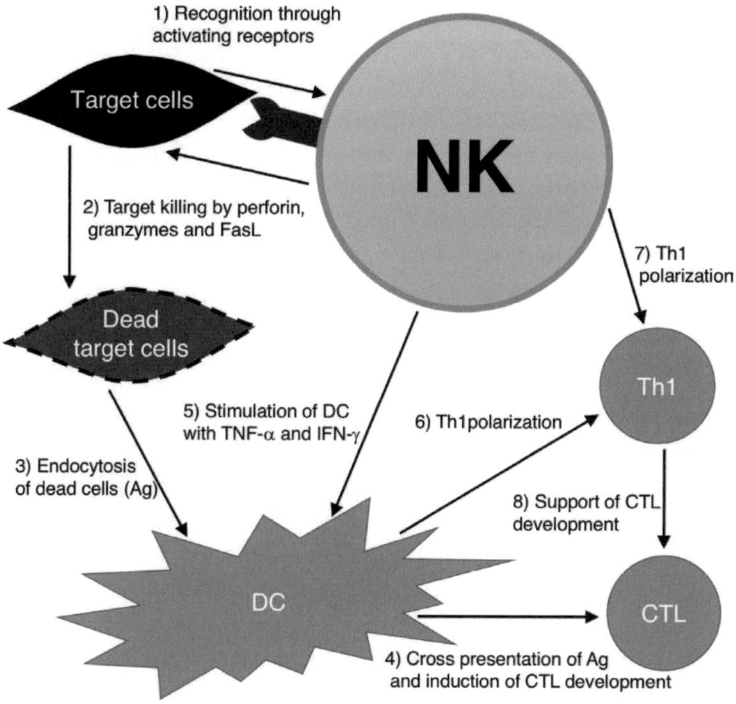


**Figure 3.** Summarized illustration of the roles executed by NK cells following the recognition of targets with activating receptors and subsequent responses in acquired immunity. (1) NK cells recognize target cells with activating receptors including NKG2D and NKp46, which trigger the machinery for target cell injury. (2) NK cells exert the action of killing targets by perforin/granzymes, FasL or TRAIL. (3) Dead target cells are endocytosed as antigen (Ag) by DCs. (4) The particular subset of DCs which have endocytosed lysed target cells play a role in "cross-presentation" to stimulate naïve $CD8^+$ T lymphocytes to develop into mature CTLs. (5) The stimulated NK cells also produce cytokines including TNF-$\alpha$ and IFN-$\gamma$, (6)–(8) which stimulate DCs to produce IL-12 and other proinflammatory cytokines, thereby promoting Th1 cell polarization and CTL development.

immunity as well as function in innate immunity by themselves. Secondly, the production of cytokines including TNF-$\alpha$ and IFN-$\gamma$ by NK cells after recognition of targets also plays an important role in DC maturation [43, 44]. Those cytokines stimulate DCs to produce IL-12 and other proinflammatory cytokines, which promote Th1 cell polarization and CTL development with specificity against target cells. Additionally, IFN-$\gamma$ produced by NK cells is able to effect Th1 polarization directly. Those findings relating to the production of cytokines by NK cells, in particular, as IFN-$\gamma$ is a key cytokine which is produced by NK cells and supports tumor immunity, leads us to hypothesize that the production of IFN-$\gamma$ by NK cells in an individual might be utilized alone to estimate the performance of natural cytotoxicity in those cells. However, it is known that NK cells can be divided into two populations comprising $CD56^{bright}$ and $CD56^{dim}$ cells, which show different natural cytotoxicity and production of IFN-$\gamma$. $CD56^{bright}$ NK cells have high production of IFN-$\gamma$ and low natural cytotoxicity, whereas $CD56^{dim}$ NK cells have low production of IFN-$\gamma$ and high natural cytotoxicity [45, 46]. Those findings demonstrate that measurement of IFN-$\gamma$ production by NK cells is insufficient to estimate the natural cytotoxicity of those cells and that determination of multiple parameters related to NK cells is necessary in order to effectively evaluate the performance of natural cytotoxicity in an indirect manner. All of this information indicates that the performance of NK cells is reflected by the strength of stimulation through cell surface activating receptors as well as the subsequent production of functional molecules as described above.

## 5. The development of a new index: non-incubating natural killer (NINK) score

The findings concerning NK cells described above led our research group to surmise that calculation of a prediction score based on several factors that play a role in NK cells might be utilized as an effective index to determine the performance of NK cell activity of PBMCs in an individual without the need to prepare target cells. Therefore, we statistically analyzed factors that may correlate with the NK cell activity of human PBMCs using multiple regression analysis with linear regression model, and in doing so attempted to arrive at a formula to calculate the prediction score of NK cell activity (**Figure 4**) (manuscript of an original article under preparation). In that analysis, the following parameters were used as independent variables for NK cell activity: the percentage of $CD3^{-}CD56^{+}$NK cells (NK%) in PBMCs and mRNA levels of NKp46, granzyme B, FasL, TNF-$\alpha$ and IFN-$\gamma$ relative to GAPDH mRNA levels in isolated NK cells, which were measured by flow cytometry and real-time PCR, respectively.

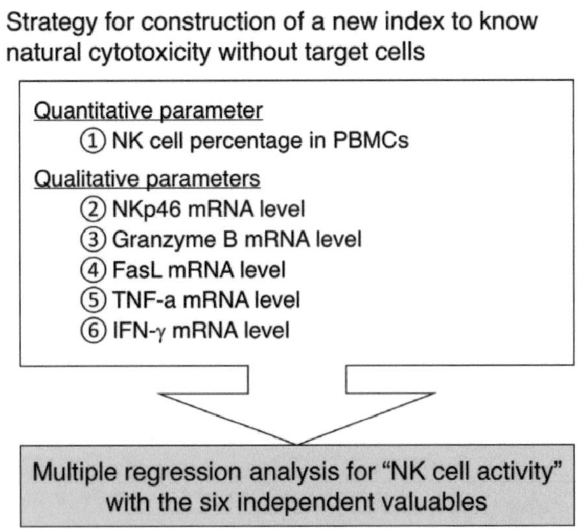


**Figure 4.** Scheme of strategy for construction of a new index to determine natural cytotoxicity without the use of target cells. The upper box shows six candidate parameters which we selected to explore the new index in an effort to determine natural cytotoxicity. The percentage of NK cells in PBMCs represents the amount of NK cells as a quantitative parameter, while mRNA expression levels of NKp46, granzyme B, FasL, TNF-$\alpha$ and IFN-$\gamma$ are thought to function or interfere with the strength of lytic activity of NK cells as qualitative parameters. We analyzed the relationship of those parameters with respect to NK cell activity using multiple regression analysis.

http://dx.doi.org/10.5772/intechopen.71912

The value of the mRNA level, being ΔCq obtained from real-time PCR, was log-transformed (base-10) and used for the multiple regression analysis. The NK% and other parameters were examined as quantitative and qualitative parameters, respectively, and related to the performance of NK cell activity, the reason why those parameters were chosen for that analysis. The conventional index of NK cell activity of PBMCs was assayed using the K562 cell line as the target cells. The results of the multiple regression analysis showed a significant correlation between NK cell activity and NK%, NKp46 mRNA and IFN-γ mRNA, and the prediction formula obtained from the statistical analysis comprises the aforementioned three correlation factors as shown below.

$$\begin{aligned}\text{NINK score} &= \text{a} + \text{b[NK\%]} + \text{c}\left[\text{NKp46 mRNA in NK cells}\right] \\ &\quad + \text{d}\left[\text{IFN-gmRNA in NK cells}\right]\end{aligned} \tag{2}$$

The score calculated using the prediction formula with values of each parameter derived from each individual showed a better Pearson's correlation coefficient with NK cell activity than using either NK%, NKp46 mRNA or IFN-γ mRNA levels alone. These results indicate that this prediction score, named the non-incubating natural killer (NINK) score, can reflect the performance of natural cytotoxicity without the use of target cells to measure NK cell activity (patent pending). Finally, we confirmed the feasibility of the NINK score using another group of individuals. In this experiment, blood in collection tubes was stored overnight in a

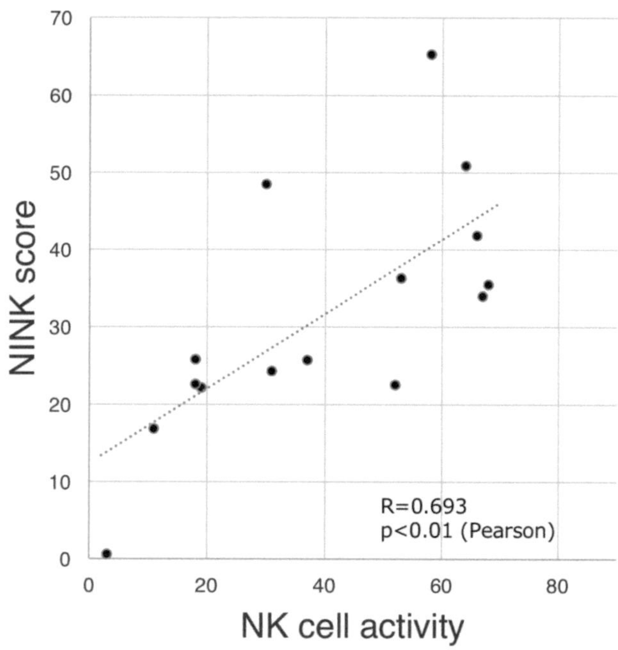


**Figure 5.** The positive correlation of the NINK score with NK cell activity. The NINK score was calculated using the prediction formula comprising NK% in PBMCs and mRNA levels of NKp46 and IFN-γ in isolated NK cells derived from PBMCs from each individual, and then examined for a correlation with NK cell activity using Pearson's correlation test. The graph shows a significantly positive correlation of the NINK score with NK cell activity. The correlation coefficient and statistical significance of the p value are shown in the graph.

container box at 22°C prior to executing the assays outlined below, since the actual procedures involving PBMC preparation, NK% measurement and isolation of CD56$^+$ NK cells, followed by subsequent measurement of mRNA levels, may need to be performed on the following day after the blood is collected at a distant clinic and then transported to the institute where the subsequent procedures are performed. The results of that experiment clearly demonstrated that the NINK score calculated with values comprising NK% and mRNA levels of NKp46 and IFN-γ in NK cells obtained even from blood stored for 1 day show good correlation with NK cell activity (**Figure 5**). When individuals were divided into groups comprising low and high NK cell activity or groups comprising low and high NINK score using the averages as cut-off values, most of the low NINK score group (87.5%) showed low NK cell activity, while most of the high NINK score group (85.7%) showed high NK cell activity. Taken together, these findings indicate that the NINK score is an effective measure of the natural cytotoxicity of specimens and obviates the need to assay for NK cell activity using target cells.

## 6. Discussion

Our demonstration indicates that the NINK score can be employed as a new index to determine the performance of natural cytotoxicity of PBMCs without the use of target cells or cell culture equipment for incubation. **Figure 6** shows the difference between the conventional index of NK cell activity and our new index of the NINK score. The conventional index of NK cell activity is useful since it can be determined by only using fluorescence or radioisotope-labeled target cells. However, it is often difficult to maintain good conditions of NK sensitivity in target cells. Technicians need to pre-culture cells under the same cell density and culture period (days) conditions in an effort to maintain good NK sensitivity of the cells. If daily measurement of NK activity is required, many pre-culture lines need to be prepared, which is unrealistic in a small institute. Additionally, since measurement of NK cell activity is based on a "bioassay", this traditional index is prone to variation between assays. This problem often troubles researchers since the altered sensitivity of target cells creates difficulties when combining results obtained from multiple assays. Similar to the measurement of NK cell activity by examining the release of $^{51}Cr$ or fluorescence labeling, the lactate dehydrogenase (LDH) release assay has a problem in terms of the bioassay. In the LDH release assay, the activity of LDH derived from lysed target cells in media is measured as an absorbance following incubation of effector cells with target cells [47–49]. As an alternative approach, the level of degranulation induced by stimulation with activating receptors was assayed to assess the lytic activity of NK cells *in lieu* of using target cells [50]. In this method, the increase in cell surface expression of LAMP1/CD107a is examined by flow cytometry following stimulation. The expression of LAMP1/CD107a is high on the membrane of lytic granules but increases on the plasma membrane as a result of degranulation. However, even this method is unable to avoid the use of incubated effector cells to assay the lytic activity, which can lead to difficulties resulting from the "bioassay". In contrast, determination of the NINK score does not require the use of target cells or cell culture equipment, and is therefore free of the potential complications associated

http://dx.doi.org/10.5772/intechopen.71912

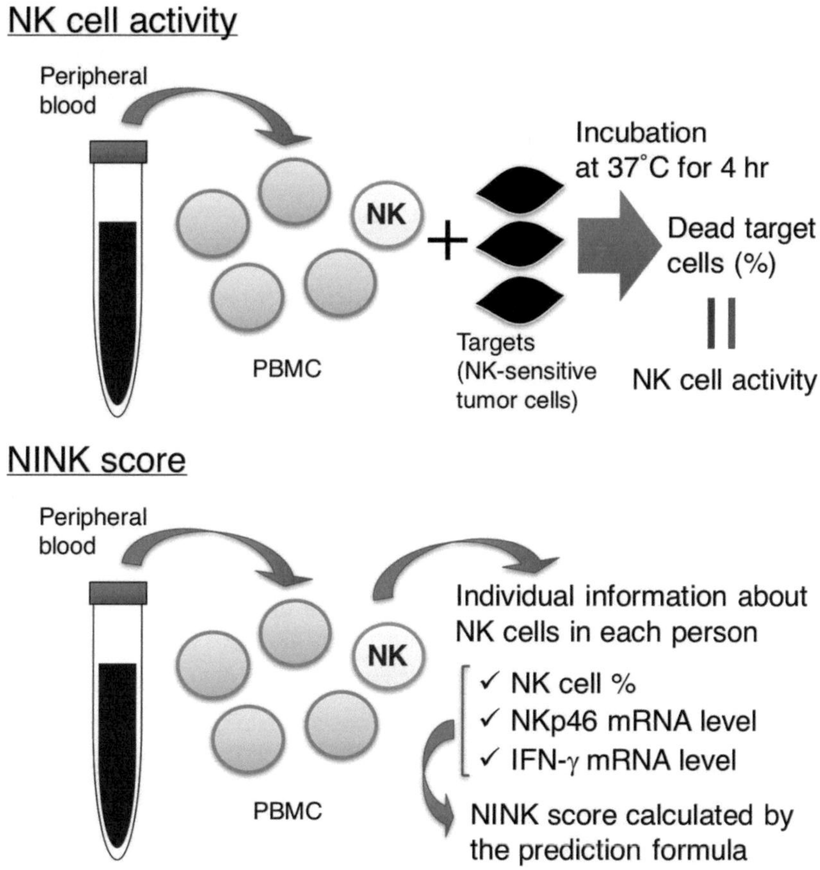


**Figure 6.** Illustration of differences between the conventional NK cell activity index and new NINK score index. To measure the NK cell activity, NK-sensitive target cells such as K562 cells need to be prepared and appropriately maintained prior to use in the assay, and then PBMCs need to be incubated with the target cells for 4 h, which is often troublesome and can cause large variation between assays. In contrast, a determination of the NINK score does not require the use of target cells or cell culture equipment for incubation. Technicians simply have to measure NK% and isolate NK cells from PBMCs. Messenger RNA levels of the two genes in the NK cells (retrieved from frozen storage) can then be determined and the NINK score calculated using the prediction formula with the measure values of the three parameters.

with the inappropriate preparation of those cells. Additionally, on any given day, technicians will measure NK%, isolate NK cells from PBMCs by flow cytometry or magnetically, and then store the NK cells frozen before subsequent assays are performed. At some later time, mRNA levels of NKp46 and IFN-γ can be determined in the frozen cells by real-time PCR and the NINK score calculated using the prediction formula with the measured values of the three parameters. Thus, employing our new approach based on the NINK score can free the technician from continuous pre-culture of target cells required in the traditional NK activity assay, and provides a stable tool to measure the performance of NK cells in each individual and independent bioassay. The NINK score is beneficial as a measure of NK cell performance in each individual, and is a requirement for clinicians working in the field of cancer therapy as well as for the assessment of healthy individuals interested in preventive medicine and health promotion. Since NK cells are linked to the CTL response in acquired immunity as mentioned above, it may be valuable for clinicians to assess the progress of the functional status of NK cell activity in a patient following cancer therapy in a steady manner by using the NINK score. It would be better if the NK cell activity could be checked in terms of a solid parameter such as bone density or body fat percentage, which can be achieved by measuring the NINK score. A vast amount of data concerning the relationship between NK cell activity and various kinds of factors related to lifestyle can be collected using the NINK score, the results of which might lead to new insights concerning healthier and disease-preventive lifestyles from an immunological perspective. The ability to store isolated NK cell specimens temporarily in a frozen state provides a benefit in that the following measurements of mRNA levels can be performed simultaneously, which allows for an accurate comparison of NINK scores among specimens. Additionally, the NINK score may be useful as a screening device to identify NK cell-activating natural compounds from within a compound library using *in vitro* experiments of PBMC cultures. An actual effect of some compound on NK cell activity can then be examined using animal experiments (mice), even where a modified method of the NINK score may be utilized to measure the performance of NK cell activity *in lieu* of using the method with NK cell-sensitive murine targets such as YAC-1 cells [51, 52]. In contrast, the traditional method involved in the NK assay using target cells is unsuitable for these purposes given the lower stability resulting from the use of bio-assays as mentioned above. The NINK score might contribute to an assessment of the efficacy of a drug at different stages of cancer treatment in patients, as well as an assessment of the effectiveness of different lifestyles, exercise and food consumption in maintaining good health in individuals. We hope that the NINK score would be utilized in various fields to facilitate the promotion of general health in the population.

## Acknowledgements

The authors thank Ms. Tamayo Hatayama, Shoko Yamamoto and Miho Ikeda for their technical help. The authors declare that there is no conflict of interests regarding the publication of this paper.

## Author details

Yasumitsu Nishimura*, Naoko Kumagai-Takei, Suni Lee, Hidenori Matsuzaki,
Kei Yoshiotme and Takemi Otsuki

*Address all correspondence to: yas@med.kawasaki-m.ac.jp

Department of Hygiene, Kawasaki Medical School, Kurashiki, Japan

## References

[1] Nishimura Y, Miura Y, Maeda M, Kumagai N, Murakami S, Hayashi H, et al. Impairment in cytotoxicity and expression of NK cell- activating receptors on human NK cells following exposure to asbestos fibers. International Journal of Immunopathology and Pharmacology. 2009;**22**(3):579-590

[2] Nishimura Y, Maeda M, Kumagai N, Hayashi H, Miura Y, Otsuki T. Decrease in phosphorylation of ERK following decreased expression of NK cell-activating receptors in human NK cell line exposed to asbestos. International Journal of Immunopathology and Pharmacology. 2009;**22**(4):879-888

[3] Nishimura Y, Kumagai-Takei N, Maeda M, Matsuzaki H, Lee S, Yamamoto S, Hatayama T, Yoshitome K, Otsuki T. Suppressive effects of asbestos exposure on the human immune surveillance system. In: Otsuki T DGM, Petrarca C, editor. Allergy and Immunotoxicology in Occupational Health. Tokyo: Springer Japan; 2016. p. accepted

[4] Nishimura Y, Kumagai-Takei N, Matsuzaki H, Lee S, Maeda M, Kishimoto T, et al. Functional alteration of natural killer cells and cytotoxic T lymphocytes upon asbestos exposure and in malignant mesothelioma patients. BioMed Research International. 2015;**2015**:1-9

[5] Nishimura Y, Maeda M, Kumagai-Takei N, Matsuzaki H, Lee S, Miura Y, et al. Effect of asbestos on antitumor immunity and immunological alteration in patients with mesothelioma. In: Belli C, editor. Malignant Mesothelioma. Rijeka: InTech d.o.o; 2012. pp. 31-48

[6] Imai K, Matsuyama S, Miyake S, Suga K, Nakachi K. Natural cytotoxic activity of peripheral-blood lymphocytes and cancer incidence: An 11-year follow-up study of a general population. Lancet. 2000;**356**(9244):1795-1799

[7] Takahashi K, Otsuki T, Mase A, Kawado T, Kotani M, Ami K, et al. Negatively-charged air conditions and responses of the human psycho-neuro-endocrino-immune network. Environment International. 2008;**34**(6):765-772

[8] Takahashi K, Otsuki T, Mase A, Kawado T, Kotani M, Nishimura Y, et al. Two weeks of permanence in negatively-charged air conditions causes alteration of natural killer cell function. International Journal of Immunopathology and Pharmacology. 2009;**22**(2):333-342

[9] Nishimura Y, Takahashi K, Mase A, Kotani M, Ami K, Maeda M, et al. Exposure to negatively charged-particle dominant air-conditions on human lymphocytes in vitro activates immunological responses. Immunobiology. 2015;**220**(12):1359-1368

[10] Nishimura Y, Takahashi K, Mase A, Kotani M, Ami K, Maeda M, et al. Enhancement of NK cell cytotoxicity induced by long-term living in negatively charged-particle dominant indoor air-conditions. PLoS One. 2015;**10**(7):e0132373

[11] Brunner KT, Mauel J, Cerottini JC, Chapuis B. Quantitative assay of the lytic action of immune lymphoid cells on 51-Cr-labelled allogeneic target cells in vitro; inhibition by isoantibody and by drugs. Immunology. 1968;**14**(2):181-196

[12] Vainio T, Koskimies O, Perlmann P, Perlmann H, Klein G. In vitro cytotoxic effect of lymphoid cells from mice immunized with allogeneic tissue. Nature. 1964;**204**:453-455

[13] Yokoyama WM, Plougastel BF. Immune functions encoded by the natural killer gene complex. Nature Reviews. Immunology. 2003;**3**(4):304-316

[14] Moretta A, Bottino C, Vitale M, Pende D, Cantoni C, Mingari MC, et al. Activating receptors and coreceptors involved in human natural killer cell-mediated cytolysis. Annual Review of Immunology. 2001;**19**:197-223

[15] Moretta L, Moretta A. Unravelling natural killer cell function: Triggering and inhibitory human NK receptors. The EMBO Journal. 2004;**23**(2):255-259

[16] Vivier E, Tomasello E, Baratin M, Walzer T, Ugolini S. Functions of natural killer cells. Nature Immunology. 2008;**9**(5):503-510

[17] Leong CC, Chapman TL, Bjorkman PJ, Formankova D, Mocarski ES, Phillips JH, et al. Modulation of natural killer cell cytotoxicity in human cytomegalovirus infection: The role of endogenous class I major histocompatibility complex and a viral class I homolog. The Journal of Experimental Medicine. 1998;**187**(10):1681-1687

[18] Arase H, Mocarski ES, Campbell AE, Hill AB, Lanier LL. Direct recognition of cytomegalovirus by activating and inhibitory NK cell receptors. Science. 2002;**296**(5571):1323-1326

[19] Sutherland CL, Chalupny NJ, Cosman D. The UL16-binding proteins, a novel family of MHC class I-related ligands for NKG2D, activate natural killer cell functions. Immunological Reviews. 2001;**181**:185-192

[20] Sutherland CL, Chalupny NJ, Schooley K, VandenBos T, Kubin M, Cosman D. UL16-binding proteins, novel MHC class I-related proteins, bind to NKG2D and activate multiple signaling pathways in primary NK cells. Journal of Immunology. 2002;**168**(2):671-679

[21] Cosman D, Mullberg J, Sutherland CL, Chin W, Armitage R, Fanslow W, et al. ULBPs, novel MHC class I-related molecules, bind to CMV glycoprotein UL16 and stimulate NK cytotoxicity through the NKG2D receptor. Immunity. 2001;**14**(2):123-133

[22] Raulet DH. Roles of the NKG2D immunoreceptor and its ligands. Nature Reviews. Immunology. 2003;**3**(10):781-790

[23] Bauer S, Groh V, Wu J, Steinle A, Phillips JH, Lanier LL, et al. Activation of NK cells and T cells by NKG2D, a receptor for stress-inducible MICA. Science. 1999;**285**(5428):727-729

[24] Wu J, Song Y, Bakker AB, Bauer S, Spies T, Lanier LL, et al. An activating immunoreceptor complex formed by NKG2D and DAP10. Science. 1999;**285**(5428):730-732

[25] Garni-Wagner BA, Purohit A, Mathew PA, Bennett M, Kumar V. A novel function-associated molecule related to non-MHC-restricted cytotoxicity mediated by activated natural killer cells and T cells. Journal of Immunology. 1993;**151**(1):60-70

[26] Valiante NM, Trinchieri G. Identification of a novel signal transduction surface molecule on human cytotoxic lymphocytes. The Journal of Experimental Medicine. 1993; **178**(4):1397-1406

[27] Endt J, Eissmann P, Hoffmann SC, Meinke S, Giese T, Watzl C. Modulation of 2B4 (CD244) activity and regulated SAP expression in human NK cells. European Journal of Immunology. 2007;**37**(1):193-198

[28] Veillette A. NK cell regulation by SLAM family receptors and SAP-related adapters. Immunological Reviews. 2006;**214**:22-34

[29] Veillette A, Cruz-Munoz ME, Zhong MC. SLAM family receptors and SAP-related adaptors: Matters arising. Trends in Immunology. 2006;**27**(5):228-234

[30] Chen X, Trivedi PP, Ge B, Krzewski K, Strominger JL. Many NK cell receptors activate ERK2 and JNK1 to trigger microtubule organizing center and granule polarization and cytotoxicity. Proceedings of the National Academy of Sciences of the United States of America. 2007;**104**(15):6329-6334

[31] Chen X, Allan DS, Krzewski K, Ge B, Kopcow H, Strominger JL. CD28-stimulated ERK2 phosphorylation is required for polarization of the microtubule organizing center and granules in YTS NK cells. Proceedings of the National Academy of Sciences of the United States of America. 2006;**103**(27):10346-10351

[32] Krzewski K, Coligan JE. Human NK cell lytic granules and regulation of their exocytosis. Frontiers in Immunology. 2012;**3**:335

[33] Sivori S, Pende D, Bottino C, Marcenaro E, Pessino A, Biassoni R, et al. NKp46 is the major triggering receptor involved in the natural cytotoxicity of fresh or cultured human NK cells. Correlation between surface density of NKp46 and natural cytotoxicity against autologous, allogeneic or xenogeneic target cells. European Journal of Immunology. 1999;**29**(5):1656-1666

[34] Trapani JA, Smyth MJ. Functional significance of the perforin/granzyme cell death pathway. Nature Reviews. Immunology. 2002;**2**(10):735-747

[35] Smyth MJ, Hayakawa Y, Takeda K, Yagita H. New aspects of natural-killer-cell surveillance and therapy of cancer. Nature Reviews Cancer. 2002;**2**(11):850-861

[36] Zamai L, Ahmad M, Bennett IM, Azzoni L, Alnemri ES, Perussia B. Natural killer (NK) cell-mediated cytotoxicity: Differential use of TRAIL and Fas ligand by immature and mature primary human NK cells. The Journal of Experimental Medicine. 1998;**188**(12):2375-2380

[37] Takeda K, Hayakawa Y, Smyth MJ, Kayagaki N, Yamaguchi N, Kakuta S, et al. Involvement of tumor necrosis factor-related apoptosis-inducing ligand in surveillance of tumor metastasis by liver natural killer cells. Nature Medicine. 2001;**7**(1):94-100

[38] Smyth MJ, Cretney E, Takeda K, Wiltrout RH, Sedger LM, Kayagaki N, et al. Tumor necrosis factor-related apoptosis-inducing ligand (TRAIL) contributes to interferon gamma-dependent natural killer cell protection from tumor metastasis. The Journal of Experimental Medicine. 2001;**193**(6):661-670

[39] Hildner K, Edelson BT, Purtha WE, Diamond M, Matsushita H, Kohyama M, et al. Batf3 deficiency reveals a critical role for CD8alpha+ dendritic cells in cytotoxic T cell immunity. Science. 2008;**322**(5904):1097-1100

[40] Cresswell P, Ackerman AL, Giodini A, Peaper DR, Wearsch PA. Mechanisms of MHC class I-restricted antigen processing and cross-presentation. Immunological Reviews. 2005;**207**:145-157

[41] Kurts C, Robinson BW, Knolle PA. Cross-priming in health and disease. Nature Reviews. Immunology. 2010;**10**(6):403-414

[42] Guermonprez P, Saveanu L, Kleijmeer M, Davoust J, Van Endert P, Amigorena S. ER-phagosome fusion defines an MHC class I cross-presentation compartment in dendritic cells. Nature. 2003;**425**(6956):397-402

[43] Ferlazzo G, Morandi B. Cross-talks between natural killer cells and distinct subsets of dendritic cells. Frontiers in Immunology. 2014;**5**:159

[44] Van Elssen CH, Oth T, Germeraad WT, Bos GM, Vanderlocht J. Natural killer cells: The secret weapon in dendritic cell vaccination strategies. Clinical Cancer Research. 2014;**20**(5):1095-1103

[45] Cooper MA, Fehniger TA, Turner SC, Chen KS, Ghaheri BA, Ghayur T, et al. Human natural killer cells: A unique innate immunoregulatory role for the CD56(bright) subset. Blood. 2001;**97**(10):3146-3151

[46] Poli A, Michel T, Theresine M, Andres E, Hentges F, Zimmer J. CD56bright natural killer (NK) cells: An important NK cell subset. Immunology. 2009;**126**(4):458-465

[47] Konjevic G, Jurisic V, Spuzic I. Association of NK cell dysfunction with changes in LDH characteristics of peripheral blood lymphocytes (PBL) in breast cancer patients. Breast Cancer Research and Treatment. 2001;**66**(3):255-263

[48] Konjevic G, Jurisic V, Spuzic I. Corrections to the original lactate dehydrogenase (LDH) release assay for the evaluation of NK cell cytotoxicity. Journal of Immunological Methods. 1997;**200**(1-2):199-201

[49] Korzeniewski C, Callewaert DM. An enzyme-release assay for natural cytotoxicity. Journal of Immunological Methods. 1983;**64**(3):313-320

[50] Alter G, Malenfant JM, Altfeld M. CD107a as a functional marker for the identification of natural killer cell activity. Journal of Immunological Methods. 2004;**294**(1-2):15-22

[51] Kiessling R, Klein E, Wigzell H. "natural" killer cells in the mouse. I. Cytotoxic cells with specificity for mouse Moloney leukemia cells. Specificity and distribution according to genotype. European Journal of Immunology. 1975;**5**(2):112-117

[52] Kiessling R, Klein E, Pross H, Wigzell H. "Natural" killer cells in the mouse. II. Cytotoxic cells with specificity for mouse Moloney leukemia cells. Characteristics of the killer cell. European Journal of Immunology. 1975;**5**(2):117-121